Organ
Histology

Colin Hinrichsen

University of Tasmania

Organ Histology
A Student's Guide

World Scientific
Singapore • New Jersey • London • Hong Kong

Published by

World Scientific Publishing Co. Pte. Ltd.

P O Box 128, Farrer Road, Singapore 912805

USA office: Suite 1B, 1060 Main Street, River Edge, NJ 07661

UK office: 57 Shelton Street, Covent Garden, London WC2H 9HE

British Library Cataloguing-in-Publication Data
A catalogue record for this book is available from the British Library.

.

ORGAN HISTOLOGY: A STUDENT'S GUIDE

ISBN   981-02-2612-8
ISBN   981-02-2613-6 (pbk)

Printed in Singapore.

Preface

Histology is an exciting and rapidly developing discipline. Many biochemical processes of the body can now be accurately located not only in particular cells but in particular organelles of those cells. A number of diseases once pooled under a single heading are now understood at a cellular level and this has led to refinement of treatment with better directed therapy and less generalized and undesirable side effects.

In the study of Histology, I have always found lecture notes and teach yourself types of books extremely useful to capture the essence of content and organization of a subject. Perhaps it is because of the dedication of the author(s) to concentrate on isolating the pertinent principles of the subject since their intent is to provide both text and teacher. The degree of success with which an author achieves his goal varies greatly but in most cases notes are an invaluable adjunct to gain an overview of the subject which is the key to productive, in depth study from reference texts, original sources and practical laboratory training.

While good texts in this style become true student's companions, I have always felt uncomfortable when in the pursuit of brevity. Some topics are treated so briefly that students become lulled into a sense of false security as to what is a workable knowledge in the field.

This book attempts to present a compact but comprehensive guide to organ histology that helps the student to appreciate the structure, function and where helpful, development of the major organs of the body.

The format is to present information and principles of the microscopic structure of the major organ systems in point form similar to those that might be covered in lectures so that functional as well as structural correlations are emphasized. The text is meant to be a study guide and should complement a laboratory course in Histology and Embryology.

I should like to thank all those who helped, stimulated and encouraged me in my graduate studies of Histology which has led to a very satisfying career in teaching. In particular, I am grateful to Professor James Yaeger, Professor Luis Larramendi, Professor Milton Engel and the late Professor Maury Massler from my days at the University of Illinois in Chicago. I also owe a debt of gratitude to Dr. Albert Forage for compiling the flow charts. I wish to thank the Lions Club of North Hobart, Tasmania who supported me with a personal computer upon which the text was written and all of the students who have shared the fascination of the subject with me.

Colin Hinrichsen. MDS., MSc., PhD., FRACDS.
Hobart , May 1995.

Contents

Chapter 1

INTEGUMENTARY SYSTEM
1. SKIN

OBJECTIVES

After reading this chapter, you should be able to:
1. Define what structures comprise the integumentary system.
2. List at least eight functions of skin.
3. Describe the composition of the two major layers of skin.
4. Outline the process by which a keratinocyte becomes keratinized and relate this to the histologic layers of the epidermis.
5. Distinguish between thick and thin skin.
6. Discuss the histological basis of skin color.
7. Describe the structure and significance of the fine vascular supply of the dermis.
8. Describe at least five types of sensory receptor associated with skin.
9. Briefly give the salient features of fetal skin development from a single layer of ectoderm.

CHAPTER OUTLINE

Skin

General. Composition of the integumentary system (skin, hair, nails, glands). Functions of skin (protection, temperature regulation, excretion, sensation, vitamin D). Physical examination of skin. Fingerprints (dermatoglyphics).

Epidermis.   Epidermal layers (thick and thin skin). Cell replacement in the epidermis. Keratinization. Melanocytes (melanin and other factors effecting skin color. Langerhans cells. Merkel cells. Development of the epidermis.

The dermal-epidermal junction.

Dermis.   Papillary layer. Reticular layer. Ground substance. Vascular supply of the dermis.

Hypodermis.

Nerve supply.   Sensory receptors. Dermatomes.

KEYWORDS, PHRASES, CONCEPTS

Integument
Ectoderm
Epidermis
Dermis (corium)
  Papillary layer
Reticular layer
Hypodermis
Keratinocytes
Layers of epidermis
  Stratum germinativum
  Stratum spinosum
  Stratum granulosum
  Stratum lucidum
  Stratum corneum
Melanocytes
  Melanin
  Eumelanin
  Pheomelanin
Cristae
Secondary dermal ridges
Dermatomes
Attachment plaques
Desquamation

Langerhans cells
Merkel cells
Periderm
Dermal-epidermal junction
Ground substance
Vascular supply of dermis
Cutaneous sensory receptors
Unencapsulated:
  Free endings
  Tactile disks
Encapsulated:
  Glomeruli
  Tactile corpuscles
  Lamellar corpuscles
Dermatoglyphics
Primary epidermal ridges
Vernix caseosa
Primary dermal (papillary) ridges

Basal lamina
  Lamina lucida
  Lamina densa
  Lamina fibroreticularis

Sulci
Dense homogeneous deposit
Keratohyaline granules
Desquamation
Thick (glaborous) skin
Melanosomes
Melanophores

Interpapillary (epidermal) pegs

Lamellar granules
Thin skin
Epidermal proliferative unit
Epidermal melanin unit

1. General

1.1. The *integument* system (in (L) on, and tegmen (L) a roof) includes the skin and its derivatives, nails, hair and associated glands.

1.2. *Skin* (cutis (L) surface, hence the adjective cutaneous) has a double origin:
Epidermis (epi (Gk) upon and derma (Gk) skin), the outermost covering layer derived from the ectoderm; and
Dermis (from derma (Gk) skin, officially the corium from corium (L) skin, hide or leather), the true skin is the vascular connective tissue subjacent to the epidermis (cf. the lamina propria of a mucous membrane) derived from the mesoderm. When tanned, the dermis gives rise to leather.

1.3. *Hypodermis*, the *subcutaneous layer or tela subcutanea* (cf. the submucosa of a mucous membrane) is the *superficial fascia* of gross anatomy. It is a deepest layer of loose fibrous tissue usually containing adipose tissue.

1.4. The skin is the heaviest organ of the body. It weighs about 4 kg, and varies in thickness from 0.5–5 mm and it covers a surface area of about 1.8 square meters.

2. Functions of Skin

2.1. *Protection* against trauma, dessication, water absorption, ultraviolet radiation and absorption of noxious gases and fluids.

2.2. *Excretion* of water, fat and catabolic wastes.

2.3. *Regulation of body temperature* (thermoregulation) by insulation, sweating and conduction of heat from the rich vascular supply of the dermis.

2.4. *Sensory reception* interpreted as pain, thermal sensation or tactile sense.

2.5. *Storage* of glycogen, cholesterol and water.

2.6. *Production of vitamin D3* or 7-dehydrocholesterol, a sterol in skin acted upon by sunlight to produce vitamin D3 (cholecalciferol), the fat soluble anti-rachitic vitamin.

3. Physical Examination of Skin

3.1. The examination of skin is an important part of physical diagnosis. It requires no invasion and is the basis of the medical speciality of *Dermatology*. It provides information about:

A. *Age.* Important also in forensic and other legal investigations.

B. *Hair distribution.* The active hair bulb is one of the most mitotically active regions of the body and is disturbed in some severe illnesses.

C. *Systemic disease.* Color of skin is changed in a variety of conditions such as jaundice (yellow to green), glandular deficiencies (bronze), silver poisoning (grey) or cyanosis (blue).

D. *Vitamin deficiency.* Vitamin A controls the degree of cornification of skin. In deficiency of vitamin A, the extensor surfaces of the limbs lose hair and become rough (excessively keratinized). There is also plugging of hair shafts and sebaceous gland ducts with keratin (*follicular keratosis*).

E. *Infectious diseases.* Such as scarlet fever, measles and chicken pox are accompanied by characteristic skin lesions.

F. *Allergy.* May result in a contact dermatitis — a local reaction to a compound with which the skin has come into contact or systemic sensitivity, a generalized eruption in reaction to systemically administered allergens.

G. *Superficial injuries.* Such as cuts, frost-bite or burns.

4. Fingerprints (Dermatoglyphics)

4.1. The free surface of skin is furrowed by criss-crossing system of fine creases which are genetically determined, individual and permanent. They can be used in personal identification.

4.2. On the palmar/plantar surfaces of the fingers/toes are a series of parallel ridges (*cristae*) and furrows (*sulci*).

4.3. The patterns of loops and whorls are individual and specific in details although closest in identical twins.

4.4. These *primary epidermal ridges or cristae* follow the contours of underlying *primary dermal (papillary)* ridges. They are adaptations to mechanical demands and appear in the third month of embryonic development.

4.5. *Secondary dermal ridges (papillae)* are subdivisions of the primary dermal ridges separated by *interpapillary (epidermal) pegs* of epithelium. The latter appear in the fourth month when ducts of sweat glands sprout as solid buds from the deep aspect of the epidermis in the region of the primary ridges.

4.6. Some 40 disorders have been linked with abnormal finger and/or palm prints.

4.7. *Flexure lines* or skin joints appear in relation to joints where skin is adherent to underlying deep fascia.

5. Epidermis

5.1. The *epidermis* comprises mostly *keratinocytes* arranged as a stratified squamous epithelium. The layer is 0.1–1.5 mm thick but it is thicker in areas of friction or where exposed to radiation of the sun.

5.2. *Keratinocytes* originate from progenitor cells in the deepest layer of the epidermis. They transform to scales (*squames*) undergoing a process of cornification or *keratinization* and are lost from the surface. The process requires about one month.

5.3. Keratinocytes are packed in vertical interlocking columns around a central stem cell and their laterally displaced progeny. These columns represent an *Epidermal Proliferative Unit*.

5.4. Skin thickness varies regionally, *thick skin* and *thin (general body) skin* refers to the thickness of epidermis rather than thickness of skin as a whole.

5.4.1. *Thin skin* has a thin granular layer (about 2 cells thick), no lucid layer and a thin cornified layer. It differs from thick skin in that it contains hair follicles and has no pattern of ridges and grooves. Grooves connect depressed openings of hair follicles.

5.4.2. *Thick (glaborous) skin* (from glaber (L) smooth) lacks hair and sebaceous glands and is found only on the palms of hands and soles of feet.

5.5. Epidermis is avascular. Its deepest layer derives nutrition from the underlying dermis.

5.6. Layers of the epidermis. from deep to superficial are:

    5.6.1. *Stratum Germinativum (Basal layer or Stratum Cylindricum)* comprises columnar or cuboidal, basophilic cells (*keratinocytes* also called basal *epidermocytes*) attached to the basal lamina by hemidesmosomes and to surrounding cells by desmosomes through lateral cell processes.

        A. The cytoplasm of basal cells contains scattered tonofilaments and free ribosomes.

        B. After division, daughter cells either remain in the basal layer (*progenitor or stem cells*) or begin to keratinize and move outward toward the surface.

    5.6.2. *Stratum Spinosum (Prickle cell layer)*, the next most superficial layer, contains large polygonal *keratinocytes* (also called *spinous epidermocytes*). These cells are less basophilic than basal cells and divide less frequently than cells of the basal layer.

        A. Cells of stratum spinosum have cytoplasmic processes (spines or prickles) which contact similar extensions of adjoining cells through a desmosome.

        B. Cytoplasmic tonofibrils are part of the precursor of keratin. Tonofibrils converge on desmosomes, but do not cross from one cell to another.

        C. In the upper spinous layer, cells accumulate irregular, non-membrane bound electron dense granules.

    5.6.3. *Stratum Granulosum* consists of a layer of 3–5 flat keratinocytes in thick skin (but the layer may be absent from thin skin).

        A. Cytoplasm of keratinocytes in this layer contains *dense homogeneous deposit (DHD)*, small deposits rich in SH groups, and *keratohyaline granules (KG)* which are a larger, irregular and granular mixture of protein, polysaccharide and lipid. Tonofilaments react with keratohyaline granules and loose definition.

        B. In the uppermost granular layer, cells show a sudden transition:

    (i) All organelles including nuclei vanish.

    (ii) The remaining cells are filled with tightly packed filaments surrounded by dense matrix.

    (iii) The inner cell membrane (cornified envelope) forms a proteinaceous (*involucrin*) skeleton.

    (iv) Round to oval membrane-bound *lamellar granules* (*or keratinosomes*) 100–500 nm in diameter appear in the peripheral cytoplasm. They are secreted by keratinocytes between cells to form the primary intercellular barrier to water.

5.6.4. *Stratum lucidum* is seen in light microscopy as a thin, lightly stained band only in very thick skin. It represents a layer of dead keratinocytes undergoing karyolysis. Cytoplasmic shells in this layer contain prekeratin filaments in amorphous protein.

5.6.5. *Stratum corneum* contains cornified cellular shells (*squames*) from which cytoplasmic organelles disappear. They are replaced by an amorphous matrix containing prekeratin filaments.

5.7. *Desquamation* is the process of shedding of keratinocytes. It is inherent in the maturation process occurring even in protected areas. It may be assisted by intercellular liberation of lipolytic enzymes. The *stratum disjunctum* is the name given to the outermost layer from which cells are lost.

5.8. *Melanocytes* are pigment-containing cells which arise from neural crest. They migrate to the dermis at 10 weeks and are found in the basal layer of the epidermis at 12–14 weeks.

5.8.1. The density of melanocytes varies from 1–2000 per square millimeter where they account for one quarter to one tenth of basal cells.

5.8.2. Melanocytes are small cells sitting on the basal lamina. They have many dendritic processes which extend into more superficial epidermal layers. They are attached to the basal lamina by hemidesmosomes but are not attached in any way to surrounding keratinocytes.

5.8.3. Melanocytes produce *melanin* in granules (*melanosomes*) which contain tyrosinase. Melanocytes distribute melanosomes to keratinocytes and in the process, the entire tip of the melanocyte containing melanosomes is phagocytosed by the keratinocyte.

5.8.4. An *Epidermal-Melanin Unit* is the population of keratinocytes supplied by one melanocyte.

5.8.5. Melanins are derived from tyrosine, dopa-quinone then dopa (deoxyphenylalanine) and in humans exist in two forms: *Eumelanin* which is brown or black (hydroxyindole polymers) or *Pheomelanin* which is red or yellow (sulphur containing polymers of cysteinyl dopa).

5.8.6. *Pigmentation* of the skin is controlled by:

　(i) *The hereditary size of epidermal-melanin units.* The pattern of aggregation of melanosomes and the production of melanin.

　(ii) *Hormones.* Melanocyte Stimulating Hormone (MSH), estrogen and progesterone influence skin pigmentation.

　(iii) *Environmental factors.* Including infections and exposure to ultra-violet light.

　(iv) *Fibroblast-like melanin-containing cells* (*melanophores*) which also exist in the dermis. These cells do not synthesize melanin but take up melanosomes from melanocytes.

5.9. *Langerhans cells* (*Non-pigmented granular dendrocytes or Clear cells* in light microscopy) are detectable by stains for ATPase. They contain specific plate-like cytoplasmic bodies known as *Langerhan's bodies* or Birbeck's granules whose function is unknown.

5.9.1. They originate in bone marrow and, like monocytes and macrophages, carry surface receptors for immunoglobulin (Fc) and complement (C3).

5.9.2. Langerhans cells belong to a system able to fix and process cutaneous antigen (*Antigen Presenting Cells*). They present antigen to T helper cells and contribute to the initiation of contact hypersensitivity reactions.

5.10. *Merkel cells* are round cells found in thickened regions of the epidermis adjacent to some hair follicles (*hair discs* or *tactile toruli*).

5.10.1. Their cytoplasm contains dense osmiophilic granules as do the *APUD* (*amine precursor and decarboxylation*) cell group which includes cells in the epithelium of the gastrointestinal tract, chromaffin cells, pancreatic A, B and D cells, and C cells in the thyroid. They may share a common origin from the neural crest.

5.10.2. Merkel cells are scattered among basal keratinocytes to which they are attached by desmosomes.

5.10.3. A discoidal enlargement of a nonmyelinated afferent (sensory) nerve ending (*terminal disk*) is associated with the base of the cell.

5.10.4. Merkel cells are considered to be receptor cells or *paraneurons*.

6. Development of the Epidermis

6.1. At first the ectoderm is a single-cell layer.

6.2. In the fifth week, a second layer is added so that the epidermis comprises:
An inner or basal layer (*stratum germinativum*).
A transient non-keratinized outer layer (*periderm*).

6.3. Mitotic activity ceases in periderm cells in the second trimester. Cells enlarge and show surface microvilli.

6.4. Periderm plays a role in secretion, conditioning and uptake of amniotic fluid. It is shed at 160 days.

6.5. The basal layer produces several cell layers (*stratum intermedium*).

6.6. By the third month skin appendages begin to form.

6.7. *Vernix caseosa* is a pasty mixture of cast-off epidermal cells, lanugo hairs and sebaceous secretions covering fetal skin which prevents maceration of the fetus by amniotic fluid.

7. The Dermal-Epidermal Junction

7.1. Keratinocytes form *hemidesmosomes* with the basal lamina. Tonofilaments in the basal epithelial cytoplasm insert onto thickenings of the inner leaflet of the basal cell membrane called *attachment plaques*.

7.2. The *basal lamina* stains with PAS in light microscopy, indicating a rich content of glycosylated proteins (laminin and entactin). It also contains proteoglycans (chiefly heparan sulphates) and type IV collagen.

7.3. In electron micrographs, the basal lamina is a complex comprising:

7.3.1. *Lamina lucida*. An electron lucent amorphous layer adjacent to epithelium containing loosely arranged cords of type IV collagen (*anchoring filaments*) encased in an adhesive glycoprotein, laminin;

INTEGUMENTARY SYSTEM

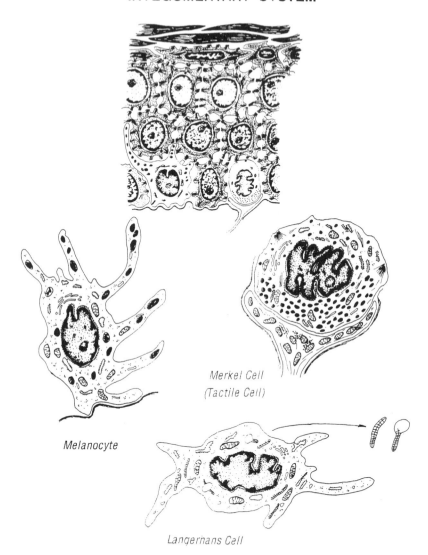

Merkel Cell
(Tactile Cell)

Melanocyte

Langernans Cell

7.3.2. *Lamina densa*. An electron dense layer comprising a fine meshwork of type IV collagen; and

7.3.3. *Lamina fibroreticularis* (*reticular lamina*), which connects the basal lamina to underlying connective tissue. It consists of condensed ground substance containing reticular fibrils which make loops and intermingle with neighboring connective tissue.

7.4. *Functions of the basal lamina* include:

  7.4.1. Binding the epidermis to dermis (it is defective in some diseases).

  7.4.2. Preventing the transport of some substances across the junction.

SKIN

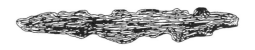

Keratinocyte (Stratum Corneum)

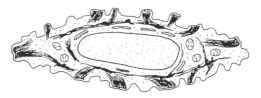

Keratinocyte (Stratum Granulosum)

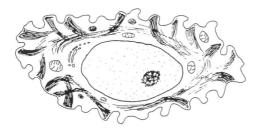

Keratinocyte (Stratum Spinosum)

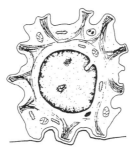

Keratinocyte (Stratum Basale)

It provides a selective barrier to the passage of some cells (fibroblasts) but not others (lymphocytes and macrophages).

7.4.3. Providing a scaffold for migration of epithelial cells in repair after damage to the skin.

7.4.4. Directing morphogenesis during development.

8. Dermis

8.1. The *dermis* varies in thickness from 0.3 mm (in the eyelid) to 4 mm (on the back). It contains collagen, elastin fibers and ground substance all produced by fibroblasts. In some regions (near hair, in the dermis of the scrotum, penis and nipple), there are smooth muscle bundles. In the head, striated muscles of facial expression insert into the dermis.

8.2. The *papillary layer* of the dermis is loosely packed fine fibrous tissue forming the dermal papillae. Papillae provide a mechanical interlocking with the epidermis.

8.2.1. Papillae may contain either:
  A. Meissner's corpuscles (*tactile papillae*); or
  B. Tufts of capillaries (*vascular papillae*).

8.3. The *reticular layer* of the dermis is the main fibrous bed of the dermis. It contains dense interlacing fibers of collagen and elastic fibers whose orientation gives rise to lines of extensibility (Langer's lines). These lines should be followed in surgical incisions to reduce gaping of a wound. Cells found in the reticular layer include fibroblasts, macrophages, mast cells and fat cells.

8.4. *Ground substance* comprises proteoglycans and other plasma constituents, metabolic products of dermal cells, water and ions.

8.4.1. Major constituents of ground substance are glycosaminoglycans, hyaluronic acid, chondroitin sulphate and dermatan sulphate.

8.4.2. There is no free fluid in the ground substance as it is a hydrophilic gel.

9. Vascular Supply of the Dermis

9.1. There are two vascular networks (or dermal arterial rete), one at the level of the dermal-subcutaneous junction and the other, more superficially, in the papillary layer of the dermis.

9.2. From the flat vascular network at the base of dermal papillae (*rete subpapillare*), small capillary loops enter dermal papillae.
9.3. The vessel leaving papillae has the characteristics of venous vessels. White cell diapedesis occurs in the postcapillary loop and histamine, serotonin and bradykinin act on this segment. In some cutaneous diseases, the venous part of the circulation increases.
9.4. The blood supply of the dermis far exceeds metabolic demands of skin. In heat regulation, the prime function of the rich dermal blood supply, blood can be shunted at two levels:
   A. Through *arteriovenous anastomoses* involving arteries deep in the dermis.
   B. In the more superficial dermis, *precapillary sphincters* close so that anastomoses from arterioles to venules bypass capillary loops.

10. Hypodermis (Subcutaneous Layer or Superficial Fascia)

10.1. The *hypodermis* gives the skin mobility.
10.2. It is a loose network of connective tissue and septa which contains blood vessels, lymphatics, nerve fibers and scattered corpuscles (of Vater-Pacini), hair bulbs and a variable amount of adipose tissue.
10.3. Where fat deposits are continuous, the layer is called the *panniculus adiposus* (panniculus (L) a piece of cloth).
10.4. There is no fat in the hypodermis of the eyelids, scrotum and penis.

11. Nerve Supply

11.1. The skin is the largest sensory organ in the body.
11.2. A *subcutaneous plexus* forms a network at the dermal-subcutaneous junction. The plexus is a mixture of sensory nerves and post-ganglionic autonomic nerves to blood vessels and appendages.
11.3. A dermal plexus is located just below the epidermis.
11.4. Sensory nerve endings associated with the skin (exteroceptors) are classified morphologically on the basis of whether or not they are encapsulated.
   11.4.1. Unencapsulated nerve endings include:
      A. *Fine myelinated nerve fibers* branch to form plexuses, then loose their Schwann cell sheath and penetrate the epidermis

or end in the dermis as *free nerve endings*. These endings respond to several modalities but in particular to cold or heat, light touch or pain.

B. *Tactile discs* are sole-shaped expansions of nerve endings applied to the base of Merkel cells in the basal layer of epidermis.

11.4.2. *Encapsulated nerve endings* have a fibrous capsule continuous with the endoneurium of the nerve fiber surrounding the nerve terminal.

A. *Glomeruli, Corpuscles or End Bulbs (of Kraus)* found in dermal papillae have a circular capsule and core of lamellated Schwann cells among which an unmyelinated nerve branches repeatedly. They are thought to respond to cold and mechanical stimuli.

B. *Corpuscles of Ruffini* are flattened encapsulated endings in the dermis of hairy skin of the fingers and toes. Several nerve fibers loose their myelin sheaths on entering the capsule and branch profusely before ending in knob-like expansions. These receptors are thought to respond to temperature and possibly to pressure.

C. *Corpuscles of Meissner (tactile corpuscles)* are cylindrical organs situated in the tip of dermal papillae, especially in the finger tips, front of the forearm, lips and palpebral conjunctiva. The core of the corpuscle consist of tactile cells (modified Schwann cells) stacked parallel with the epidermal surface. Several unmyelinated nerves loose their sheaths, then enter the corpuscle, branch and ramify among the tactile cells. Meissner's corpuscles are rapidly adapting mechanoreceptors.

D. *Corpuscles of Vater-Pacini* (lamellar corpuscles) are large, oval bodies 2–5 mm long and 100–500 μm across located in the hypodermis particularly in the palm of the hand and sole of the foot. The capsule is continuous with the perineurium. The core of the corpuscle consists of up to 60 bilaterally arranged concentric lamellae of flattened (0.2 μm thick) fibrocytes separated by a narrow fluid filled space which also contains collagen. A single (rarely two) thick myelinated nerve looses its myelin sheath on entering the corpuscle, courses axially as the inner core and may branch before ending in an expansion. These receptors are rapidly adapting mechanoreceptors.

11.5. The area of skin supplied by a segmental nerve is known as a *dermatome*. The boundaries of areas supplied for some sensations differ somewhat and there is some overlap of the areas supplied by adjacent segmental nerves.

Chapter 2
INTEGUMENTARY SYSTEM
2. SKIN APPENDAGES

OBJECTIVES

After reading this chapter, you should be able to:

1. Describe the histological features of eccrine sweat glands and explain how they differ from the so called apocrine sweat glands.
2. Describe the composition of sweat and list its functions.
3. Describe the wall of the hair follicle, relating its structure to the layers of dermis and epidermis.
4. Describe the structure of the hair shaft and list the differences between soft and hard keratin.
5. Give an account of the histological structure and function of muscle and glands associated with skin.
6. List the histological features of nails and the area concerned with growth of the nail.

CHAPTER OUTLINE

Eccrine Sweat Glands

General.

Detailed structure. Secretory tubule (Gland cells, Myoepitheliocytes). Excretory duct.

Composition of sweat.

Functions of sweat.

Development of sweat glands.

Apocrine sweat glands.

Hair

General.

Detailed structure. Hair shaft and root (medulla, cortex and cuticle)

Hair follicle. Dermal root sheath. Epidermal root sheath.

Functions of hair.

Development of hair. Shedding and replacement.

Associated muscle and glands. Arrector pili muscle. Sebaceous glands.

Nails

General.

Detailed structure. Nail groove, nail bed and nail plate.

Functions of nails.

Development of nails.

Growth of nails.

KEY WORDS, PHRASES, CONCEPTS

Eccrine (merocrine) secretion
Sudoriferous glands
Myoepitheliocytes
Apocrine secretion
Cerumen
Sweat (composition)
Sweat (functions of)
Lanugo hair
Dermal root sheath

Glassy membrane
Epidermal root sheath
Outer root sheath
Inner root sheath
Hair bulb
Hair shaft
Vellus
Soft keratin
Hard keratin

Arrector pili muscle

Sebaceous glands

Holocrine secretion

Nail fold

Germinal matrix

Nail bed

Sterile matrix

Hyponychium

Eponychium

Lunule

Nail wall

Sebum

Sebaceous cells

ECCRINE SWEAT GLANDS

1. General

1.1. *Eccrine sweat glands*, or *Sudoriferous (sudor L. sweat) glands,* are unbranched, coiled, simple tubular cutaneous glands comprising a *body* or secretory portion and an *excretory duct*.

1.2. The secretory portion is located deep in the dermis or in the hypodermis. The duct fuses with the basal layer of the epi dermis and continues as a spiralling cleft lined by keratinocytes opening on the crest of an epidermal ridge.

1.3. The regional distribution of sweat glands varies from approximately $460/\text{cm}^2$ in the palm to being totally absent from the lips, clitoris, glans penis and inner prepuce.

2. Detailed Structure

2.1. Gland cells form a single layer of two types of cuboidal to columnar secretory cells:

A. *Dark (Mucoid or Dense)* Cells have a basophilic cytoplasm rich in RNA and contain mucopolysaccharide granules.

B. *Clear Cells* have an abundant cytoplasmic glycogen content and an extensive intercellular canalicular system between adjacent cells.

2.2. Secretion (*sweat*) is eccrine (merocrine) by exocytosis without loss of gland cell cytoplasm.

2.3. Gland cells are innervated by sudomotor (sympathetic autonomic) nerves which release acetyl choline.

2.4. *Myoepitheliocytes* are slender, flat, stellate, acidophil cells situated between the bases of secretory cells and the basal lamina. Ultrastructurally, they resemble smooth muscle cells but are of ectodermal origin. Their contraction helps to empty the gland and they may regulate the flow of metabolites to secretory cells.

2.5. The excretory duct is bistratified at its beginning, containing two cell types:

    A. *Peripheral Cells* are cuboidal cells whose cytoplasm contains many mitochondria; and

    B. *Superficial Cells* which form the luminal surface of the duct. These cells are poor in organelles but they have a well-developed terminal web and cytoplasm interlaced with tonofilaments.

    2.5.1. The duct joins the germinative layer of epidermis at its thickest part where it dips between dermal papillae. It continues as a tunnel (intercellular cleft) to the surface opening on the crest of epidermal ridges at a *sweat pore*.

3. Sweat

3.1. *Sweat* contains water, sodium chloride, potassium, urea and lactate. Sodium is actively pumped between cells in the excretory duct and water passively transported to restore isotonicity. Some sodium is reabsorbed by duct cells under the influence of *aldosterone* levels in blood. The relative composition of sweat depends on environmental temperature.

3.2. Functions of sweat include:

    A. *Body temperature control*. Evaporation of sweat from the skin accounts for 15% of body temperature loss under normal conditions. Sweat loss is 0.57–1.14 liters/day (300–530 cal) to a maximum of 11 liters/day (7000 cal).

    B. *Excretion*. Of water, salt and some lipid. Acclimatization results in reduced salt loss in sweat and in urine.

4. Development of Sweat Glands

4.1. Sweat glands begin to develop from deep epidermal ridges as solid ingrowths of the epidermis at 4 months.

4.2. The secretory portion twists at 6 months and develops a lumen by 7 months.

5. Apocrine Sweat Glands

5.1. *Apocrine sweat glands* are sac-like tubulo-alveolar glands located in the axilla, pubic region, labia majora, scrotum, perineal and circumanal region, and areola of the breast. The composition of their secretion varies with the anatomical position of the gland.

5.2. *Apocrine glands* open into the upper part of hair follicles and become functional at puberty. Secretion occurs between microvilli and is more accurately described as merocrine (eccrine).

5.3. *Myoepitheliocytes* surround secretory alveoli.

5.4. Apocrine "sweat" glands are under dual autonomic control but are not responsive to temperature changes; hence, they differ from the eccrine type. Other apocrine glands include:

A. *Axillary glands* which secrete a proteinaceous, milky secretion which becomes odoriferous with bacterial decomposition.

B. *Ciliary glands* (of Moll) open into the distal end of hair follicles (eyelashes) or onto the free surface of the epidermis.

C. *Areolar glands* (*of Montgomery*) are intermediate in structure between mammary glands and sweat glands. They lubricate the nipple.

D. Apocrine glands in the labia majora show involutionary changes in relation to the menstrual cycle.

E. *Ceruminous glands* (cera (L) wax) in the external auditory meatus produce a yellowish secretion which, with sebaceous gland secretion and desquamated epithelium, contributes to *cerumen*, a brownish, waxy substance.

HAIR

1. General

1.1. *Hairs* (pili (L) hairs) are specialized epidermal threads resting on sunken papillae of the corium. They are only found in mammals, However, in man, the insulating function of hair is largely compensated for by subcutaneous fat.

1.2. *Lanugo* (lanugo (L) down) is the first generation of fine fetal hair shed at or just after birth. The shaft lacks a medulla.

1.3. *Vellus* (vellus (L) fleece) is the fine prepubertal hair replacing lanugo.

1.4. *Hard keratin* in hair (and nails) is relatively unreactive, contains more cystine and disulphide bonds than soft keratin in skin and, unlike soft keratin, is not desquamated.

1.5. The *root or radix* of the hair is the part implanted in the skin.

1.6. The *shaft* or *scapus* is the part of a hair projecting from the surface of the skin.

1.7. The *bulb* is a proximal enlargement of the root. It comprises matrix cells which give rise to the layers of the hair follicle and hair shaft.

1.8. The *hair follicle* is an invagination of the epidermis and corium into which the hair is set. It may extend into the subcutaneous tissue.

1.9. The *papilla* is a conical vascular invagination of the bulb which is continuous with the dermal layer of the follicle.

2. Detailed Structure

2.1. The *shaft and root* arising from matrix cells in the bulb are constructed of epidermal cells in 3 concentric layers:

A. The *medulla* comprises the core of the hair. It is two or three cells thick and is found in hair of the axilla, beard and eyebrows but not in fine hair and head hairs. Cells are cornified, cuboidal and contain refractile (trichohyaline) granules and pigment. Grey hair has a prominent medulla and loss of pigment.

B. The *cortex* is the chief part of the shaft comprising long, flat spindle-shaped cornified cells with pigment in and between cells.
Melanin granules (eumelanin) in the cortex accounts for brown and black hair color while the presence of air vacuoles can modify the color. Eumelanin produced by melanocytes and transferred to cortical and medullary cells. Pheomelanin is a yellow pigment accounting for red hair. Grey hair results from inability of melanocytes to produce pigment.

C. The cuticle is an outermost single layer of cornified squames overlapping one another from below upwards. They interdigitate with downward oriented cuticular cells of the inner root sheath.

2.2. The *hair follicle* comprises:

2.2.1. The *Epidermal Root Sheath*, the innermost sheath of the follicle, which comprises layers equivalent to those of the epidermis:

A. The *Inner Root Sheath*, situated only below the opening of the sebaceous gland, is equivalent to the specialized superficial layers of epidermis. It comprises:

    (i) The *cuticle* (cf. cornified layer of epidermis), a single cell layer of overlapping squames interlocking with the epidermal sheath.

    (ii) *Huxley's layer,* also known as the granular epithelial stratum (cf. stratum granulosum), is one to three layers of cornified cells.

    (iii) *Henle's layer*, also known as the pale epithelial stratum (cf. stratum lucidum), is a single layer of elongated cells.

B. The *Outer Root Sheath* also arises from matrix cells and is equivalent to the less modified deeper layers of epidermis.

    (i) The *prickle cell layer* (*Stratum spinosum*), the most internal cell layer, is several cells thick; and

    (ii) The *columnar layer*, a single cell layer adjacent to the basal lamina (*Glassy membrane*).

    Peritrichial or Lanceolate sensory nerve endings surround the hair root in contact with the glassy membrane.

2.2.2. The *Dermal Root Sheath* (*bursa*) is a condensation of connective tissue around the epidermal sheath developed in the lower two thirds of the root and comprises:

    (i) *Inner layer* of type IV collagen and laminin (cf. basal lamina).

    (ii) *Middle layer*, a thick cellular layer (cf. papillary layer of dermis).

    (iii) *Outer layer*, a poorly defined layer (cf. reticular layer of dermis).

3. Functions of Hair

3.1. Provision of some warmth by insulation, a function largely replaced in man as opposed to other mammals by adipose tissue.

3.2. Hairs are tactile organs. Follicles are surrounded by specialized *peritrichial or lanceolate nerve endings*.

3.3. Hairs provide some degree of protection against trauma.

3.4. Follicles are a source of new epidermal cells when superficial layers of skin are damaged by trauma.

4. Development of Hair

4.1. Hairs first appear at 3 months as a crowded and elongated cluster of germinative cells in the epidermis of the eyebrows, upper lip and chin (*primary hairs*).

4.2. Germinative cells of the epidermis grow into the dermis as an epithelial peg surrounded by a mesenchymal sheath with a condensed base (the future *papilla*).

4.3. Basal epidermal cells near the papilla give rise to the inner epithelial sheath and shaft of the hair.

4.4. Peripheral cells of the downgrowth give rise to the outer epithelial sheath.

4.5. Hair growth is cyclic, follicles alternating between growing and resting phases. Growth phases vary from 4 years for scalp hairs to 3–4 months for eyelashes. Hair loss in man is continuous and irregular.

4.6. Scalp hair reaches an average length of 1 meter growing at an average rate of 0.25 mm per day.

4.7. Male sex hormone (androgen) stimulates growth of terminal hair but in the presence of an autosomal dominant gene predisposing to baldness, contributes to expression of the gene.

4.8. Baldness is more common in males (6:1) and is a trait with both sex hormone and heredity components.

5. Associated Muscle and Glands

5.1. *Arrector pili muscles* (arrigere (L) to raise and pilus (L) a hair) are small bundles of smooth muscle fibers which originate in the superficial layer of corium and are inserted into the outer coat of the hair follicle below the entrance of the duct of the sebaceous gland.

5.1.1. Muscle fibers are placed on the side towards which the hair slopes. With contraction, they decrease the obliquity of the follicle elevating the hair. Skin over the origin is depressed and around the hair, elevated, producing "goose bumps". Sebaceous glands are squeezed by the contraction which aids the expulsion of sebum from sebaceous glands. ⸴

5.1.2. Arrectores are supplied by sympathetic nerves and respond in cold, fear and anger.

5.2. *Sebaceous glands* are small, sacculated, alveolar glands in the substance of the dermis especially in the scalp, face, apertures of the nose, mouth and anus. They are absent from the palms of the hand and soles of the feet.

5.2.1. The glands have a single duct serving a cluster of 2–5 alveoli.

5.2.2. Epithelial cells of the glands (sebaceous cells) are continuous with cells lining the duct. They undergo fatty degeneration passing toward the center of the lumen where they break down and are shed (holocrine secretion) to produce a mixture of cellular debris and fatty material (sebum).

5.2.3. *Sebum* is a natural lubricant which protects skin from the effects of dessication and hairs from becoming brittle.

5.2.4. Sebaceous glands have no nervous control but are stimulated by hormonal action (especially androgen).

5.2.5. The first sebaceous glands appear at 5 months as an epithelial swelling of the outer epithelial root sheath of hair follicles.

5.2.6. Some develop neonatally independently of hair follicles in the genitalia, nostrils, eyelids and lips.

NAILS

1. General

1.1. *Nails* are flattened, horny plates of hard keratin on the distal dorsal surfaces of fingers and toes.

1.2. The nail is analogous to the keratinized layer of thick skin but squames are hard, strongly coherent and not shed.

2. Detailed Structure

2.1. The *root* is the proximal part of the nail implanted in a groove of skin.

2.2. The *body* is the exposed part of nail.

2.3. The *free border* is the distal end of the nail. The epidermal thickening under the free edge of the nail plate is the *hyponychium* (hypo (Gk) under and onyx (Gk) a nail).

2.4. The *nail fold* is a fold of skin overlapping the root. It is prolonged as the *eponychium* (epi (Gk) upon and onyx (Gk) a nail), a thin fold of cuticle.

2.5. The *lunule* (lunula (L) a little moon) is the white, opaque, crescent-shaped proximal part of the nail resulting from the greater thickness of the proximal part of the nail plate.

2.6. The *nail wall* is a fold of skin overlapping each collateral border of the nail and separated from it by the *nail groove*.

2.7. The *nail bed* or *lectulum* comprises:
   A. Germinative layers of epidermis, smooth in contact with the nail plate but ridged longitudinally in contact with the dermis, lacks glands or hair follicles.
   B. Corium which is thick and also raised in very vascular longitudinal dermal ridges.

2.8. *Germinal matrix* is the part of the nail bed beneath the nail root and lunule. It is the thickest part of the bed and contains dividing cells of the stratum germinativum. These cells undergo keratinization without showing keratohyalin granules.

2.9. *Sterile matrix* is the part of the nail bed beneath the remainder of the nail. It is thinner than the germinal matrix, does not contribute to growth of the nail but provides a sliding surface for the growing nail.

3. Function of Nails

3.1. Nails are *supportive* and *protective*, acting as a rigid background for support of the digital pads.

4. Development of Nails

4.1. Epidermis on the dorsal surface of digits (the *nail field*) thickens at 10 weeks.

4.2. Local cornification of the nail field gives rise to a "false nail".

4.3. Nail matrix begins to form in the epidermis of the proximal nail fold at 5 months.

4.4. The *eponychium* (periderm and epidermis) covers the first nail but the layer is largely lost in late fetal development.

5. Growth of Nails

5.1. The average nail grows 0.5 mm per week but grows more quickly in summer and fastest on the largest digit. Fingernails grow approximately four times faster than toe-nails.

5.2. Nail growth is commonly disturbed in illness and by trauma.

5.3. Flecks or opacities in nails are caused by minute air bubbles in the nail substance.

SKIN APPENDAGES

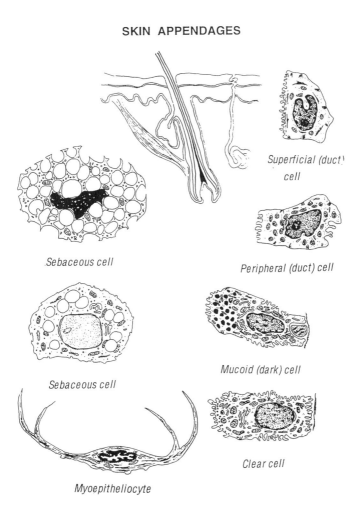

Superficial (duct) cell

Sebaceous cell

Peripheral (duct) cell

Sebaceous cell

Mucoid (dark) cell

Myoepitheliocyte

Clear cell

Chapter 3

ENDOCRINE SYSTEM
1. HYPOPHYSIS, DIFFUSE NEUROENDOCRINE AND CHROMAFFIN SYSTEMS

OBJECTIVES

After reading this chapter, you should be able to:
1. Distinguish between the anatomical subdivisions of the hypophysis.
2. Give an account of the development of the hypophysis.
3. Describe histological features and secretory products that distinguish between cells of the pars distalis.
4. Give an account of the structure of the neurohypophysis and of the origin and path followed by its hormones.
5. Describe the anatomy and functional significance of the blood supply of the hypophysis.
6. Describe the features of the chromaffin and diffuse neuroendocrine systems.

CHAPTER OUTLINE

Characteristics of Endocrine Glands

General. Ductless glands/Glands of internal secretion. Hormones. Target organs. Adenohypophysis, the focus of neuroendocrine integration. Diffuse Neuroendocrine System. Paracrine secretion.

Hypophysis.

Development of the hypophysis.

General structure.

Detailed structure (including products of individual cell types). Pars distalis. Pars intermedia. Pars tuberalis.

Secretion of adenohypophyseal hormones.

Hypothalamic regulation of the adenohypophysis.

Neurohypophysis.

Blood supply of the hypophysis.

Histophysiology. Hyposecretion. Hypersecretion.

Diffuse Neuroendocrine System

KEY WORDS, PHRASES AND CONCEPTS

Ductless glands
Glands of internal
 secretion
Endocrine secretion
Pars Nervosa
Releasing Factors
Paracrine secretion
APUD cells
Rathke's pouch
Infundibulum
Adenohypophysis
Pars distalis
Pituicytes
Panhypopituitarism
Gigantism
Acromegally
Hypopituitarism
Thyrotrops

Pars Intermedia
Neurohypophysis
Pars Tuberalis
Homeostasis.
Target organs
Infundibular stalk
Median eminence
Anterior lobe
Posterior lobe
Chromophobes
Chromophils
Somatotrops
Lactotrops
Blood supply of
 the hypophysis
Dwarfism
Hyperpituitarism
Diabetes insipidus

Gonadotrops (Type I-FSH cell
  and Type II-ICSH cell)
Melanocyte Stimulating Hormone
Hypothalamo hypophyseal tract
Neurophysin
Herring bodies
Hypothalamus
Adrenocorticotrophic Hormone
  (ACTH)
Thyroid Stimulating Hormone (TSH)
Luteinizing Hormone (LH)
Interstitial Cell Stimulating Hormone
  (ICSH)
Proopiomelanocortin

Adrenocorticotrops
(Corticotrops)
Tanycytes
Acidophils
Basophils
Growth Hormone
Prolactin (Lactogenic Hormone)

Lipotropic Hormone (LPH)
Follicle Stimulating Hormone (FSH)

Tuberoinfundibular tract
Supraoptico and
Paraventriculohypophyseal tracts

1. General

1.1. *Endocrine glands* are "ductless" glands or "glands of internal secretion". Their parenchymal cells secrete specific products known as *hormones* usually directly into the bloodstream but in some cases via lymphatics.

1.2. Endocrine glands have in common:
   A. No ducts, parenchymal cells abut blood or lymph vessels.
   B. An exceptionally rich blood supply.
   C. Cells which contain clear vacuoles filled with lipid (e.g., steroid hormones in suprarenal cortex) or granules with specific affinity for certain dyes (e.g., peptide or protein hormones in adenohypophysis).

1.3. Glands universally recognized as endocrine are the *hypophysis, thyroid gland, parathyroid glands, suprarenal glands, gonads, pancreatic islets* and the *placenta*. Other organs (e.g., intestine and kidney) have endocrine functions in addition to their dominant activity.

1.4. The number of hormones produced by endocrine glands ranges from one (parathyroid) to more than 10 (hypophysis).

1.5. *Hormones* act as chemical regulators of specific tissues elsewhere in the body or of somatic cells in general.

1.6. A *target organ* is the specific organ affected by the hormone concerned whose cells (*target cells*) possess either specific surface or intracellular hormone receptors.

1.7. The focus of neuroendocrine integration is the *adenohypophysis* (ade (Gk) an acorn, hypo (Gk) under, and physis (Gk) growth) which regulates the function of a number of target organs.

1.8. The function of the hypophysis is controlled by the *hypothalamus* in the diencephalon at the base of the brain. Cells of the hypothalamus produce *releasing factors* (or *hypophyseotrophic hormones*) and are stimulated to release them by afferent signals from several brain centers. Releasing factors are conveyed to the adenohypophysis by blood vessels and control adenohypophyseal function.

1.9. Hormones of the hypophysis may not only modulate the function of other organs but the brain's function, in particular that of the hypothalamus, by feedback through the bloodstream.

1.10. Endocrine glands constitute one of the great coordinating mechanisms of the body. The other mechanism is the nervous system. The two systems are intimately linked in their functions.

1.11. The *Diffuse Neuroendocrine System* is a system of peptide-producing cells derived from neuroectoderm scattered throughout the epithelium of organs. Composite cells have the ability to decarboxylate amine precursors (are known as *Amine Precursor Uptake and Decarboxylation or APUD cells*), producing peptide hormones similar or identical to those found in some endocrine and nerve cells. They secrete their products into the immediate environment and thereby control the function of nearby cells (*paracrine secretion*).

1.12. Both nervous and endocrine systems maintain steady physiological state (*homeostasis*).

2. Development of the Hypophysis

2.1. At 3 weeks, the ectoderm from the roof of the *stomodeum* immediately in front of the oro-pharyngeal membrane invaginates, forming *Rathke's pouch* which grows dorsally towards the base of the brain. Connection of the invagination with the oral cavity is lost by the end of the second month.

2.2. The *infundibulum* is a thickening of the floor of the diencephalon which grows downward towards Rathke's pouch.

2.3. Rathke's pouch becomes vesicular and contacts the infundibulum.

2.4. Cells of the anterior wall of Rathke's pouch proliferate, forming the glandular pars distalis of the hypophysis.

2.5. From the upper part of the anterior wall, a small extension (*pars tuberalis*) envelops the stem of the infundibulum.

2.6. Cells of the posterior wall of Rathke's pouch proliferate relatively less but form the thin, poorly defined *pars intermedia*.

2.7. The cavity of Rathke's pouch becomes the *residual lumen* which is greatly reduced after childhood.

2.8. The infundibulum develops into the *infundibular stalk* and the *pars nervosa*.

2.9. Cellular differentiation in the hypophysis is advanced by 3–4 months.

3. General Structure

3.1. The *hypophysis* is the size and shape of a flattened grape attached to the base of the diencephalon and located in the hypophyseal fossa (sella turcica of the sphenoid bone). It comprises:

   3.1.1. *Adenohypophysis*, the pinkish glandular tissue subdivided by the residual lumen of Rathke's Pouch into very unequal parts.

      A. *Pars Distalis*. The larger part in front of the residual lumen plus its extension surrounding the neural stalk (*pars tuberalis*). Both contain epithelial cords separated by sinusoids.

      B. *Pars Intermedia*. The smaller part of the adenohypophysis behind the residual lumen.

   3.1.2. *Neurohypophysis*, the whitish, posterior part comprising:

      A. *Pars Nervosa* generally fused to the epithelial part.

      B. *Infundibular Stalk*. A narrow stalk of non-myelinated axons connecting pars nervosa with the hypothalamus.

      C. *Median Eminence*. A circumventricular organ in the floor of the third ventricle comprising ependymal cells and tanycytes, neurosecretory axons of supraoptic and paraventricular neurons and blood capillaries.

3.2. *Lobes* of the hypophysis relate historically to gross anatomical dissection where a cleft through the residual lumen caused the hypophysis to divide into:

    A. *Anterior Lobe.* The portion anterior to the residual lumen (pars distalis and pars tuberalis) and

    B. *Posterior Lobe.* The portion posterior to the residual lumen (pars intermedia and pars nervosa).

4. Detailed Structure

4.1. The framework of the *adenohypophysis* includes:

    4.1.1. A fibrous *capsule*, the innermost layer of dura mater.

    4.1.2. *Trabeculae*-carrying blood vessels which radiate into the pars distalis.

    4.1.3. Reticular fibers which support epithelial cords.

4.2. *Pars Distalis* is in bulk, three quarters of the gland.

    4.2.1. Epithelium of pars distalis is arranged in anastomosing cords separated by thin-walled sinusoids. Epithelial cells are of two main types of unequal number and distribution which may vary with some physiologic conditions, e.g., pregnancy.

        A. *Chromophobes* stain faintly, are small and located axially within cell cords not bordering capillaries. Ultrastructurally, these cells appear to be metabolically inactive and represent a non-secretor phase in the activity of other glandular cell types.

        B. *Chromophils* have a granular cytoplasm and are distinguished by various staining methods since some form proteins, some form glycoproteins and others form polypeptides. Degree of staining depends on the functional state of the cell. Chromophils are classified by their differential affinities for mixtures of acidic and basic dyes. More recently, immunocytochemistry, ultrastructure and cell fractionation techniques have better identified sites of synthesis of individual hormones.

    4.2.2. *Acidophils (Alpha cells)* represent 40% of all cells or three times the number of other stainable cells. These cells stain with acid dyes but also stain with certain basic dyes.

A. *Somatotrops or Growth Hormone Cells (Alpha cells or Orangeophils)* contain dense secretory granules (300–350 nm) of protein (MW 21000) which fill most of the cell. Somatotrops produce *Growth Hormone* which stimulates body growth but particularly growth of long bone.

B. *Lactotrops or Mammotrops (Epsilon cells or Carminophils)* contain large secretory granules (600–900 nm) of a protein (MW 25000). Lactotrops produce *Prolactin or Lactogenic Hormone (LTH)* which promotes mammary gland development and lactation. When these cells enlarge in response to estrogen, they stain more deeply.

4.2.3. *Basophils (Beta cells)* are incorrectly named since the analine blue component of trichrome stain is in fact acidic. Basophils are sometimes called mucoid cells because their glycoprotein granules stain with PAS.

A. *Adrenocorticotrops (Adrenocorticolipotrops, ACTH/LPH or Beta 1 cells)* contain a large eccentric nucleus and small (200 nm) granules of a polypeptide (MW 4500). They predominate among cells invading the pars nervosa. Adrenocorticotrops produce *Adrenocorticotropic Hormone (ACTH)* which stimulates production of glucocorticoids by cells of the suprarenal cortex The function of *Lipotropic Hormone (LPH)* also produced by these cells is thought to stimulate liberation of fatty acids from stored triglycerides via cyclic AMP.

B. *Thyrotrops (Beta 2 cells)* are small, angular or irregular cells with flattened nuclei and small dense cytoplasmic granules (120–150 nm) containing a glycoprotein (MW 10 000–30 000). These cells produce *Thyroid Stimulating Hormone (TSH or Thyrotropin)* which stimulates the production of thyroid hormones by the thyroid gland.

C. *Gonadotrops (Delta basophils or FSH/LH cells)* are small cells with coarse cytoplasmic granules staining with aldehyde thionine (less well with PAS). *Type 1* cells produce *Follicle Stimulating Hormone* and *Type 2* cells produce *Luteinizing Hormone* but it is possible that these cells can produce both hormones. *Follicle Stimulating Hormone (FSH)* stimulates the growth of ovarian follicles in the female and activates spermatogenesis in the male. *Luteinizing Hormone (LH or Luteotropin)* in the female is essential for ovulation, formation of the corpus luteum and stimulation of steroid production by the follicle and corpus luteum. In the male (where it is known as Interstitial Cell Stimulating Hormone (ICSH), Luteinizing Hormone stimulates interstitial cells (of Leydig) in the testis to produce androgens especially testosterone.

4.3. *Pars Intermedia* contains numerous beta cells and chromophobe cells as well as follicles of PAS staining colloid.

    4.3.1. Cells of pars intermedia contain pro-opiomelanocortin from which peptides *beta lipotropin* and *beta endorphin* are derived.

    4.3.2. *Alpha Melanocyte Stimulating Hormone (MSH)*,is probably not produced in the human pars intermedia. *Gamma Melanocyte Stimulating Hormone*, which has similar functions, is derived from ACTH.

4.4. *Pars Tuberalis* comprises short cords mostly of basophils (gonadotrops) and some follicles.

    4.4.1. It is traversed by a large number of capillary loops upon which neurosecretory fibers of the *tuberoinfundibular tract* end.

5. Secretion of adenohypophyseal hormones occurs by exocytosis of vesicular contents of cells into perivascular spaces. They pass through fenestrated endothelium of sinusoids into the circulation.

6. Hypothalamic Regulation of the Adenohypophysis

6.1. Regulation of the secretion of cells in the adenohypophysis is controlled by polypeptides (*Releasing Factors*) produced by neurons in the dorsomedial, ventromedial and infundibular nuclei of the hypothalamus. Axons of these neurons down which the polypeptides travel, collectively form the *Tubero-infundibular tract*.

6.2. *Releasing Factors* are released from nerve endings into portal vessels which drain the median eminence and infundibulum. They are carried from the bloodstream to the adenohypophysis where they act on cells with the appropriate receptors as the signal for secretion.

6.3. Releasing Factors known at present are:
Adrenocorticotropic Hormone RF or Corticotropin RF(ACTH-RF or CRF), Growth Hormone RF, Somatotropic Hormone RF or Somatotropin RF (GH-RF, STH-RF or SRF), , Luteotropic Hormone or Prolactin RF (LTH-RF or PRF), Gonadotropin RF (originally called Luteinizing Hormone RF (LH-RF)), Melanotropin RF and Thyroid Stimulating Hormone RF or Thyrotropin RF (TSH-RF or TRF).

7. Tanycytes (tanyo (Gk) to stretch) are specialized ependymal cells lining the wall of the third ventricle and the infundibular recess. They have a single long basal process and terminal foot ending on a capillary basal lamina within the median eminence.

7.1. Tanycytes may transport hormones from the CSF to capillaries of the portal system of the hypophysis and from hypothalamic neurons to the CSF.

8. Neurohypophysis

8.1. The neurohypophysis contains unmyelinated axons of neurosecretory neurons of the supraoptic and paraventricular nuclei of the hypothalamus (which form the *Supraoptico- and Paraventriculo-Hypophyseal tracts*). The *Hypothalamo-Hypophyseal tract* is a combination of these tracts and of the Tuberoinfundibular tract

8.2. Hormones produced by Supraoptic and Paraventricular neurons pass from their perikarya along axons and are released from nerve terminals.

8.3. Neurosecretion comprises polypeptides associated with carrier glycoprotein (*Neurophysin*) from which they are split once they enter the bloodstream.

8.4. Collections of neurosecretion in axons and terminals are visible in the light microscope as *Herring Bodies*.

8.5. Proximally axons of hypothalamic neurons entering the neurohypophysis are covered by astrocytes but toward the neurohypophysis by specially differentiated *Pituicytes*.

    8.5.1. *Pituicytes* are dendritic cells with processes ending near capillaries between nerve endings. They have roles in support and possibly secretory control.

8.6. Capillaries in the neurohypophysis are fenestrated.

8.7. Nerve terminals in the neurohypophysis are of at least three types:
   A. Terminal axons containing hormones bound to glycoproteins adjacent to capillaries.
   B. Sympathetic nerve endings containing dense core vesicles.
   C. Axons containing clear core vesicles which contact hormone-containing endings and presumably control their release.

9. Hormones Released by the Neurohypophysis

9.1. *Vasopressin or Antidiuretic Hormone* (*ADH*) controls the reabsorption of water by kidney tubules.

9.2. *Oxytocin* promotes the contraction of uterine and mammary smooth muscle.

10. Blood Supply of the Hypophysis

10.1. *Superior hypophyseal arteries* from the internal carotid arteries form capillary loops in the pars tuberalis and penetrate the median eminence and infundibulum. These are drained by portal vessels which open into sinusoids of the pars distalis.

10.2. A branch of the superior hypophyseal artery by-passes the portal vessels but forms similar smaller loops in the pars intermedia before opening into sinusoids of pars distalis.

10.3. *Inferior hypophyseal arteries* also from the internal carotid arteries form capillary networks in pars nervosa. There is some communication between superior and inferior hypophyseal vessels and reversal of blood flow can occur between the two.

10.4. The *portal system* of vessels carries hormone-releasing factors from the parvocellular hypothalamic neurons which control secretory cycle of cells of pars distalis.

10.5. Hypophyseal hormones to leave in the blood stream for target organs.

10.6. Adenohypophyseal hormones may pass to the neurohypophysis before entering the systemic circulation.

10.7. Venous drainage of the neurohypophysis is by three possible routes:
   A. To the adenohypophysis via portal vessels.
   B. To the systemic circulation via inferior hypophyseal veins to dural sinuses.

C. To the hypothalamus via small capillaries between hypothalamus and median eminence.

10.7.1. This pattern of venous drainage allows:

A. Feedback control of secretion.

B. Reversed flow from neurohypophysis to hypothalamus provides a route for neurohypophyseal hormones to reach the CSF via tanycytes.

11. Histophysiology of the Hypophysis

11.1. *Hypopituitarism* usually results from overall failure of adenohypophyseal function (*panhypopituitarism or Simmond's Disease*).

11.1.1. The etiology is commonly post-partum necrosis (*Sheehan's syndrome*). The hypophysis enlarges in pregnancy and when severe obstetric shock follows post-partum hemorrhage, an infarct occurs in the adenohypophysis. The neurohypophysis is spared.

11.1.2. Clinical features relate to deficiency of target gland hormones. Post-partum occurrence is followed by absence of lactation and menstruation, lassitude, intolerance to cold, failure of sexual function and lack of sweating.

11.1.3. *Selective hypopituitarism* involves failure of secretion of a single hormone (most commonly gonadotrophin). In children this presents as dwarfism which may have contributing genetic, endocrine or nutritional components. In the latter, associated chronic disease depresses hypophyseal function.

11.1.4. *Diabetes insipidus* results from deficiency of *ADH (Vasopressin)*. Intracranial tumor or infiltration with granulomatous tissue may cause extensive destruction of the neurohypophysis before diabetesensues. There is an abrupt onset of polyuria (urine output may reach 5–10 liters/day) and polydipsia or thirst keeping pace with water loss. Urine is of low specific gravity but plasma osmolality is only slightly increased.

11.2. *Hyperpituitarism*:

11.2.1. *Acromegally* results from an acidophil adenoma producing excess STH. The epidermis is thickened, subcutaneous fluid and tissue increased and there is an increase of new subperiosteal bone formation (particularly in the jaw, frontal bones and terminal phalanges).

11.2.2. *Gigantism* is associated with more generalized stimulation of growth and results from an adenoma appearing in childhood.

12. The Diffuse Neuroendocrine System (Amine Precursor Uptake and Decarboxylation or Apud Cells)

12.1. The *diffuse neuroendocrine system* comprises isolated groups of hormone secreting cells widely scattered throughout body tissues and derived from ectoderm or entoderm.

12.2. They do not stain with routine histologic stains and have been referred to as "clear cells".

12.3. Characteristically, these cells produce structurally related peptides which act as *hormones* or as *neurotransmitters*.

12.4. The neurotransmitters which they release are slower in onset and longer in duration of action. For these reasons, they are also known as *neuromodulators*.

12.5. Neuromodulators may act on contiguous cells, on groups of nearby cells (*paracrine secretion*) or on distant cells.

12.6. The *APUD system* is complementary to and links the nervous and endocrine systems. Cells of the system modulate or amplify the action of the autonomic or somatic nervous systems or of each other.

13. The Chromaffin System

13.1. *Catecholamines* in cytoplasmic granules of some cells are oxidized by potassium bichromate, giving a brown reaction product (*adrenochrome*), the *chromaffin reaction*.

13.2. After reacting with formaldehyde vapor, cells containing catecholamines (*chromaffin cells*) also fluoresce yellow-green in ultraviolet light.

13.3. Groups of chromaffin cells associated with the sympathetic nervous system are located in the suprarenal medulla, para-aortic bodies, autonomic ganglia and some cells in the carotid bodies.

13.4. Chromaffin cells have common features in that they are derived from neural crest, innervated by preganglionic sympathetic nerves, and synthesize and secrete catecholamines (dopamine, epinephrine or norepinephrine).

13.5. Three main groups of cells give a positive chromaffin reaction:

  13.5.1. *Sympathetic neurons*

  13.5.2. *Enterochromaffin cells* in epithelial tissue lining the gastro-intestinal and respiratory tracts.

  13.5.3. *Mast cells* in connective tissue of the gut, pancreas and liver.

HYPOPHYSIS

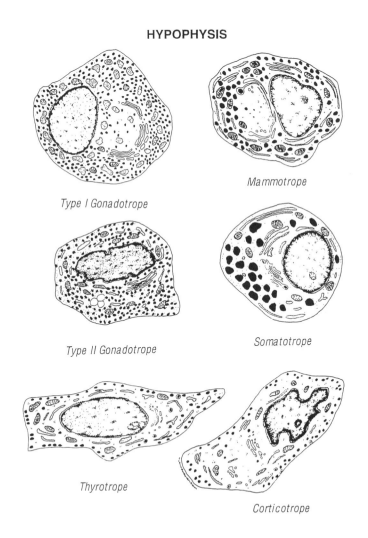

Type I Gonadotrope

Mammotrope

Type II Gonadotrope

Somatotrope

Thyrotrope

Corticotrope

Chapter 4

ENDOCRINE SYSTEM
2. THYROID, PARATHYROID AND ENDOCRINE PANCREAS

OBJECTIVES

After reading this chapter, you should be able to:

1. Explain on developmental grounds why ectopic thyroid tissue is found in the midline along a line between the tongue and front of the larynx.
2. Describe the histology of thyroid follicular cells and how this alters in response to circulating TSH or thyroid hormones.
3. Describe the developmental origin, histology and product of parafollicular cells.
4. Give an account of the developmental origin of the parathyroid glands.
5. Draw a feedback diagram demonstrating the factors that control and are controlled by parathyroid gland secretion.
6. Describe the detailed histology of the parathyroid glands.
7. Describe the developmental origin of the pancreas, including development of islets.
8. Give an account of the histology and histophysiology of the pancreatic islets.
9. Describe the blood supply and innervation of pancreatic islets and how this affects the function of the pancreas.

CHAPTER OUTLINE

— Thyroid Gland

Development.

General structure.

Detailed structure. Follicular cells: Morphologic changes in response to TSH. Thyroglobulin synthesis and degradation. Sites of iodine incorporation. Parafollicular cells: Thyrocalcitonin.

Histophysiology of the thyroid gland.

— Parathyroid Glands

General structure. Superior and Inferior Parathyroids.

Detailed structure. Chief (Principal) cells. Oxyphil (Eosinophil) cells.

Histophysiology of Parathyroid hormone (PTH).

— Pancreas

General structure.

Development of the pancreas.

Detailed structure of pancreatic islets. Alpha cells (Glucagon). Beta cells (Insulin). Delta cells (Somatostatin, Gastrin). PP cells (Pancreatic polypeptide). D1 cells (Vasoactive Intestinal Polypeptide). Enterochromaffin cells.

Blood supply.

Hormones of pancreatic islets.

Control of islet secretion.

Histophysiology.

KEY WORDS, PHRASES AND CONCEPTS

Thyroid diverticulum
Thyroglossal duct
Ultimobranchial bodies
Thyroid follicle
Thyroid follicular cells
Thyroglobulin
Triiodothyronine (T3)
Tetraiodothyronine (T4)
Thyroid Stimulating Hormone
Parafollicular cells
Thyrocalcitonin
Chief (Principal) cells
Oxyphil (Eosinophil) cells
Parathyroid Hormone
Diabetes

Dorsal pancreas
Ventral pancreas
Pancreatic islets
Beta cells
Alpha cells
Delta cells
D1 cells
PP cells
Insulin
Glucagon
Somatostatin
Gastrin
Pancreatic Polypeptide
Vasoactive Intestinal
Polypeptide (VIP)

THE THYROID GLAND

1. Development

1.1. The *thyroid gland* (thyreos (Gk) a shield and oeides (Gk) shape) is the earliest glandular structure to develop (at 2 mm or 6 somites).

1.2. A thickening of entoderm on the floor of the foregut becomes the *thyroid diverticulum* which protrudes ventrally between the first pair of pharyngeal pouches.

1.3. The diverticulum becomes a bilobed sac but remains attached to the pharynx by a narrowing neck. This neck of tissue elongates into the *thyroglossal duct* which connects the thyroid to the developing tongue at a site between the *tuberculum impar* (impar (L) unpaired) and copula (copula (L) a bond), the swelling formed by joining or bonding the second and third branchial arches.

1.4. The *thyroglossal duct*, a solid epithelial stalk, breaks up at 6 weeks. The site of origin of the thyroid is indicated by a median pit, the *foramen caecum* (caecum (L) blind), in the adult at the junction of the anterior two thirds and posterior third of the tongue.

1.5. The developing thyroid remains a solid mass of cells closely approximated to the aortic sac.

1.6. By the 7th week, the *ultimobranchial bodies* from the 5th pharyngeal pouches contact the thyroid and fuse with it.

THYROID GLAND

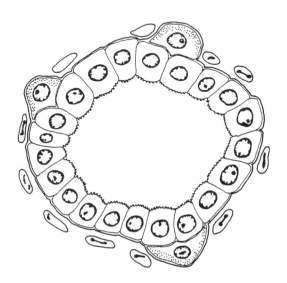

THYROID FOLLICLE

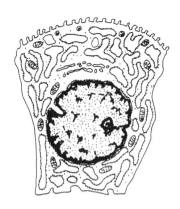

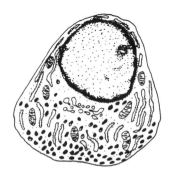

Follicular Cell

Clear Cell

1.7. At the 8th week, thyroid follicles begin to appear as discontinuous cavities among solid plates of *thyroid cells*. New follicles appear by partial subdivision of those already present.

1.8. *Colloid*, an amorphous, gelatinous substance secreted by follicular cells into the core of follicles, appears in the third month and the gland is functional soon after.

1.9. The capsule and stroma of the thyroid arise from local mesenchyme.

2. General Structure

2.1. An inner (true) connective tissue thyroid *capsule* sends *septa* inwards to partially enclose *lobules*.

2.2. Within lobules are rounded or elongated bodies (follicles) surrounded by a highly vascular loose stroma. Surrounding vessels are fenestrated, anastomosing blood capillaries and lymphatic capillaries.

2.3. Sympathetic nerves supply both arterioles and follicular cells.

3. Detailed Structure

3.1. *Thyroid follicles* appear in sections to be closed epithelial sacs 0.02–0.9 mm in diameter. Reconstructions show that they are not separate units but aggregates with a shared sheet of epithelial cells linking them together.

3.2. The central core of the follicle contains *colloid* which is acidophilic if dense or basophilic if dilute. Colloid comprises an iodinated glycoprotein (thyroglobulin), a precursor of thyroid hormones, *triiodothyronine (T3)* and *tetraiodothyronine or thyroxine (T4)*, products of follicular cells surrounding the colloid.

3.3. *Follicular cells* vary from squamous to columnar depending on their level of activity controlled by circulating *thyrotropin (TSH)* from the pars distalis of the hypophysis.

    3.3.1. In the absence of TSH, follicular cells are squamous ("resting") and colloid is voluminous and dense, indicating increased storage.

    3.3.2. In the presence of TSH, there is uptake of colloid by follicular cells from the lumen of the follicle by endocytosis at the luminal aspect of the cell. Cavities then appear where luminal colloid abuts epithelium. There is progressive resorption of colloid and increased stromal vascularity.

3.3.3. Follicular cells are linked by junctional complexes which prevents the leakage of antigenically active thyroglobulin from the follicle. They have an infolded basal plasma membrane and secretory vesicles above the Golgi zone which transport glycoprotein from the RER. Apical microvilli are short in resting cells but longer and branching after stimulation with TSH.

3.3.4. Ultrastructurally, there is evidence of functional polarity in follicular cells. Concurrently, two oppositely directed processes occur:

(i) Apically (luminally) directed thyroglobulin synthesis and exocytosis activated by TSH or adrenergic nerves.

(ii) Basally directed thyroglobulin endocytosis, degradation and liberation of thyroid hormones to capillaries.

3.3.5. In thyroglobulin synthesis, iodine, as iodide from capillaries, enters the base of follicular cells by active transport across the plasma membrane. It is quickly located luminally and is oxidized to iodine by peroxidase in the apical plasma membrane. Iodine is then attached to tyrosyl groups of secreted glycoprotein made by follicular cells producing mono and diiodotyrosyls. Their coupling produces iodothyronyl groups (thyroid hormones in peptide linkage) and completes the formation of iodinated thyroglobulin (the large precursor of thyroid hormones).

3.3.6. In thyroglobulin degradation, long cytoplasmic processes of follicular cells extend into luminal colloid which is taken into the follicle cell. Lysosomes fuse with intracellular colloid droplets, producing secondary lysosomes (phagolysosomes) which migrate to the base of the cell. Acid proteases and peptidases in lysosomes degrade the thyroglobulin. T3 and T4 pass through the cell base to surrounding capillaries. 3 monoiodotyrosine and 3–5 diiodotyrosine are deiodinated by a dehalogenase and the iodine released migrates apically to be reused.

3.4. *Parafollicular cells* (*C, Clear or Light cells*) are a type of APUD cells. They are larger than follicular cells and occur singly or in small groups within the basal lamina but do not reach the lumen of the follicle.

3.4.1. The cytoplasm contains organelles of a secretory cell in amount depending on the level of activity of the cell. In addition, membrane-bound secretory granules store the peptide hormone, thyrocalcitonin.

3.4.2. Parafollicular cells do not appear to have a direct nerve supply.

4. Histophysiology

4.1. *Triiodothyronine* is the chief agent stimulating and increasing rate of cellular metabolism. Its effect is powerful and immediate.

4.2. *Tetraiodothyronine* (*Thyroxine*) has a powerful but delayed action.

4.3. Thyroid hormones also increase sensitivity of body tissues to the effects of adrenalin and noradrenalin (produced by the suprarenal medulla).

4.4. Follicular cell function is controlled by:

A. TSH released by thyrotrops in the hypophysis under the influence of TRF from the hypothalamus; and

B. Sympathetic nerves.

Both activate adenyl cyclase which increases cyclic AMP production and increased release of thyroid hormones.

4.5. An enlarged thyroid is called a *goitre*; however, there is a normal physiological enlargement which occurs during menstruation and pregnancy. *Thyrotoxicosis* (*exophthalmic goitre*) results from overproduction of thyroid hormones.

4.6. *Myxedema* results from hyposecretion in the adult. It is characterized by dry, brittle hair and coarse, dry, scaling skin, lethargy, memory impairment, and slow cerebration. There is edema of the face and eyelids and thickening of the tongue with slow speech. Sensation of coldness is accompanied by diminished perspiration. There may be enlargement of the heart and frequent hypertension, ascites and generalized weakness.

4.7. *Cretinism* results from hyposecretion in the immediate postnatal period. In addition to the changes seen in myxedema, it is characterized by failure of skeletal growth and maturation, marked retardation and deficiency in intellect and characteristic facies.

4.8. *Grave's disease or Diffuse Hyperthyroidism* results from *human thyroid stimulating immunoglobulin* (*HTSI*) antibodies binding to TSH receptor sites on follicular cells, resulting in excessive thyroid hormone production. It is characterized by goitre and exophthalmos, nervousness, excitability, emotional instability and insomnia. There is muscular weakness and tremor, palpitation, rapid pulse and shortness of breath. Gynecomastia occurs in males and oligomenorrhea, in females. Gastrointestinal disturbances include increased appetite and, occasionally, diarrhea; however, there is loss of weight.

4.9. The concentration of serum calcium controls the release of *thyrocalcitonin*. A rise stimulates secretion and a fall suppresses secretion (Note that this is in reciprocal relationship with the secretion of parathyroid hormone).

4.10. The exact role of thyrocalcitonin is unclear because it is difficult to detect in serum and there is no disease state attributable to its deficiency.

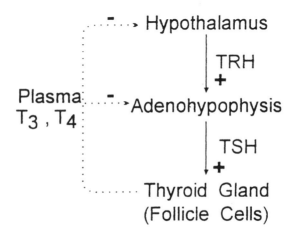

Control of Thyroid Hormone secretion

PARATHYROID GLANDS

1. General

1.1. *Parathyroid glands* (para (Gk) beside) are named because of their close proximity to the thyroid gland. Usually, four small ovoid parathyroid glands are situated between the posterior borders of the thyroid lobes and its capsule. Each measures 6 mm by 3–4 mm by 1–2 mm and weighs about 50 mg.

1.2. The four parathyroid glands are:
Superior parathyroid glands (2) at the middle of the posterior border

of the lobe of the thyroid gland. These arise from the fourth pharangeal pouches and are also known as *Parathyroids 4*.

Inferior parathyroid glands (2) are found in either of various positions:

A. In the fascial sheath of the thyroid below the inferior thyroid artery, near the inferior pole of the thyroid gland.

B. Behind the thyroid, outside of its fascial sheath, in front of the inferior thyroid artery; or

C. In the substance of the thyroid gland near the end of its inferior border. The inferior parathyroid glands develop from the third pharyngeal pouches and are often known as *Parathyroids 3*.

Note that the parathyroids develop in relation to the thymus and may descend with it into the thorax or they may not descend at all.

1.3. The function of the parathyroid glands is to raise blood calcium by multiple actions on several organ systems, including bone, kidney and the gut.

2. Detailed Structure

2.1. Parathyroids are surrounded by a *capsule* from which *septa* radiate but do not divide the glands into distinct lobules.

2.2. The *parenchyma* comprises:

    2.2.1. *Chief (Principal) cells*, light, dark or clear types arranged in wide, irregular anastomosing columns or cords separated by sinusoidal capillaries.

      (i) In contrast with other endocrine gland cells, these cells pass through their secretory cycles independently.

      (ii) They contain a large Golgi zone, small membrane-bound vesicles, glycogen and lipofuscin. However, their general appearance depends on their level of activity. Inactive cells outnumber active cells by 35:1.

      (iii) Chief cells secrete *parathyroid hormone (PTH)*.

    2.2.2. *Oxyphil (Eosinophil) cells* appear before puberty and increase in number thereafter. They are larger than Chief cells and their cytoplasmic eosinophilic granules result from an abundance of mitochondria. They do not appear to be involved in parathyroid hormone synthesis; however, in some rare cases of hyper-parathyroidism, tumors have been shown to contain oxyphil cells.

PARATHYROID GLAND

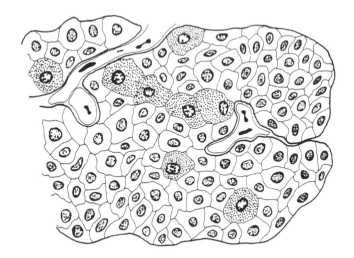

Parathyroid gland (light micrograph)

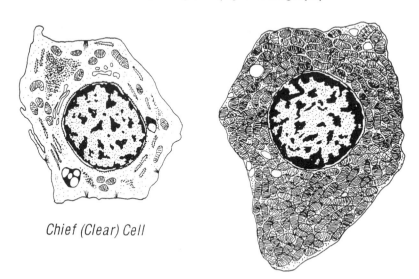

Chief (Clear) Cell

Oxyphil Cell

3. Histophysiology

3.1. *Parathyroid hormone* (*PTH*) is a polypeptide of 84 amino acids which maintains extracellular fluid calcium concentration by raising blood calcium.

3.2. PTH acts:

A. directly on osteocytes and osteoclasts stimulating osteolysis.

B. by increasing excretion of phosphate, sodium and potassium which decrease calcium excretion.

C. by effecting intestinal synthesis of 1 alpha, 25-dihydroxyvitamin D, which acts to increase serum calcium.

3.3. Removal of the parathyroids results in convulsive spasms of muscles (tetany from tetanus (Gk) stiffness) which, when it includes laryngeal muscles, results in death.

3.4. Excessive secretion of PTH by tumors results in *Generalized Osteitis Fibrosa Cystica* in which calcium ions pass from bones to blood, resulting in hypercalcaemia.

Clinical symptoms include polyuria, excessive thirst, nausea and anorexia, as well as bone rarefaction, cyst formation and spontaneous fractures, absence of the lamina dura from around teeth and diffuse "salt and pepper" decalcification of the skull. Calcium may be deposited in blood vessel walls and in a semicircular form around the limbus of the cornea (limbus keratopathy). Excess calcium is excreted in urine and may result in calcification of renal tubules (nephrocalcinosis) and kidney stone formation (nephrolithiasis).

THE PANCREAS

1. General

1.1. The *pancreas* (pan (Gk) all, and kreas (Gk) flesh) combines exocrine and endocrine functions. It is a compound tubuloalveolar serous gland covered with thin connective tissue (areolar tissue) from which septa radiate to divide the gland into lobules.

1.2. The parenchyma is supported by a long, branched, axial duct system, collagenous septa and reticular tissue embedding individual alveoli and epithelial islets.

1.3. The predominant *exocrine part* comprises serous alveoli and a duct system which drains into the duodenum.

1.4. The *endocrine part* comprises some 800,000–1,200,000 scattered epithelial masses (*pancreatic islets*) each penetrated by a rich capillary network.

2. Development

2.1. The pancreas first appears at 3–4 mm as two entodermal outpockets on opposite sides of the duodenum. A *dorsal pancreas* develops just rostral to the hepatic diverticulum and a *ventral pancreas* in the angle between the gut and hepatic diverticulum.

2.2. The *dorsal pancreas* grows more rapidly while the ventral pancreas remains smaller.

2.3. The *ventral pancreas* is carried away from the duodenum by lengthening of the common bile duct.

2.4. Unequal growth of the duodenal walls shifts the bile duct dorsally. This brings the ventral pancreas into the dorsal mesentery.

2.5. By 7 weeks, the two primordia interlock.

2.6. The dorsal pancreas produces part of the head, and all of the body and tail or splenic portion of the definitive pancreas. The ventral pancreas forms part of the head and all of the uncinate process.

2.7. Pancreatic islets develop from cells within duct epithelium at the time of fusion of the ducts of the ventral and dorsal pancreas. Mitoses result in disruption of tight junctions between duct and islet cells so that most islet cells detach from duct epithelium. It is possible that islet cells are derived from neuroectoderm cells randomly embedding in the exocrine part of the pancreas.

3. Cells of Pancreatic Islets

3.1. Islet cells are pale in haematoxylin and eosin stained sections and contain granules which differ in alcohol solubility, staining characteristics and binding of antisera.

3.2. A (*Alpha*) *cells*:

3.2.1. These polygonal shaped cells located mostly at the periphery of

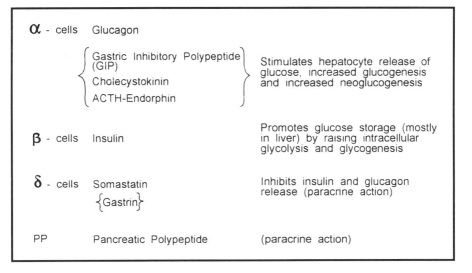

α - cells	Glucagon	
	Gastric Inhibitory Polypeptide (GIP) Cholecystokinin ACTH-Endorphin	Stimulates hepatocyte release of glucose, increased glucogenesis and increased neoglucogenesis
β - cells	Insulin	Promotes glucose storage (mostly in liver) by raising intracellular glycolysis and glycogenesis
δ - cells	Somastatin {Gastrin}	Inhibits insulin and glucagon release (paracrine action)
PP	Pancreatic Polypeptide	(paracrine action)

Cells of Pancreatic Islets.

the islet, represent 20% of all islet cells.

3.2.2. They stain with phosphotungstic acid, Orange G or Mallory Azan but not aldehyde fuchsin and are argyrophilic with the Grimelius technique.

3.2.3. Cytoplasmic granules are fixed by alcohol and are uniform in size (300 nm) with a dense core surrounded by a less densehalo.

3.2.4. Immunocytochemistry indicates that A cells produce *glucagon* as well as other peptides (Gastric Inhibitory Peptide, Cholecystokinin Pancreozymin and ACTH-Endorphin).

3.2.5. Alpha cells originate from neural crest ectoderm.

3.3. *B (Beta) cells*:

3.3.1. B cells are polygonal-shaped cells representing up to 75% of all cells in an islet. They are located mostly toward the center of the islet.

3.3.2. Their cytoplasm contains alcohol-soluble granules which stain with aldehyde fuchsin. In electron micrographs, cytoplasmic vesicles are 200 nm in diameter with a halo around rhomboidal crystalloids. Other cytoplasmic granules in B cells with no subunit structure may be the same granules at a different stage of maturation.

3.3.3. Granules react immunocytochemically with anti-*insulin* serum.

3.3.4. Granules of insulin are released by exocytosis into the pericapillary space.

3.4. *D (Delta or Type III) cells*:

3.4.1. D cells are oval or polygonal in shape, staining blue with Mallory Azan. They comprise up to 8–14% of islet cells and are located toward the periphery of the islet.

3.4.2. The cytoplasm contains vesicles of variable sizes filled with a fine granular homogeneous matrix. They react with anti-*somatostatin* serum (*Somatotrophin Releasing Inhibitory Factor* or *SRIF*).

3.4.3. Granules of the peptide are released into the pericapillary space.

3.5. *D1 (Delta or Type IV) cells*:

3.5.1. Cells are ovoid or comma-shaped and occur singly throughout the islet. They are argyrophilic with the Grimelius stain.

3.5.2. The cytoplasm contains small secretory vesicles with a homogeneous granular interior surrounded by a narrow electron lucent space. These cells react with anti-*vasoactive intestinal peptide* (*VIP*) serum.

3.6. *PP(F) cells*:

3.6.1. PP cells are not confined to islets and may be associated with alveolar cells or located within the epithelium of small ducts of the exocrine pancreas.

3.6.2. The cytoplasm contains small secretory vesicles with a homogeneous granular core. They react with antibodies to *Human Pancreatic Polypeptide* (*PP*).

3.7. *Enterochromaffin (EC)* cells:

3.7.1. These cells are infrequently found in islets.

3.7.2. They stain with silver without reduction of tissue.

3.7.3. The cytoplasm contains pleomorphic vesicles with a pale homogeneous matrix of variable density. They react with anti-sera to *serotonin (5HT)*, *motilin* and *substance P*.

4. Blood Supply of the Pancreas

4.1. The superior and inferior pancreaticoduodenal arteries and pancreatic branch of the splenic arteries divide into interlobular and intralobular arteries which contribute one or more arterioles (vasa afferentia) to each islet.

4.2. Blood enters the mantle of the islet to reach both poles of A and D cells before reaching B cells.

4.3. Capillary walls in islets are fenestrated, allowing rapid translocation of islet products.

4.4. Efferent capillaries (vasa efferentia) radiate from islets to perialveolar networks of the exocrine pancreas.

4.5. Blood flow is controlled by central nervous system directed redistribution resulting from the presence of plasma glucose.

5. Hormones of the Pancreatic Islets

5.1. Many islet cells have now been shown to have structural and functional counterparts in the gastro-intestinal endocrine system; hence, they are grouped with them as the *Gastroentero-Pancreatic Endocrine System*. Their interrelation extends to their origin and development (except for B cells).

5.2. *Insulin* is functionally and quantitatively the major hormone produced. It stimulates the uptake and utilization of sugars by target tissues (liver, adipose tissue and skeletal muscle).

5.3. At the cell membrane, insulin enhances transport of glucose into the cell.

5.4. Within the cell, insulin stimulates phosphorylation of glucose by glucokinase and activates glycogen synthase.

5.5. The overall effect of insulin is to lower blood sugar by favoring storage and utilization of energy substrates.

5.6. Insulin is also known as the "anabolic hormone" as it stimulates protein and triglyceride synthesis in some target tissues.

5.7. *Glucagon* stimulates glycogenolysis by initiating events that leads to activation of glycogen phosphorylase.

5.8. It is a "catabolic hormone" in that it affects proteolysis and a "gluconeogenic hormone" in that it stimulates glucose synthesis.

5.9. It stimulates hepatic lipase activity and fat mobilization in adipose tissue.

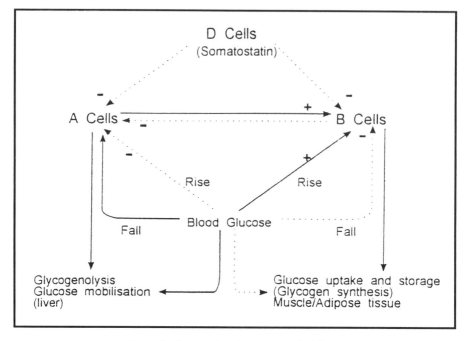

Control of secretion in pancreatic islets.

5.10. Peptides in A cells have an as yet unknown role.

5.11. *Somatostatin (SRIF)* is identical with hypothalamic somatostatin and inhibits the secretion of both insulin and glucagon.

5.12. *Vasoactive Intestinal Polypeptide (VIP)* resembles glucagon in that it is hyperglycaemic and glycogenolytic. VIP also acts as a neurotransmitter regulating muscle tone, motility and secretory activity of the gastrointestinal tract.

5.13. *Pancreatic Polypeptide (PP)* stimulates gastric enzyme secretion and opposes the action of CCK inhibiting bile secretion and intestinal motility.

6. Control of Islet Secretion

6.1. Islet cell secretion is controlled by:

A. *Activity of the autonomic nervous system.* Unmyelinated efferent sympathetic and parasympathetic nerve terminals end in close association with islet cells but only 10% or less islet cells receive

PANCREATIC ISLETS

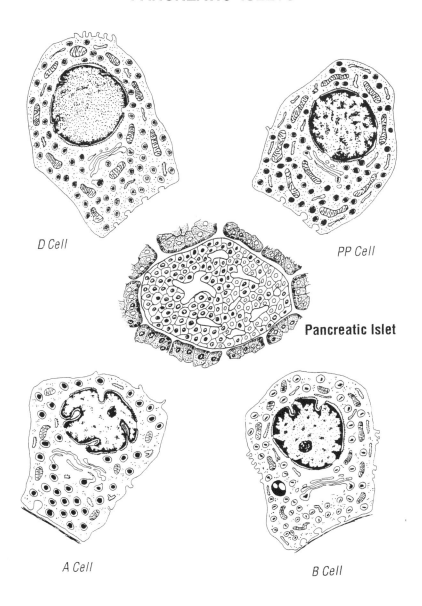

D Cell

PP Cell

Pancreatic Islet

A Cell

B Cell

direct innervation. Cell junctions spread excitation from directly innervated to non-innervated cells. Cholinergic stimulation favors release of all four peptides while adrenergic (or noradrenergic) stimulation inhibits B, D and PP cells only. Stress or catecholamines increase release of glucagon from A cells while A cell breaking is through paracrine or intercellular mechanisms.

B. *Concentration of nutrients in blood,* e.g., sugars, fatty acids or amino acids.

C. *Other islet and gastrointestinal hormones.* Islets show short range (paracrine) control over their own secretion, e.g., insulin inhibits glucagon release and glucagon stimulates insulin release. Somatostatin inhibits the secretion of both.

7. Histophysiology

7.1. *Diabetes Mellitis* is caused by a deficiency of circulating insulin. This may result from B cells which are either:

A. Functionally deficient;

B. Numerically decreased; or

C. Totally absent.

7.2. Less often, the cause may be related to:

A. Resistance of target organs to circulating insulin; or

B. Production of abnormal insulin or proinsulin by B cells.

7.3. Two types of diabetes are described:

A. *Growth onset (insulin dependent) diabetes* is a life threatening, auto-immune disease striking suddenly in childhood or early adulthood. Few B cells survive and treatment requires continued insulin injection therapy.

B. *Maturity onset (non-insulin dependent) diabetes* is less severe and manageable by diet, drugs and exercise. This form may go clinically undetected.

8. **Exocrine Pancreas** (See Section on Gastrointestinal Tract).

Chapter 5
ENDOCRINE SYSTEM
3. SUPRARENAL GLANDS

OBJECTIVES

After reading this chapter, you should be able to:
1. Describe the origin and the fetal development of the suprarenal glands.
2. Describe the histology and products of cells of the suprarenal cortex.
3. Describe the histology and products of cells of the suprarenal medulla.
4. Give an account of the blood supply of the suprarenal glands, including the fine structure of cortical sinusoids.
5. Show, on a feedback diagram, the factors that control secretion of cells of the suprarenal cortex.
6. Describe the histophysiology of the suprarenal cortex in response to hypophysectomy, ACTH or exposure to stress or maintenance on a sodium deficient diet.
7. Give an account of the chromaffin system.
8. Give an outline of what is understood by the diffuse neuroendocrine system.

CHAPTER OUTLINE

The Suprarenal Glands

General structure. Development. Detailed structure of the suprarenal cortex.

Zona Glomerulosa. Zona Fasciculata. Zona Reticularis.

Blood supply of the suprarenal cortex.

Histophysiology of the cortex Aldosterone Cortisol.

Dehydroandosterone.

Effects of Suprarenel medulla ACTH

Detailed structure of the suprarenal medulla.

Histophysiology of the medulla.

The Chromaffin System.

KEY WORDS, PHRASES AND CONCEPTS

Fetal (Provisional) cortex
Permanent cortex
Norepinephrine
Zona Fasciculata
Chromaffin system
Aldosterone
Mineralocorticoids
Cortisol

Chromaffin cells
(Pheochromocytes)
Zona Glomerulosa
Epinephrine
Zona Reticularis
Cushing's syndrome
Glucocorticoids
Addison's disease
Dehydroandosterone

1. General Structure

1.1. Cut in cross section, *suprarenal glands* (supra (L) above and renes (L) kidneys) comprise an outer *cortex* which is yellow in fresh specimens and forms the main mass of the gland, and central medulla, which is dark red and forms one tenth of the total mass.

1.2. The *medulla* is completely enclosed except at the hilum where the suprarenal vein emerges.

1.3. The gland is enclosed in a thick collagenous *capsule* from which trabeculae radiate into the cortex.

2. Development

2.1. The suprarenal gland has a double origin comprising two glands secondarily combined in a common capsule.

2.2. The *fetal (provisional) cortex* is derived from mesoderm. It first appears at 8 mm beneath peritoneal mesothelium, at the base of the mesentery near the cephalic pole of the mesonephros.

2.3. Surface mesothelium first appears in direct continuity with subjacent mesenchyme. These mesenchymal condensations enlarge and project from the dorsal body wall into the coelom between the urogenital organs laterally and dorsal mesentery medially.

2.4. *Provisional cortex* forms the bulk of the gland but it declines (involutes) in the first weeks after birth. It produces corticosteroids during fetal life and cooperates with the placenta to produce estrogen.

2.5. A more compact cortical primordium (*permanent cortex*) originating from the same proliferative focus envelops the original provisional cortex.

2.6. The *medulla* develops from migratory (neuroectoderm) cells which leave ganglia of the celiac plexus and invade the medial side of the gland at 7 weeks. Cells reach the center of the gland by mid-fetal life.

2.7. Medullary cells group into cords and masses which are invaded by a profuse network of capillaries.

2.8. Suprarenal glands are relatively large organs at birth. They are one third of the weight of the kidney at birth compared with one twenty-eighth of the weight of the kidney in the adult.

3. Detailed Structure of the Suprarenal Cortex

The *suprarenal cortex* is divided into three zones:

3.1. *Zona Glomerulosa*, the outermost 15% of total cortical volume, is relatively poorly developed in man.

    3.1.1. Cells are ovoid to columnar arranged in spherical masses or arcades.

    3.1.2. Nuclei are deeply staining.

    3.1.3. The cytoplasm is weakly basophilic and contains a few lipid droplets, microtubules, elongated mitochondria and abundant agranular endoplasmic reticulum, characteristic of steroid-producing cells.

3.2. *Zona Fasciculata*, the middle layer, comprises 78% of total cortex.

    3.2.1. Cells of zona fasciculata (*spongiocytes or clear cells*) are polyhedral, larger than those of the other zones, and arranged in straight columns one or two cells thick.

    3.2.2. The cytoplasm is basophilic and contains lipid droplets, phospholipids, fats, fatty acids and cholesterol (extracted in routine histologic preparation). Organelles include agranular endoplasmic reticulum in a complex arrangement, an extensive Golgi complex and spherical mitochondria with characteristic tubular cristae.

    3.2.3. Adjacent cell cords are separated by fenestrated capillaries.

3.3. *Zona Reticularis*, the innermost zone, is characterized by anastomosing cords of smaller rounded cells.

    3.3.1. Cells are smaller and more compact than those of other zones, contain agranular endoplasmic reticulum, relatively few small lipid inclusions, lysosomes and large accumulations of lipofuscin pigment.

4. Blood Supply of the Suprarenal Cortex

4.1. A subcapsular vascular plexus from branches of *suprarenal, inferior phrenic and renal arteries* opens into the cortical capillaries.

4.2. Most capillaries which have a fenestrated lining pass centripetally between anastomosing cords of cortical cells to reach medullary venules.

4.3. Some major vessels (perforating arterioles) by-pass the cortex to supply the medulla directly.

4.4. Muscular cushions in the wall of venules at the cortico-medullary junction may regulate blood flow through the cortex.

5. Histophysiology of the Suprarenal Cortex

5.1. The suprarenal cortex is essential to life and its removal or destruction is lethal unless replacement therapy is instituted.

5.2. *Zona glomerulosa* produces *aldosterone*, a corticoid influencing electrolyte and water balance (hence aldosterone is known as a mineralocorticoid).

5.3. *Aldosterone* has the effects of:

    A. Promoting resorption of sodium ions in the distal convoluted tubules of the kidney.

B. Increasing potassium excretion by the kidney.

C. Causing lowered sodium concentration in sweat, saliva and intestinal secretion.

5.4. Aldosterone secretion is regulated by:

A. The *renin-angiotensin system*. A fall in renal blood pressure or blood volume causes discharge of the enzyme renin by juxtaglomerular cells. Renin converts plasma angiotensinogen to angiotensin I in the lung and subfornical organ. Angiotensin I is modified to angiotensin II which stimulates the cells of the zona glomerulosa to release aldosterone.

B. *Natriuretic factor*, a peptide which promotes renal sodium (and potassium) excretion is secreted by atrial muscle cells in response to stretch of the atrial wall.

C. Plasma concentrations of potassium and sodium.

5.5. Sodium deficiency leads to hypertrophy of zona glomerulosa with increased aldosterone secretion. This results in sodium and water reabsorption from the distal convoluted tubules of the kidney.

5.6. ACTH does not cause hypertrophy of zona glomerulosa nor increase secretory rate of aldosterone except when given in large doses.

5.7. Zona fasciculata produces hormones effecting carbohydrate metabolism (*glucocorticoids*) most prominently *cortisol*.

5.8. Blood levels of glucocorticoids inhibit the release of *corticotropin releasing factor* (CRF) by the arcuate nucleus of the hypothalamus (negative feedback).

5.9. Glucocorticoids have broad effects, for example, they:

A. Combine with cytoplasmic receptors on a wide variety of cells to form a complex which interacts with nuclear chromatin to modify DNA transcription of mRNA.

B. Promote catabolism in muscle, stimulating the conversion of protein to carbohydrate. They also promote catabolism in skin, adipose and lymphoid tissues.

C. In the liver, they promote carbohydrate production from protein and protein precursors (anabolism) without taking glucose from blood.

D. Inhibit protein synthesis (amino acids are used in gluconeogenesis in the liver).

    E. Decrease uptake of glucose by somatic cells.

    F. Are necessary for lipolysis to occur.

    G. Depress the inflammatory response (suppress fibroblast proliferation) and cause wounds to heal poorly.

    H. Depress the immune response by inhibiting DNA synthesis/mitosis necessary for lymphocyte proliferation and plasma cell differentiation.

    I. Glucocorticoids are necessary for coping with stress.

5.10. The deeper part of zona fasciculata is wider during pregnancy.

5.11. *Zona reticularis*, and to a lesser extent zona fasciculata, produce weak androgens, in particular, dihydroepidandrosterone.

5.12. *Hypophysectomy* results in atrophy and injections of ACTH produce hypertrophy of zona fasciculata and zona reticularis. Neither procedure effects zona glomerulosa.

5.13. When cortical cells are stimulated, nuclei and nucleoli enlarge and the cytoplasm looses its lipid stores. With chronic stimulation, cholesterol stores are lost but not unsaturated fatty acids. With removal of the stimulation, nuclei and nucleoli shrink and lipid droplets coalesce and disappear.

5.14. Cortical atrophy occurs in old age (especially in males), mostly affecting the deepest layer of zona fasciculata.

5.15. *Addison's disease* is associated with atrophy of the suprarenal cortex or its destruction most commonly by autoantibodies or tuberculosis. Symptoms include low blood pressure, anaemia, brown skin pigmentation, changes in electrolyte and fluid balance and terminally, by circulatory and renal failure.

5.16. *Cushing's syndrome* is associated with tumors or hyperplasia of the suprarenal cortex. Symptoms include obesity, excessive hairiness of the face and trunk and diabetes mellitis.

    A. In women, there is amenorrhea and possibly masculinization of secondary sex characteristics (virilism).

    B. In men, there is impotence, hypogonadism and feminization (breast enlargement).

    C. In children, there is precocious body growth, development of genital organs and early menstruation in females.

    D. In the female fetus, cortical hyperplasia produces female pseudohermaphrotidism. Excessive androgen secretion causes the urethra and vagina to open into a persistent urogenital sinus. The clitoris enlarges.

E. In the male fetus, cortical hyperplasia causes excessive development of the genital organs.

SUPRARENAL MEDULLA

1. General Structure

1.1. The suprarenal medulla comprises groups and columns of *chromaffin cells* (*pheochromocytes*) in close contact with capillaries.

1.2. Postganglionic sympathetic neurons related to vascular innervation also appear in groups or singly among chromaffin cells.

2. Detailed Structure

2.1. *Chromaffin cells* (*pheochromocytes*) are large columnar or polyhedral cells arranged in cords one cell thick in close contact with capillaries.

2.2. Cells synthesize and secrete norepinephrine and epinephrine.

2.3. Their cytoplasm is basophilic, has an extensive RER and contains secretory granules. *Norepinephrine* granules are round or ellipsoidal and electron dense while *epinephrine* vesicles are paler and surrounded by a clear zone.

2.4. Secretion, under preganglionic sympathetic control, occurs into a perivascular space and reaches the bloodstream through fenestrated capillaries.

2.5. Cholinergic nerve terminals synapse directly on chromaffin cells.

2.6. Glucocorticoids in blood, draining through the suprarenal cortex, induce the synthesis of an enzyme (PNMT) needed for the synthesis of epinephrine and norepinephrine by cells in the medulla.

3. Histophysiology of the Medulla

3.1. Under normal conditions, medullary cells secrete very little but the amount of secretion increases with fear, stress or anger.

3.2. Norepinephrine causes cardiac acceleration, vasoconstriction and increased blood pressure.

3.3. Epinephrine has a greater effect on carbohydrate metabolism.

3.4. *Pheochromocytoma* is a tumor of cells of the suprarenal medulla. It is accompanied by excessive production of epinephrine and norepinephrine. Clinical symptoms include palpitations, excessive sweating, skin pallor, hypertension, headaches, retinitis and vascular changes in the kidney.

4. The Chromaffin System

4.1. Catecholamines in cytoplasmic granules of some cells are oxidized by potassium bichromate resulting in a brown reaction product (adrenochrome). This is known as the *chromaffin reaction*.

4.2. After reacting with formaldehyde vapor, chromaffin cells also fluoresce yellow-green in ultraviolet light.

4.3. Groups of chromaffin cells associated with the sympathetic nervous system are located in the suprarenal medulla, para-aortic bodies, autonomic ganglia and some cells in the carotid bodies.

4.4. *Chromaffin cells* have common features in that they are derived from the neural crest, are innervated by pre-ganglionic sympathetic nerves and synthesize catecholamines (dopamine, epinephrine or norepinephrine).

4.5. Three main groups of cells give a positive chromaffin reaction:

A. *Sympathetic neurons*.

B. *Enterochromaffin cells* in epithelial tissue lining the gastrointestinal and respiratory tracts.

C. *Mast cells* in connective tissue of the gut, pancreas and liver.

SUPRARENAL GLAND

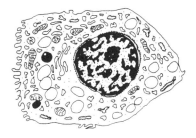

Zona Glomerulosa cell

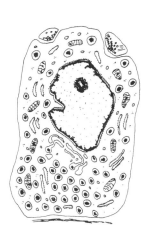

Epinephrocyte

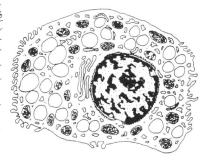

Zona Fasciculata cell
(Spongiocyte)

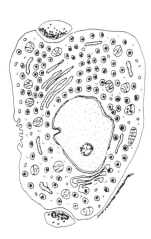

Norepinephrocyte

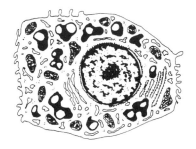

Zona Reticularis cell

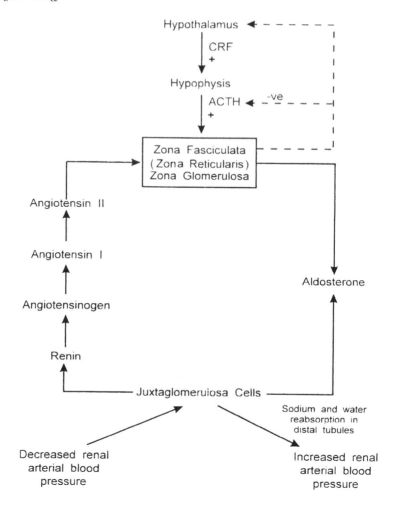

Control of secretion in the suprarenal cortex.

CHAPTER 6

IMMUNE SYSTEM
1. CELLS OF THE IMMUNE RESPONSE

OBJECTIVES

After reading this chapter, you should be able to:
1. Give an account of the functional characteristics of B lymphocytes and describe their role in the humoral immune response.
2. Discuss the different functional subsets of T lymphocytes and describe their role in the immune response.
3. Describe the structure of macrophages and give an account of how they participate in the defence mechanism (the Mononuclear Phagocytic System).
4. Describe what is meant by the slow and fast circulations of lymphocytes.
5. Differentiate between the primary and secondary immune responses.
6. Discuss immunological tolerance and auto-immunity.
7. Describe the structure and function of Mast cells, Langerhans cells and M cells.
8. Give an account of a current theory of the developmental origin of blood elements (CFU's) and describe the prenatal sites of hematopoiesis.

CHAPTER OUTLINE

General. Interstitial fluid. The Mononuclear Phagocytic System. The Immune System.

Terminology. Lymphoepithelial organs. Lymphopoietic organs. Lymphatic organs. Lymphatic tissue. Bursa analogue. Mucosa Associated Lymphoid Tissue (MALT). Primary (Central) Lymphoid Organs. Secondary (Peripheral) Lymphoid Organs.

Lymphocytes. Small Lymphocytes, Large Lymphocytes. B Lymphocytes, T Lymphocytes, Immunoblasts, Null cells, NK cells, K cells.

Origin of lymphocytes.

Plasma cells. Classes of antibodies.

Functions of antibodies. Immune responses. Immunological tolerance. Autoimmunity.

Circulation of lymphocytes.

Macrophages. Reticuloendothelial system. Mononuclear Phagocytic System.

Antigen Presenting Cells.

Mast Cells.

Polymorphonuclear Leucocytes or Granulocytes (Polymorphs)

KEY WORDS, PHRASES, CONCEPTS

Interstitial fluid
Lymphocytes (T&B)
Antibodies (Immunoglobulins)
Plasma cells (Plasmacytes)
Immunoblasts
Cell mediated immunity
Lymphokines
Helper cells
Suppressor cells
Memory cells
Immunological tolerance
Lymphoepithelial organ
Lymphatic organ
Mucosa Associated Lymphoid Tissue
Secondary Lymphoid Organs

Primary immune response
Secondary immune response
Humoral immunity
Mononuclear Phagocytic System
Monocytes
Activated lymphocytes
Complement
M cells
Langerhans cells
Circulation of lymphocytes
Lymphopoiesis
Lymphoietic organ
Lymphatic tissue
Primary Lymphoid Organs
Small Lymphocytes

Large Lymphocytes
Natural Killer cells
Immunoglobulins
Autoimmunity
Fast circulation
Follicular Dendritic Cells
Macrophages (Histiocytes)

Null cells
K (killer) cells
Immunological tolerance
Slow circulation
Antigen Presenting Cells
Mast cells
Bursa analogue

1. General

1.1. Tissue comprises cells in a fluid medium. *Interstitial fluid* (Claude Bernard's milieu interieur) varies in composition, containing nutrients transported to cells and waste products transported from cells.

1.2. Higher vertebrates have evolved a second "circulation", *the lymphatic system* to recirculate interstitial fluid back to the bloodstream.

1.3. *Lymphatic capillaries* begin as blind channels in connective tissue and are permeable to substances of greater molecular weight than those that can pass through the walls of blood capillaries.

1.4. Along the path of lymphatic capillaries, *lymph nodes*, which are filtering beds, remove particles before they can enter the blood stream.

1.5. Lymph nodes contain macrophages which are part of a protective *Mononuclear Phagocytic System (MPS)*. They ingest dead tissue, particles and bacteria.

1.6. Lymph nodes are also centers for proliferation and storage of lymphocytes which originate from elsewhere (e.g., the thymus or bone marrow).

1.7. *Lymphocytes* produce proteins (globulins also known as *antibodies*) which can inactivate foreign substances, bacteria and neoplastic cells, thereby contributing to a defence system, the immune system which complements the *mononuclear phagocytic system*.

2. Terminology

2.1. *Lymphoepithelial organs* are a group of organs in which lymphocytes contact and colonize an epithelium, e.g., tonsils, Peyer's patches, the appendix and thymus.

2.2. *Lymphopoietic organs* (lymph + poiesis (Gk) making) are tissues and organs in which the production of lymphocytes takes place, e.g., marrow, lymphatic tissue and lymphoepithelial organs.

2.3. *Lymphatic (Lymphoid or Lymphoreticular)* organs are organs formed totally of lymphatic tissue, e.g., lymph nodes and spleen.

2.4. *Lymphatic (Lymphoid or Lymphoreticular) tissue* is a category of reticular tissue forming the parenchyma of lymph nodes, the spleen and tonsils. In its meshes, there is an abundance of lymphopoietic cells and lymphocytes.

2.5. *Bursa Analogue* is an unknown organ in mammals analogous to the Bursa of Fabricius in birds which is a maturation and differentiation site for B lymphocytes. It is thought that lymph nodules and Peyer's Patches in the mammalian gut can partially assume this role.

2.6. *Mucosa Associated Lymphoid Tissue (MALT)* refers to non-encapsulated accumulations of lymphoid tissue which occur throughout the body. When associated with the gastrointestinal tract, accumulations are known as Gut Associated Lymphoid Tissue (GALT).

2.7. *Primary (Central) Lymphoid Organs* are the bone marrow, skin, Peyer's patches and thymus, major sites of lymphopoiesis where lymphocytes differentiate from stem cells, proliferate and mature into functional effector cells.

2.8. *Secondary (Peripheral) Lymphoid Organs* include the lymph nodes, spleen, tonsils and lymphoid nodules scattered throughout the body. They create an environment where lymphocytes can interact with each other and with antigens to disseminate the immune response.

3. Lymphocytes

3.1. *Lymphocytes* are the most common type of agranular leucocyte and second most numerous leucocyte ($1500-2700/mm^3$ or $25-40\%$ of circulating leucocytes). They are produced in primary lymphoid organs at a high rate ($10^9/day$).

3.2. Lymphocytes differ from other white cells in that although they arise from stem cells in marrow, they are produced in large numbers by further divisions outside bone marrow.

3.3. Lymphocytes are non-phagocytic leucocytes.

3.4. They undergo initial differentiation in central lymphoid tissues, bone marrow (B lymphocytes) or thymus (T lymphocytes).

3.5. Progeny pass in the circulation to peripheral lymphoid organs (*secondary lymphoid organs*) where they proliferate, mature and migrate into surrounding tissue or return to the circulation.

3.6. A morphological classification of lymphocytes is on the basis of cell size:

3.6.1. *Small Lymphocytes* are round cells (diameter 8 μm) with a spherical nucleus containing very condensed chromatin and 1–3 nucleoli. The cytoplasm forms a 0.2–1 μm rim with few organelles, indicating a low metabolic activity. Small lymphocytes are freely motile, passing between endothelial cells into the extravascular space or into saliva.

3.6.2. *Large Lymphocytes* are not usually found in the circulation and are either:

Immunoblasts capable of becoming small lymphocytes, a step occurring in the lymphoid system; or

Transforming cells or functionally active small lymphocytes after antigenic stimulation.

Both have a euchromatic nucleus, prominent nucleolus and basophilic cytoplasm, and are active in protein synthesis.

3.7. The life span of lymphocytes varies. One group is short lived (a few days) while another group (memory cells) is long lived (many years) and reacts rapidly to reintroduction of an antigen in the secondary immune reaction.

3.8. Lymphocytes are constantly present in the bloodstream, lymph, other body fluids, connective tissue and specialized lymphoid organs and tissues.

3.9. A functional classification of lymphocytes is on the basis of immunological capacity:

3.9.1. *B (Bursa Dependent) Lymphocytes* are defined by their ability to proliferate and produce immunoglobulins.

A. B cells originate from stem cells in marrow, mature in bursa analogue (thought to be lymphatic nodules along the gut in man), and may return to the circulation where they represent 65% of circulating lymphocytes.

B. They do not pass through the thymus but move directly via the circulation to general lymphoid tissue differentiating en route.

C. Non-activated B lymphocytes have a life span of 12 days.

D. The cell surface is covered with molecules of immunoglobulin (mostly IgM and IgD types) which can form complexes with some antigens rendered immunogenic by macrophages.

E. After interiorization of these complexes by micropinocytosis, B lymphocytes become activated under the influence of a subgroup of T Lymphocytes (Helper Cells) and differentiate into *Immunoblasts*. These are larger cells characterized by an increase in cytoplasmic volume which is rich in free ribosomes.

F. *Immunoblasts* divide every 6 hours, some differentiating into plasma cells which secrete immunoglobulin (IgG type) that neutralize circulating antigens. The process of immunity resulting from substances in a fluid is known as *humoral immunity*.

G. The remaining B immunoblasts become *Memory cells* which can react more rapidly in future when contacting the same antigen. These cells have a life span of several years.

H. B cells also have receptors on their cell membranes that bind antigens. These include *Fc receptors* that bind to the Fc regions of immunoglobulins, *complement receptors* and *insulin receptors*. The latter is used as a marker of cellular activation.

3.9.2. *T* (*Thymus Dependent*) *Lymphocytes* represent 35% of circulating lymphocytes.

A. T cells originate from stem cells in bone marrow and migrate to and colonise the *thymus* where they divide, differentiate and mature.

B. Upon re-entering the bloodstream, they migrate through the walls of *post-capillary venules* and *colonize thymus-dependent zones* of lymph nodes and spleen.

C. T Lymphocytes, in contrast to B lymphocytes, carry out a number of distinctive activities including a type of defence which does not depend directly on antibody attack. They also have a role of controlling other cells of the immune system.

D. Stimulated by antigen, defensive T cells (*effector cells*) are stimulated to reproduce and grow into large lymphocytes. These cells either:

    (i) Release cytotoxic substances (*lymphokines*) in the neighborhood of the antigenic body. Lymphokines also effect migration of macrophages, neutrophils and eosinophils, stimulate mitosis of other lymphocytes and increase capillary permeability;

    (ii) Cause destruction of the antigen by cellular adherence to it and release of toxic material at short range; or

    (iii) Arm other cells to carry out aggressive cytotoxic operation (e.g., macrophages).

E. The type of immunity mediated by T lymphocytes is directed against foreign or abnormal cells including virus infected, neoplastic and graft cells. The process of direct destruction of antigens by T lymphocytes and macrophages is known as *cell mediated immunity* (*CMI*).

F. T cells respond to *major histocompatability complex* (*MHC*) antigens expressed on foreign cells in grafts leading to graft rejection.

G. In contact with corresponding macrophage processed antigen, some T lymphocytes produce microhumoral substances or cooperate directly with B lymphocytes, stimulating their transformation to immunoblasts.

H. T cells possess surface receptors for erythrocytes (E receptor), Fc region of immunoglobulins, complement, histamine, fetoprotein (a major fetal serum protein) and transferrin (an iron binding protein).

I. Functional subpopulations of T cells also possess one or several specific cell surface antigens (CD1 etc., where CD stands for cluster of differentiation), for example helper cells have CD4 antigen, suppressor cells have CD8, while immature T cells have CD9 and CD10.

J. Other T cells proliferate and differentiate into T immunoblasts which become:

    (i) *Helper Cells* which bring a specific antigen directly or via a macrophage to a preconditioned B lymphocyte or interact with plasma cells to amplify the production of immunoglobulins.

(ii) *Killer cells* (*cytotoxic lymphocytes or graft rejection cells*) may surround bacteria, grafted cells, etc., adhere to them, and provoke their lysis by releasing cytotoxic substances such as lymphotoxins and lymphokines. These cause an irreversible alteration of the plasma membrane of the target cell. In addition, they activate passing macrophages. Killer cells have a life span of a few days.

(iii) *Suppressor cells* regulate both cellular and humoral immunity by inhibiting helper and killer cells.

(iv) *Memory cells*, the long living progeny of T immunoblasts, which react rapidly upon second exposure to the same antigen.

3.9.3. *Null cells* are lymphocytes that do not possess a characteristic set of surface markers that identifies them as either T or B cells.

A. They represent about 5–10% of peripheral blood lymphocytes.

B. Null cells include two types of cytotoxic lymphocytes:

(i) *Antibody independent natural killer* (*NK*) cells which non-specifically kill tumor cells and virally infected cells. They also play a role in regulating cells of the immune response; and

(ii) *Antibody dependent killer* (*K*) cells which also kill non-specifically but this occurs via antibodies bound to their target cells.

4. Origin of Lymphocytes

4.1. According to the monophyletic theory, *totipotent hematopoietic stem cells* (*THCS*), or a class of such cells, originate from a primitive reticular cell. THCS produce bipotential stem cells for lymphopoiesis (immunoblasts) and pluripotential myeloid restricted stem cells or *Colony Forming Units* (*CFU-S*). The latter are capable of transforming into progenitor cells of the granulopoietic (CFU-G), erythropoietic (CFU-E) monopoietic (CFU-m) and megakaryopoietic (CFU-M) series.

4.2. Prenatal hematopoiesis appears firstly within *blood islands* in the yolk sac wall (the *mesoblastic phase*) from 1–3 months. It then follows sequentially in the mesenchyme of the forming liver and spleen (the *hepatosplenic phase*) from 2–9 months, and finally within bone marrow (the *myeloid phase*) after 5 months.

5. Plasma Cells

5.1. *Plasma cells* are ovoid cells about 20 μm in diameter with a round, eccentric nucleus, small nucleolus and radial clumps of dense heterochromatin adjacent to the nuclear membrane, giving it a "cartwheel" appearance. The cytoplasm has a highly developed RER with expanded cisternae which contain immunoglobulins.

5.2. Plasma cells are produced from B lymphocytes in bone marrow, connective tissues and lymphatic tissues and have a life span of 10–30 days.

5.3. Antigenically stimulated B lymphocytes proliferate into plasma cells (*plasmacytes*) which synthesize and secrete circulating *antibodies*. These in turn recognize and bind specifically to foreign chemical substrates (*antigens*), inactivating them.

5.4. Plasma cells are weakly ameboid but are seldom seen in the circulation.

5.5. *Antibodies (Immunoglobulins)* are either:

    5.5.1. *Soluble* (circulating freely in body fluids); or

    5.5.2. *Cytophilic* (secondarily attached to defence cells).

5.6. Antibodies produced by plasma cells are proteins which contain four polypeptide chains, two long (heavy) and two shorter (light) chains joined by SH groups.

    5.6.1. The molecule is Y shaped with two arms on a central hinge.

    5.6.2. The stem of the molecule, the *Fc (Fraction, constant)* portion, has a relatively constant amino acid sequence and attaches to cell membranes via specific Fc receptors.

    5.6.3. The arms of the molecule, the *Fab (Fraction, antigen binding)* fraction, have a highly variable amino acid sequence which is responsible for specific binding to antigens.

    5.6.4. Classes of antibodies include:

        A. *Immunoglobulin G (IgG)* produced by plasmacytes represent the bulk of plasma immunoglobulins.

B. *Immunoglobulin A (IgA) or secretory antibody* is a local antibody produced by the plasma cells and lymphocytes of the lamina propria of the respiratory, urogenital and gastrointestinal tracts and is present in their secretions. During passage through the epithelium, two molecules are assembled into a dimer by a glycoprotein *secretory component (SC)* produced by epithelial cells, then released at the surface in a form resistant to proteolytic enzymes. IgA protects epithelia against viral and bacterial invasion.

C. *Immunoglobulin E (IgE) or cytophilic antibody* is fixed to the cell membrane of mast cells and basophil leucocytes. In contact with antigens, it induces the release of histamine by mast cells and leukotrienes by leucocytes, provoking some allergic reactions.

D. *Immunoglobulin M (IgM)* is a pentamer of monomers joined by their Fc end into a star shaped aggregate. IgM is produced early in an immune response and is progressively replaced by IgG.

E. *Immunoglobulin D (IgD)* is a cytophilic antibody found on the cell membrane of B lymphocytes. It may have a role in antigen triggered lymphocyte proliferation but its significance is poorly understood.

5.7. Antibodies act to:

5.7.1. Agglutinate antigens by forming cross links between them.

5.7.2. Bind with complement and with the antigenic site puncturing the cell membrane and causing lysis of bacteria.

5.7.3. Attach by Fc ends to other defence cells (macrophages or neutrophils) arming them to detect, adhere to and ingest or enzymatically damage foreign bodies. Cell bound antibodies can activate complement complex causing lysis of bacteria.

5.7.4. May coat an antigen (opsonizing antibodies or opsonins) before attaching to a macrophage and stimulating its phagocytic activity.

5.7.5. *Cytophilic antibodies* activate cells, e.g., mast cells, when they bind antigens, causing them to release their cytoplasmic products (degranulation), a reaction seen in allergy.

5.8. *Complement* is a system of proteins in serum that interacts with antibodies to kill bacteria or cells by lysis. Antibodies and complement provide finer selectivity for phagocytosis.

6. Immune Responses

6.1. The *primary response* is a series of morphological and biochemical events resulting in proliferation and differentiation of B lymphocytes to immunoblasts, memory cells and plasma cells following primary contact with appropriate antigen. The response may extend over several weeks.

6.2. The *secondary response* is a rapid, amplified reaction of memory cells accompanied by a great increase in circulating antibodies after secondary contact with the antigen that provoked the primary response.

6.3. *Immunological tolerance* refers to a specific lack of responsiveness to an antigen by either B or T cells. It results from the generation of specifically programmed T suppressor (Ts) cells but can also result from exposure to high concentrations of antigen (T Helper cells are also made non-responsive in this way).

6.4. *Autoimmunity* refers to immunological reactivity directed against "self" macromolecules. In some cases, the protein comes directly in contact with the immune system while in other cases, cross reacting immune responses eventually involve body tissues.

7. Circulation of Lymphocytes

7.1. Lymphopoietic cells and lymphocytes pass between various lymphopoietic organs and tissues via blood and lymph.

7.2. *Slow circulation* of lymphocytes requires several weeks. It involves the movement of undifferentiated lymphocytes from marrow to the thymus or bursa analogue where they mature. They return to the bloodstream, then pass into the tissues and are collected by afferent lymphatics and transported to nodes. Through efferent lymphatics, lymphocytes return to the bloodstream before the cycle repeats.

7.3. *Fast circulation* of lymphocytes involves the recirculation of B and T lymphocytes from blood to tissues and lymph organs and back into the bloodstream. Recirculation through blood requires about 0.6 h, through spleen 6 h and through lymph nodes 15–20 h. Large lymphocytes do not recirculate.

7.4. The purpose of recirculation is to have a constant population of immunocompetent lymphocytes throughout all parts of the body that informs lymphopoietic organs about the presence or absence of antigens.

7.5. In the presence of antigen, some lymphocytes settle in lymphopoietic organs, begin to divide and trigger an immune response.

7.6. Lymphocytes that are lost during recirculation are replaced by the slow circulation from production in marrow, thymus and lymphatic tissue. It is estimated that of the average number of lymphocytes (10^{10}), 10^9 new lymphocytes are produced daily from marrow and the thymus to replace effete cells.

8. Macrophages (Histiocytes)

8.1. *Macrophages* are a class of large cells capable of phagocytosing large particles, e.g., entire cells or cell debris, bacteria, foreign bodies or inert particles. They are motile when stimulated.

8.2. The nucleus is smaller and more heterochromatic than that of a fibroblast.

8.3. The cytoplasm contains conspicuous lysosomes and the cell membrane, which possesses receptors for the Fc end of IgG, has prominent surface folds, pseudopodia and microvilli.

8.4. They may group around large foreign bodies resistant to intracellular digestion and fuse to form multinucleated, syncytial *Foreign Body Giant Cells*.

8.5. The precursor cell of the macrophage is a *monocyte*.

8.6. Functions of macrophages include:

A. *Phagocytosis*. Macrophages selectively phagocytose particles previously coated by antibodies, synthesized by lymphocytes, and are the site of cytophilic antibody attachment (they have cell surface receptors for the Fc end of IgG), enabling them to recognize and attack foreign substances. Phagocytosis is also facilitated when macrophages are activated by complement.

B. *Synthesis*. Macrophages produce a wide range of products important in the reaction against microorganisms, viruses and tumor cells. These include:

(i) Some *complement* proteins.

(ii) *Lysosomal proteases, collagenases, elastases and leukotrienes* released only during the phagocytosis, degrade bacterial cell walls.

(iii) *Interferon*, an antiviral glycoprotein.

(iv) Products which *regulate the immune response*, e.g., *interleukin 1* which promotes the immune response and *plasminogen activator* which stimulates T cells. Interferon, produced by lymphocytes and prostaglandins, produced by a number of cells, tend to inhibit immune responses.

C. *Regulation of the immune response.* In two additional ways, by producing hematopoietic growth regulators, and by passing on adherent antigens to neighboring immunologically competent cells.

8.7. The Reticuloendothelial System (RES) is the name given to a diffuse system of macrophages, lymphatic organs and specialized phagocytic endothelial cells lining blood sinuses. The name has been replaced by the Mononuclear Phagocytic System (MPS) for two main reasons:

A. Cells comprising the system, although morphologically dissimilar, appear to have a common origin from a monocyte-like cell.

B. Endothelial cells lining sinuses, although once thought to be phagocytic, are not. Macrophages immediately beneath the endothelium reach processes between fenestrae in endothelial cells — a process confirmed with the improved resolution of the electron microscope.

8.7.1. Cells of the MPS include:

Monocytes in marrow and blood.

Macrophages (fixed and wandering histiocytes) in connective tissues.

Kupffer cells (stellate reticuloendothelial cells) in liver.

Reticular cells in spleen and lymph nodes.

Alveolar macrophages (dust cells, heart failure cells) in lung.

Osteoclasts in bone and possibly *odontoclasts* which resorb teeth and *chondroclasts* which resorb cartilage.

Foreign Body Giant Cells which surround inert particles and some bacteria.

Kolmer's Cells (supraependymal macrophages) on the wall of the brain ventricles.

Microglia in brain.

9. Antigen Presenting Cells (APC)

9.1. *Antigen presenting cells* are found primarily in skin, lymph nodes, spleen and thymus. Their main role is to present antigens to antigen sensitive lymphoid cells

9.2. This group includes:

    9.2.1. *Langerhans cells* (*Granular non-pigmented dendrocytes*) found in all viable layers of skin and in lymph nodes. They have slender dendritic processes and are motile. The cytoplasm contains SER, small lysosomes, lipid droplets and specific granules (Birbek's granules or Langerhan's bodies). The cell membrane possesses Fc and C3 receptors and cells contain class 2 MHC, important in presenting antigen to T cells. Langerhans cells migrate as "veiled cells" into lymph nodes where they interdigitate with T cells. They produce *interleukin 2* (*IL2*), which causes T lymphocytes to proliferate, and they promote the cutaneous *Delayed Hypersensitivity Reaction* presenting antigen to T helper cells.

    9.2.2. *Follicular dendritic cells* found in secondary follicles of B cell areas of lymph nodes and spleen.

    9.2.3. *Interdigitating follicular cells* (*IDC*) in the thymic medulla. These cells are rich in "self" antigens including Class 2 *major histocompatability complex* (*MHC*) which, carried to T cells, helps in selecting out T cells that react against self antigens.

    9.2.4. *Macrophages* (see above).

    9.2.5. *M* (*Membrane-like epithelial*) *cells or Follicle Associated Epithelial Cells* (*FAE*) are specifically differentiated absorptive cells scattered in the epithelium covering Peyer's patches in the intestine. They have loosely arranged surface microvilli and apical pits and are joined to adjacent cells by junctional complexes. M cells transport intact intraluminal antigens to subjacent intraepithelial lymphocytes or macrophages.

10. Mast Cells

10.1. *Mast cells* are large wandering cells of connective tissue generally found along blood vessels.

10.2. The cell body is extremely variable in shape and covered by small folds, invaginations and long microvilli.

10.3. The cytoplasm contains RER, microtubules, microfilaments and large metachromatic secretory granules which contain *histamine*, *heparin* (as heparin proteoglycan whose main function is to bind other granular constituents), *chimase*, *beta glucuronidase*, *eosinophilic chemotactic factor of anaphylaxis* (*ECF-A*), *neutrophil chemotactic factor* (*NCF*) and *lysosomal hydrolases*. Outside the granules are *leukotrines*, *prostaglandins*, *platelet activating factor* (*PAF*) and *hydrogen peroxide*.

10.4. Mast cells contribute to *immediate sensitivity* in cases of allergy. Fc receptors in the cell membrane have a high affinity for IgE which reacts with antigen. This causes degranulation of the cell and results in bronchospasm and edema.

10.5. The life span of mast cells is 8–18 days.

11. Polymorphonuclear Leucocytes or Granulocytes (Polymorphs)

11.1. *Polymorphonuclear granulocytes* (*leucocytes*) possess no specificity for antigens but participate in the defence mechanism by reacting with antibodies and complement coated (opsonized) foreign bodies through specific receptors on their cell membrane. Their predominant role is in acute inflammation and protection against microorganisms through subsequent phagocytosis.

11.2. Granulocytes are produced in great numbers in bone marrow and are relatively short lived.

11.3. They are classified on the basis of the staining reaction of cytoplasmic granules.

11.4. *Neutrophils*:

    A. *Neutrophils* are formed in marrow, move to the blood circulation (where they comprise 60–90% of circulating granulocytcs) then to the tissues.

    B. They are 10–20 μm in diameter with a single segmented nucleus.

    C. The cytoplasm contains little RER (indicating small reserve) and two types of granules:

      (i) *Primary* (*azurophilic*) *granules* (lysosomes) 500 nm in diameter contain *neutral and acid hydrolases*, *neutral proteases*, myeloperoxidase and lysozyme. These granules represent 20% of total cytoplasmic granules.

(ii) *Secondary (specific) granules* contain *lactoferrin, alkaline phosphatase, lysozyme* and *collagenase.*

D. Neutrophils are very motile, especially in the presence of bacterial products, factors produced by damaged cells, leukotrienes, factors produced by mast cells, opsonins, complement and some of its cleavage products.

E. Coating of the particle by opsonins or C3 (the neutrophil has receptors for both) which reduces surface negative charge is necessary before neutrophils will phagocytose.

F. The attachment of the particle to the cell membrane of the neutrophil initiates the *respiratory burst metabolic pathway*. In this pathway, hydrogen peroxide is converted to bactericidal compounds via myeloperoxidase located in primary granules. Hydrogen peroxide is catalysed in reaction with intracellular chloride to produce bactericidal hypochlorite ions.

G. Iron, which is essential for bacterial growth, is denied from bacteria by lactoferrin in secondary granules of neutrophils.

H. Neutrophils are the first cells to react to foreign antigens but do not prepare the antigen for antigen presenting cells.

11.5. *Eosinophils (Azurophilic Granulocytes)*

A. *Eosinophils* comprise 1–4% of blood leucocytes. They are released from marrow, mature in the spleen and migrate to the tissues where they have a half life of about 12 days.

B. The nucleus is bilobed and the cytoplasm contains many ribosomes and mitochondria indicating that the cell is metabolically very active.

C. In addition, the cytoplasm contains granules (lysosomes) which stain with eosin. These specific granules are membrane bound with a crystalloid core containing acid phosphatase and peroxidase.

D. Attracted by products released by T lymphocytes, mast cells (histamine) and basophils (Eosinophilic Chemotactic Factor of Anaphylaxis, ECF-A), they bind to the cell membrane of some parasites which have been coated with IgG (opsonin). They degranulate, releasing a protein (*eosinophilic basic protein*) which is toxic to the parasite.

E. Eosinophils also have a role in dampening the inflammatory allergic response. They release *histaminase*, which inactivates histamine released by mast cells, and *aryl sulphatase*, which inactivates *Slow Reactive Substance of Anaphylaxis* (*SRS-A*), a collection of leukotrienes produced by macrophages.

11.6. *Basophils*

A. *Basophils* are 10–12 μm in diameter and comprise less than 0.5% of blood leucocytes. They are not normally seen in the intercellular spaces but migrate there under the influence of T lymphocytes.

B. The nucleus is kidney-shaped and the cytoplasm contains densely staining specific basophil granules.

C. Granules contain *heparin, histamine, serotonin, Slow Reactive Substance of Anaphylaxis* (*SRS-A*) or *Leukotrienes C4, D4* and *E4* and the peptide *Eosinophil Chemotactic Factor of Anaphylaxis* (*ECF-A*). While these substances are also found in mast cells, it is unclear whether the two cell types have the same precursor cell.

D. Degranulation of basophils follows when an allergen cross links specific surface IgE molecules via Fc receptors for IgE. The result is to promote the symptoms of allergy.

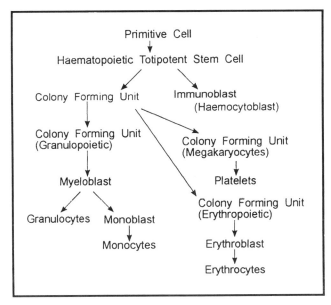

Haematopoiesis.

IMMUNE SYSTEM

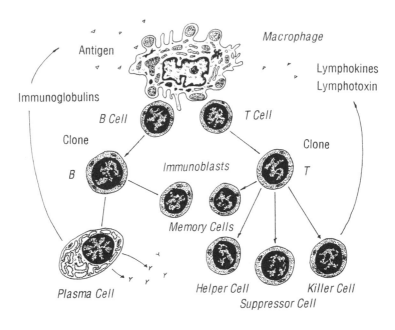

Humoral Immunity   **Cellular Immunity**

The immune response.

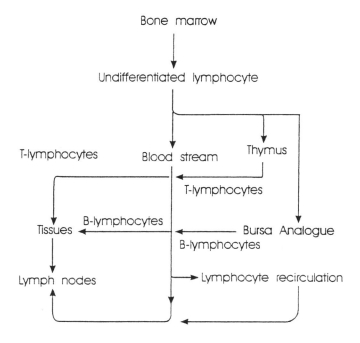

Circulation of Lymphocytes.

IMMUNE SYSTEM

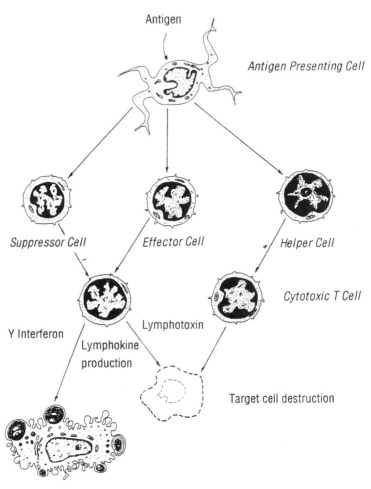

Immunological functions of T lymphocytes (after Tizard).

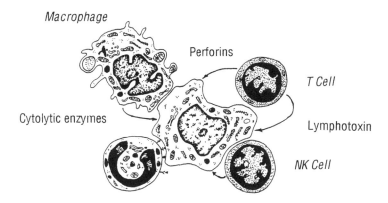

Mechanisms of cell mediated cytotoxicity.

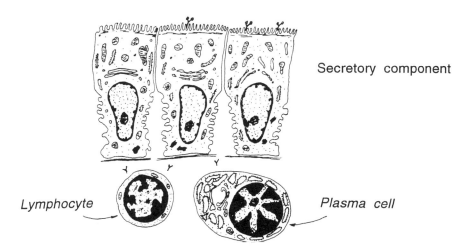

Dimers of IgA and secretory component which are resistant to proteolytic enzyme are released into the gut lumen.

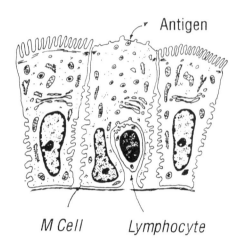

Follicle associated epithelial (M) cells particularly covering Peyer's patches transport antigens from the gut lumen to intraepithelial lymphocytes.

CHAPTER 7

IMMUNE SYSTEM
2. LYMPH, LYMPH VESSELS, LYMPH NODES AND TONSILS

OBJECTIVES

After reading this chapter, you should be able to:
1. Describe the structure of lymphatic capillaries, relating the structure to their function. You should know what factors cause movement of lymph in lymph vessels and what factors control the amount of tissue fluid.
2. Identify the salient histologic features of lymph nodes and differentiate nodes from other lymphoid organs.
3. Describe the distribution of entangled lymphocytes in nodes with reference to cell zones and distribution of B and T lymphocytes.
4. List the histological features and functions of cell types other than lymphocytes found in lymph nodes.
5. Describe the blood supply of lymph nodes and its role in the circulation of lymphocytes.
6. Give at least seven functions of lymph nodes.
7. Describe the salient histologic features which differentiate components of gut associated lymphoid tissue (GALT).

CHAPTER OUTLINE

Lymph.

Lymph vessels. General. Detailed structure of collecting lymphatic vessels. Movement of lymph. Methods of studying lymph vessels. Edema.

Lymph nodes. General. Detailed structure. Circulation of lymph through nodes. Cells entangled in the framework of nodes. Cell zones in lymph nodes. Blood supply of lymph nodes. Functions of lymph nodes.

Gut associated lymphoid tissue (GALT).

Tonsils. General. Palatine tonsils. Pharyngeal tonsils. Lingual tonsils. Tubal tonsils.

KEY WORDS, PHRASES AND CONCEPTS

Lymph
Edema
Interstitial fluid
Lymphatic capillaries
Lacteals
Lymph node
Hilum
Stroma (reticulum)
Trabeculae
Cortex
Medulla
Lymphatic nodules

Germinal centers
Diffuse cortex
Tonsils
Tubal tonsils
Palatine tonsils

Thymus dependent zone
Subcapsular sinus
Cortical sinus
Medullary sinus
Macrophages
Antigen presenting cells
Dendritic reticular cell
Fibroblasts (Reticulocytes)
Pericytes
Endothelial cells
Post capillary venules
Gut associated lymphoid
   tissue (GALT)
M cells
Langerhans cells
Pharyngeal tonsils
Lingual tonsils
Peyer's patches

1. Lymph

1.1. *Lymph* is a clear, colorless, opalescent fluid formed by continuous ultrafiltration of blood plasma through capillary walls. It is basically interstitial fluid.

1.2. It contains lymphocytes only after passing through lymphoid organs.

1.3. Lymph in vessels (*lacteals*) draining the gut is often turbid milky white (*chyle*), containing small (1–3 μm) fatty bodies (*chylomicrons*).

1.4. Lymph is carried in lymph vessels in only one direction (towards connections of major lymphatic trunks with the venous system).

2. Lymph Vessels

2.1. General

    2.1.1. Lymph vessels commence as dilated, bulb-like blind ended tubes in tissues and then form anastomosing networks in tissue spaces. The meshwork is larger than that of neighboring blood capillaries.

    2.1.2. The endothelial wall of lymphatic capillaries is permeable to substances of greater molecular size than those passing through the endothelial wall of blood capillaries.

    2.1.3. Unlike blood vessels, lymph vessels do not form a circulatory system.

    2.1.4. Lymph vessels are absent from avascular structures (epidermis, hair, nails, cornea and articular cartilage) and also from brain and spinal cord, splenic pulp and bone marrow.

2.2. Detailed Structure of Collecting Lymphatic Vessels

    2.2.1. A single layer of endothelial cells connected by occasional zonulae occludentes lines the lumen.

    2.2.2. *Anchoring filaments* run from the outer surface of the endothelium to perivascular collagen and help to keep apertures between cells open. Contractile actin filaments in endothelial cells also help to control apertures between cells.

    2.2.3. Vessels absorb fat, electrolytes and some proteins through apertures between cells or by micropinocytosis without these substances being used by the cell (*transcytosis*).

    2.2.4. Permeability of lymph vessels increases greatly under certain mild conditions including pressure, stroking, warming or histamine release.

2.2.5. The *basal lamina* of lymphatic capillaries is poorly developed and pericytes are absent.

2.2.6. The structure of larger collecting trunks is comparable with that of small veins.

    A. *Tunica intima* comprises endothelial cells and a thin layer of fibrous tissue.

    B. *Tunica media* contains smooth muscle which is mostly circularly arranged. This coat is thickest in the Thoracic Duct.

    C. *Tunica adventitia* is mainly fibrous tissue with a slight admixture of smooth muscle. This coat is thickest in the collecting vessels.

2.2.7. Lymphatic vessels possess more *valves* than veins. They are semilunar and arranged in pairs.

3. Movement of Lymph

3.1. Net filtration pressure is generated by filtration of fluid from blood capillaries.

3.2. Contraction of surrounding muscles compresses adjacent vessels. Lymph moves in a direction determined by valves toward the point of entry of the major lymph vessels into the venous system. From this, it can be understood that there is little flow in an immobilized limb while massage promotes flow.

3.3. Pulsation of nearby arteries in a neurovascular bundle rhythmically compresses lymphatics.

3.4. Respiratory movements and negative pressure in brachiocephalic veins also contributes to movement toward the thorax.

3.5. Smooth muscle in the wall of main lymph trunks most marked just proximal to valves, contributes to movement.

4. Methods of Studying Lymph Vessels

4.1. Experimental methods have included injections into vessels of India ink, neoprene latex or Prussian blue. In living animals, methylene blue or lipiodol, which is picked up by lymph vessels, is injected into tissue spaces. Radio-opaque material is detected, outlining lymph vessels by radiography (*lymphangiography*).

4.2. Clinical methods involve injection of radio-opaque dyes into tissue spaces. Nodes involved in inflammation or malignant disease can be detected macroscopically.

4.3. Blockage of lymphatics may cause valves to become incompetent and lead to retrograde spread of infection or malignancy. Direction of spread can therefore be difficult to predict.

5. Edema

5.1. Excessive accumulation of tissue fluid mainly involving the extracellular space is called *edema* which can be caused by:

A. Venous obstruction, e.g., from cardiac incompetence, causing raised intracapillary hydrostatic pressure. This forces more fluid into tissues, reducing the volume of blood collected from capillaries.

B. Injured capillary walls, e.g., from heat, resulting in increased permeability with greater egress of fluid, solutes and colloids. This lessens osmotic attraction for tissue fluid to return to the capillary.

C. Lowering systemic plasma colloids (proteins) from proteinuria (excretion of protein in urine), protein starvation or exudation from burnt skin surfaces

D. Obstruction of lymph vessels, e.g., by filaria parasites often producing massive swelling of the effected part (elephantiasis).

6. Lymph Nodes

6.1. General

6.1.1. *Lymph nodes* are small, encapsulated, ovoid or reniform bodies 5–15 mm in diameter situated in the course of lymph vessels.

6.1.2. *Lymph* passes through them on its way to the blood vascular system in a direction dictated by valves in afferent lymphatic vessels to the node and efferent lymphatic vessels from the node.

6.1.3. *Afferent lymphatic vessels* enter the node at different parts of the convex periphery.

6.1.4. Nodes have a highly cellular *cortex* and darker staining *medulla* containing many cavities. The line between cortex and medulla is indefinite. The cortex is deficient at the *hilum* where the medulla reaches the surface.

6.1.5. The *hilum* is a depression on one side of a node through which blood vessels enter and leave. One or more efferent lymph vessels also leave from the hilum.

6.1.6. The *capsule* of a lymph node is composed of dense collagen and some smooth muscle. The framework of a node is continuous with the capsule and includes *trabeculae* projecting from its inner surface and a delicate reticular fiber stroma in which cells are entangled.

6.1.7. Lymphatic channels permeate nodes, ensuring maximum exposure of lymph to entangled macrophages and lymphocytes.

6.2. Detailed Structure

6.2.1. *Lymphatic nodules* (*follicles*) in the outer cortex may be either of two types. They may contain only tightly packed small lymphocytes (then known as *primary nodules*) or, in addition, they may contain a central *germinal center* of larger, less deeply staining and more rapidly dividing cells (then called a *secondary nodule*).

6.2.2. The number and degree of isolation of *lymphatic nodules* in the cortex varies according to the degree of antigenic stimulation.

6.2.3. The number and size of germinal centers within the lymphatic nodules increases with raised rate of lymphopoiesis, proliferation of macrophages and differentiation of plasma cells.

6.2.4. Under intense antigenic stimulation, the whole lymph node increases in size and vascularity and is known as a *reactive node*.

6.2.5. The inner or deep cortex contains diffusely arranged lymphoid tissue and the area is known as the *paracortex or thymus dependent zone*.

6.2.6. The *medulla* contains loosely packed branched extensions of lymphatic tissue of the inner cortex comprising medullary cords.

6.3. Circulation of Lymph Through Nodes

6.3.1. *Afferent lymph vessels* enter lymph nodes along the periphery and open into the *subcapsular sinus*, a cavity around the periphery of the cortex (except at the hilum).

6.3.2. *Cortical sinuses* lead radially from the subcapsular sinus towards the medulla and coalesce to form larger medullary sinuses.

6.3.3. *Medullary sinuses* are confluent at the hilum, draining into the *efferent lymphatic vessels*.

6.3.4. Lymphatic sinuses are lined throughout by reticular cells whose cytoplasmic processes crisscross the lumen.

6.3.5. *Littoral cells* are squamous endothelial-like cells lining sinuses. They contain a few lysosomes and under some conditions, may become phagocytic.

6.4. Cells Entangled in the Framework of Nodes

6.4.1. Cells of germinal centers are mostly *lymphoblasts* dividing into small lymphocytes which accumulate initially in the peripheral *marginal zone (mantle or crescent)* around the germinal center.

6.4.2. *Small lymphocytes* leave the periphery of nodules, enter lymph sinuses and are conveyed through the medulla to efferent vessel(s) at the hilum.

6.4.3. *Macrophages* are plentiful in lymph nodes where they phagocytose foreign cells, cell debris and bacteria. They also secrete products important in the defense process.

6.4.4. *Antigen Presenting Cells (APC)* originate in bone marrow. They are also known as *interdigitating cells* of T cell zones or *follicular dendritic cells* of B cell zones. *Langerhans cells* which have migrated to nodes from the skin are also present. They capture antigen, thereby facilitating the immune response.

6.4.5. Other cells in lymph nodes are:
A. *Fibroblasts*.
B. *Perivascular cells* in nodes include pericytes and smooth muscle cells.
C. *Endothelial cells* in nodes are non-phagocytic.

6.5. Cell Zones in Lymph Nodes

6.5.1. Three cortical zones are established by the presence of lymph nodules in the superficial cortex.
A. *Nodular cortex* is the part of the cortex containing nodules.
B. *Internodular cortex* is the zone between nodules.
C. *Deep or tertiary cortex* is located below nodular and internodular cortex but above the medulla. Internodular and tertiary cortex are often combined as diffuse cortex.

6.5.2. B lymphocytes are concentrated in primary nodules.

6.5.3. High levels of antibody formation and B cell differentiation occur in germinal centers.

LYMPH NODE

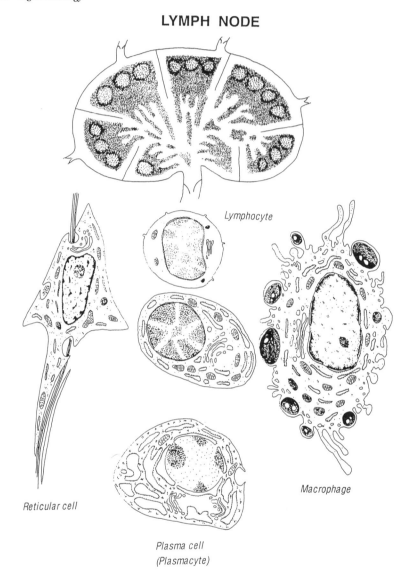

Lymphocyte

Reticular cell

Plasma cell
(Plasmacyte)

Macrophage

6.5.4. T lymphocytes are concentrated in diffuse cortex which, because it is depleted following neonatal thymectomy, is known as the *Thymus Dependent Zone*.

6.6. Blood Supply of Lymph Nodes

6.6.1. Blood vessels enter the hilum and straight branches traverse the medulla in trabeculae.

6.6.2. These vessels break up in the cortex, forming arcades of arterioles and capillaries in anastomosing loops particularly around the periphery of follicles.

6.6.3. *Post-capillary venules* (*high endothelial venules*), especially in the paracortical zones, are the important site of lymphocyte migration from blood into the parenchyma of nodes.

6.6.4. Antigenic stimulation is accompanied by increases in the capillary beds and large increases in the numbers of lymphocytes migrating to the parenchyma.

6.7. Functions of Lymph Nodes

6.7.1. Nodes *provide an intricate network* of spaces of large volume and surface area through which lymph percolates slowly.
Here, foreign material can be trapped and exposed to macrophages.

6.7.2. Nodes are *sites where phagocytes-carrying antigens can interact* with lymphocytes, resulting in either a cellular or humoral immune response.

6.7.3. They provide *centers for lymphocyte production.*

6.7.4. Nodes are *sites of transfer of blood borne lymphocytes back to lymphatic channels.*

6.7.5. *Humoral antibody production* also occurs in nodes.

7. Gut Associated Lymphoid Tissue (Galt)

7.1. The term *Gut Associated Lymphoid Tissue* is often reserved for the lymphoepithelial tissue of the appendix and of Peyer's patches although the mucosa of the intestines and tonsils contain in total more lymphoid tissue than the spleen.

7.2. *Peyer's patches* are collections of 2–400 nodules as large as 20 mm long and 12 mm wide in the submucosa of the ileum opposite the insertion of the mesentery.

7.2.1. They appear to develop from clusters of lymphocytes and macrophages within the mucosa after antigenic stimulation. Nodules may interrupt the muscularis mucosae, invade the lamina propria and erase villi.

7.2.2. *M cells* are found in the epithelium covering Peyer's patches.

7.2.3. Some Peyer's patches appear to be secondary lymphoid organs containing germinal centers in response to antigenic stimulation. Others appear to be primary lymphoid organs in that they are the site of B cell differentiation.

8. Tonsils

8.1. General

8.1.1. The *tonsils* are a group of secondary lymphoid (lymphoepithelial) organs which form a discontinuous ring around the junction of the nasopharynx and oropharynx with the nasal and oral cavities.

8.1.2. Tonsils reach their maximum development in childhood and are atrophic by adulthood, being replaced by fibrous tissue.

8.1.3. They create the environment in which lymphocytes can interact with each other and with antigens and disseminate the immune response. These functions are performed by phagocytic macrophages, antigen presenting cells and mature T and B lymphocytes.

8.1.4. Secretory IgA which is particularly resistant to proteolysis by digestive enzymes, passes out and antigen in through covering epithelium.

8.1.5. Tonsils have only efferent lymphatics.

8.2. *Palatine Tonsils*

8.2.1. The *palatine tonsils* ("*tonsils*") are situated in the tonsillar fossa between the palatoglossal and palatopharyngeal arches. They comprise 10–20 deep crypts lined by stratified squamous non-keratinizing epithelium which is infiltrated with lymphocytes.

8.2.2. The lamina propria around the crypts is non-encapsulated lymphoid tissue (mucosal associated lymphoid tissue or MALT) containing secondary nodules.

8.2.3. Mucous glands beneath the capsule have ducts opening into the crypts.

8.3. *Pharyngeal Tonsils*

8.3.1. The *pharyngeal tonsils* ("*adenoids*") are situated in the roof of the nasopharynx.

8.3.2. Epithelium covering the pharyngeal tonsils is not arranged in crypts but longitudinal folds over encapsulated lymphoid tissue containing nodules. The covering epithelium is pseudostratified columnar ciliated with goblet cells.

8.3.3. Outside the capsule are mixed seromucous glands which open into the folds.

8.4. *Lingual Tonsils*

8.4.1. *Lingual tonsils* are situated on the root of the tongue behind the vallate papillae. They comprise 30 or more epithelial pits (crypts) lined with stratified squamous epithelium surrounded by a single layer of lymphoid nodules containing germinal centers.

8.4.2. Subjacent mucous glands open into the crypts or directly onto the epithelial surface.

8.5. *Tubal Tonsils*

8.5.1. *Tubal tonsils* are collections of lymphoreticular tissue near the opening of the auditory tube.

8.5.2. They are covered with pseudostratified ciliated epithelium.

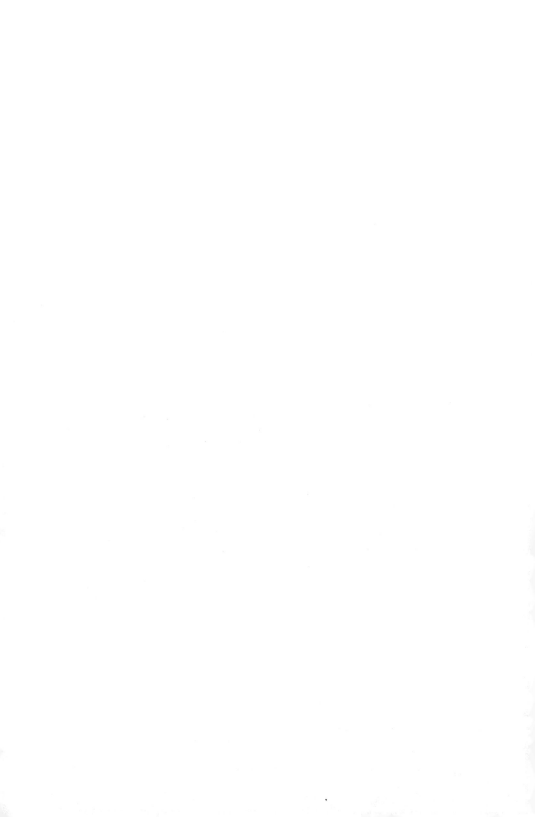

Chapter 8

IMMUNE SYSTEM
3. THYMUS AND SPLEEN

OBJECTIVES

After reading this chapter, you should be able to:
1. Identify and describe the structural histological features of the thymus and what features distinguish it from other lymphoid organs.
2. List the cell types found in the thymus and explain their functions.
3. Discuss the structural framework of the thymus with particular reference to the Blood-Thymus Barrier and its significance.
4. Discuss the causes and structural changes in thymic involution.
5. Give an account of the functions of the thymus in relation to the origin and fate of T lymphocytes and production of thymic humoral factors.
6. Identify and describe the structural histologic features of the spleen and what features distinguish it from other lymphoid organs.
7. Describe the blood circulation through the spleen.
8. Discuss the functions of the spleen.

CHAPTER OUTLINE

Thymus

Development of the thymus.

General structure. Cortex, Medulla, Lobules.

Tissue components. Epithelial reticular cells, Macrophages, T Lymphocytes, Antigen Presenting cells, Mast cells, Thymic (Hassall's Corpuscles).

Blood supply of the thymus. Blood-Thymus Barrier.

Fate of T lymphocytes.

Functions of the thymus. T lymphocyte production, Production of humoral factors, Thymopoietin, Thymosin.

Involution of the thymus.

Spleen

Development.

Structure. Capsule, Trabeculae, Reticulum Splenic pulp, White pulp, Red pulp.

Blood circulation through the spleen. Periarterial Lymphatic Sheaths (PALS), Lymphatic nodules (Malphigian bodies), Marginal Zone.
Penicillar arteries, Periarterial Macrophage Sheaths (PMS) or Ellipsoids, Endothelial (Stave) cells, Splenic cords, Sinusoids.
Open Theory of blood circulation through the Spleen.

Functions of the spleen.

Effects of splenectomy.

KEY WORDS, PHRASES, CONCEPTS

Central (Primary) lymphatic organs
Peripheral (Secondary) lymphatic organs
Thymic (Hassall's) corpuscles
Epithelial reticular cells
Macrophages
Dendritic cells
Blood supply of the thymic cortex
Blood-Thymus barrier
Cell death in the Thymus

Stave cells
Central arteries
Splenic cords
T lymphocytes
Inner cortical zone
Outer cortical zone
White pulp
Red pulp
Marginal zone

Thymosin 21
Penicillar arteries
Splenic pulp
Periarterial Lymphatic Sheaths (PALS)
Lymphatic nodules (Malphigian Bodies)
Central (Sheathed) arteries
Periarterial macrophage sheath (PMS)
Closed circulation

Thymopoietin
(Thymic hormone)
Germinal centers
Pitting function
Sinusoids
Reticular cells
Open circulation

THE THYMUS

1. Development of the Thymus

1.1. The *thymus* (thymos (Gk) feeling or sensibility from the close physical but mistaken association of the thymus to the heart) appears at the end of the 6th week as a condensation of entoderm in the *ventral sacculation of the third pharyngeal pouches*.

1.2. The epithelial pouches are hollow at first and attached to the inferior parathyroid (III). They separate from the pharynx by the 7th week.

1.3. The pouches become solid and unite with their opposite number by the 8th week. A tail portion becomes elongated and attenuated and finally fragments.

1.4. The lower ends of the thymus attach to the pericardium and sink with it into the thorax.

1.5. By the 10th week, the thymus comprises stellate epithelial reticular cells some of which begin to aggregate into *thymic corpuscles (of Hassall)*.

1.6. Stem cells of *T lymphocytes* colonize the epithelium and begin to divide from the end of the 3rd month.

2. General Structure

2.1. The thymus has two halves or *lobes* closely connected in the midline by connective tissue.

2.2. A *capsule* encloses each lobe from which interlobular septa extend inward to separate lobes into *lobules*. *Trabeculae* project from both the capsule and septa to further divide the thymic cortex.

2.3. Lobules have a *cortex* which is densely populated by lymphocytes (thymocytes). The cortex is sharply demarcated from an axial, less dense *medulla* which sends lateral projections into each lobule.

2.4. The *cortex* is divided into two zones:

A. *Outer zone* contains large lymphoblasts, many of which are undergoing mitoses.

B. Inner zone is much more extensive and houses predominantly small, more mature lymphocytes. Macrophages are present in both outer and inner zones.

Degenerating lymphocytes are numerous in the thymic cortex (90% never leave the thymus); however, they are inconspicuous in sections.

2.5. The *medulla* is lighter staining because of its relatively rich population of *epithelial reticular cells* and more sparse *large lymphocytes*. It also contains *macrophages*, *plasma cells* and occasional *eosinophils*. Beginning in mid fetal life, *thymic (Hassall's) corpuscles* (see below) become prominent in the medulla.

2.6. No lymphatics enter the thymus.

3. Tissue Components

3.1. Principal cells and tissue components of the thymus are:

3.1.1. *Epithelial reticular cells* are branched, stellate cells forming a network of incomplete, anastomosing sheets throughout the thymic parenchyma. These cells contain lysosomes and secretory granules and produce polypeptide (*thymosins*). They are not members of the reticuloendothelial system.

In the cortex, as well as providing a framework, epithelial reticular cells form a continuous layer covering the inner surface of the capsule, trabeculae and blood vessels.

In the medulla, they form a more widely branched network with larger interstices. Outer layers of the epithelial framework form a partial *blood-thymus barrier* which permits passage of nutrients and migrating lymphocytes into the cortex but not antigens. Those antigens that do cross the barrier are collected by macrophages.

3.1.2. *Macrophages* are fewer in number than in the spleen. They are located near vessels of the capsule and trabeculae and phagocytose products of lymphatic destruction in the cortex. They also restrict access of macromolecules to developing lymphocytes.

3.1.3. *T Lymphocytes* belong to two pools:
- A. Lymphocytes that arise mainly in the outer cortex by division of stem cells originally migrated there from bone marrow. Most have a short life span of 3–5 days and degenerate in the thymus. The remainder leave the thymus through blood vessels while immunologically immature to lodge in *thymus dependent zones* of peripheral (secondary) lymphoid organs and form part of the circulating pool of lymphocytes.
- B. Lymphocytes in the medulla belong to the circulating pool and exchange via post capillary venules and the circulatory system with those in other lymphatic organs.

3.1.4. *Plasma cells* are relatively few in the cortex but present in the medulla, arising from activated B lymphocytes from the circulation.

3.1.5. *Antigen presenting cells* similar to those in the spleen, lymph nodes or in epidermis are present in the medulla.

3.1.6. *Mast cells* are more plentiful in older persons. The thymus contains stem cells for mast cells.

3.1.7. *Thymic (Hassall's) corpuscles* are first formed in the fetus and continue to form throughout life. They arise primarily from medullary epithelial cells which enlarge and degenerate. Further cells add to the periphery, forming concentric lamellae around the central degenerate mass which may keratinize, become swollen and necrotic and may calcify. Corpuscles may also contain degenerating lymphocytes or macrophages. They increase in number and size to puberty but after the onset of involution. They then decrease in number but those that remain increase in size. The function of Hassall's corpuscles is unknown.

4. Blood Supply

4.1. Arteries run in the septa and as arterioles enter the parenchyma in the depths of septa to follow the corticomedullary junction. These arterioles give capillaries to the cortex. Some capillaries drain directly into veins in the septa but the bulk drain to post capillary venules at the corticomedullary junction. Mature T lymphocytes reach the blood circulation by passing through the walls of post capillary venules. Relatively few capillaries supply the medulla.

4.2. A functional and selective barrier separates the blood of cortical capillaries from developing lymphocytes. This *"Blood-Thymus Barrier"* comprises:

A. Endothelium and pericytes.

B. Endothelial basal lamina.

C. Perivascular space and connective tissue.

D. Basal lamina of epithelial reticular cells.

E. Epithelial reticular cells.

4.3. The blood-thymus barrier is incomplete in the medulla but better in the cortex where any small substances crossing it are phagocytosed by macrophages. The barrier has two major functions:

A. It prevents particulate matter from crossing from medulla to cortex and;

B. It shields developing T lymphocytes from high concentrations of antigens, allowing their untroubled differentiation.

4.4. Lymph vessels and veins run in septa carrying T lymphocytes from the thymus but there are no afferent lymphatics to the thymus.

5. Fate of T Lymphocytes

5.1. It is estimated that 90% of the progeny of T lymphocyte stem cells in the thymic cortex die within a few days. Cells capable of producing antibodies to the body's own tissues are suppressed in the thymus.

5.2. It is possible that rapidly proliferating lymphocytes may be non-viable mutants.

6. Functions of Thymus

6.1. *T Lymphocyte production*: Stem cells pass from bone marrow to the thymus and undergo final maturation in the spleen where they meet antigens. They circulate and recirculate through blood and lymph and spend time in thymus dependent zones in lymphoid organs. T lymphocytes require priming by macrophages which have ingested antigenic material. Neonatal thymectomy is accompanied by severe immunological defects from impaired cellular immunity (runt disease in animals).

6.2. Production of *thymopoietin* by epithelial reticular cells which induces the formation of specific receptors on immature T lymphocytes capable of recognizing foreign proteins or antigens (maturation). In addition, they are immuno regulatory increasing suppressor cell populations or

THYMUS

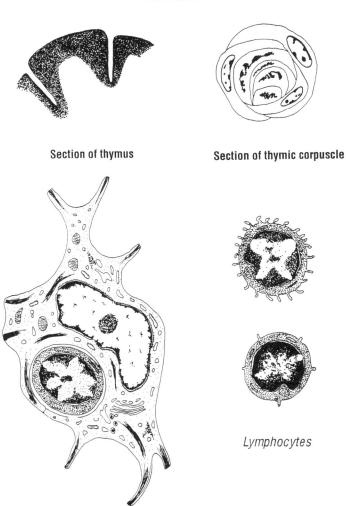

Section of thymus   Section of thymic corpuscle

Lymphocytes

Epithelial reticular cell

restoring immune competency.

6.3. Production of *thymosin* a polypeptides produced by epithelial reticular cells which stimulates the differentiation and maturation of T lymphocytes.

6.4. *Thymic Humoral Factor* (*THF*) is a peptide that can restore immune responsiveness in neonatally thymectomized rats or immune suppressed humans.

7. Involution of the Thymus

7.1. The thymus undergoes a normal gradual age dependent *involution* beginning at puberty. Fat accumulates in the cortex, the number of lymphocytes and epithelial cells in the cortex decreases and Hassall's corpuscles in the medulla decrease in number but increase in size.

7.2. The process can be accelerated (*accidental involution*) by stress (infections, poisoning, radiation or dietary deficiencies) or hormonal factors (in particular steroids and ACTH) which lyse immature T cells.

7.3. The thymus nevertheless remains an important source of lymphocytes into late adulthood.

THE SPLEEN

1. Development

1.1. The rudiment of the *spleen* (splen (Gk) spleen) first appears at 8 mm as an accumulation of mesenchymal cells beneath the mesothelium on the left side of the *dorsal mesogastrium*.

1.2. It acquires its characteristic form by 3 months mostly by proliferation of cells of its reticular framework.

1.3. Lymphocytes colonize the sheaths around arteries within the spleen.

1.4. Formation of white cells in the spleen is supplemented from 5–8 months by red cell formation.

1.5. *Splenic corpuscles* form ovoid nodules about arterioles from 6 months.

1.6. The spleen remains a potential site of haematopoiesis throughout life.

2. Structure

2.1. An external *serous coat* is a single layer of mesothelial cells (peritoneum).

2.2. The fibroelastic *capsule* is predominantly dense white connective tissue with some elastic tissue but little smooth muscle in man (in contrast with the capsule of some animals).

2.3. From the capsule, *trabeculae* of the same structure as the capsule subdivide the spleen into communicating compartments.

2.4. *Reticular fibers* which blend with the trabeculae, capsule and vessels form a spongework throughout the enclosed tissue (*splenic pulp*). *Reticular cells* are closely associated with reticular fibers.

2.5. Interstices of the reticulum are occupied by *splenic pulp* which is either

    2.5.1. *White Pulp* comprising:

        A. Zones of tightly packed lymphocytes distributed along the axial *central arteries* (*periarterial lymphatic sheaths or PALS*) radiating into the splenic parenchyma. PALS mostly contain T lymphocytes.

        B. *Lymphatic* (*splenic or Malphigian*) *nodules* which lie within the periarterial sheaths. Splenic nodules, contain B lymphocytes and with antigenic stimulation may contain germinal centers. Each nodule is surrounded by a layer of T lymphocytes in a *mantle zone*.

    2.5.2. The *marginal zone* is a condensation of reticular fibers and cells (many of which are macrophages, antigen presenting cells and slowly recirculating B cells) at the boundary between white and red pulp. Many branches of the central arteries end in the marginal zone which is the site of first contact between blood borne antigens and effector cells.

    2.5.3. *Red Pulp* is red because of the predominant presence in the region of erythrocytes. Red pulp contains venous *sinusoids* separated by *splenic cords* (*of Billroth*), perivascular tissue rich in macrophages and reticulum and continuous throughout the spleen.

        A. *Sinusoids* of the red pulp have walls of flattened, greatly elongated endothelial cells. These cells (*Stave cells*) contain two longitudinal bands of cytoplasmic microfilaments, one central and the other basal to maintain the shape of the cell.

        B. *Stave cells* are surrounded by a fenestrated basal lamina and are separated from one another by gaps which allow blood to pass into or out of surrounding cord tissue.

C. The sieve-like structure of sinusoid walls enables stave cells to carry out a *"pitting function"* in which undeformable inclusions are squeezed out of cells as they pass through intercellular clefts.

D. Reticular fibers also encircle the endothelial cell wall, maintaining the shape of the sinusoid and controlling the dimensions of separating intercellular crevices.

3. Blood Circulation Through the Spleen

3.1. The *splenic artery* enters the hilum and divides into trabecular arteries which follow trabeculae.

3.2. Branches leave the trabeculae and become *central or sheathed arteries* where the adventitial coat is replaced by *periarterial lymphatic sheaths* (*PALS*). Within the PALS and distributed along their length are *lymphatic* (*splenic*) *nodules* (*Malpighian Bodies*).

3.3. *Sheathed arteries* (or central arteries which are in fact eccentric with respect to cross sections of white pulp) give many small branches to:

3.3.1. White Pulp.

3.3.2. Germinal centers and mantle zones of secondary nodules.

3.3.3. Most empty into marginal sinuses or near the marginal zone.

3.4. The main stem of the central artery divides into short, straight, non-anastomosing vessels (penicilli) which empty into cords of the red pulp.

3.5. Some terminal branches of the central arteries penetrate the marginal zone and acquire a *periarterial macrophage sheath* (*PAMS*) or *ellipsoid*. These segments house the major population of macrophages in the spleen and the cells, in addition to their phagocytic activity, may have a role in controlling blood flow.

3.6. Blood passes directly into cord tissue then between endothelial cells and into sinusoids (the "Open Theory" of circulation). It is unlikely that blood passes directly into sinusoids from branches of the central arteries (the "Closed Theory" of circulation). In this theory, flow between sinusoids and cords depends upon opening and closing of vessels at either end of the sinusoid bed.

3.7. Segments of the spleen are supplied by branches of the splenic artery which have no apparent anastomoses. Occlusion of a branch produces a large, wedge-shaped area of dead tissue (an *infarct*).

3.8. *Trabecular veins* drain the sinusoids to splenic veins.

3.9. Efferent lymphatics from the white pulp drain toward trabecular vessels.

4. Functions of the Spleen

4.1. The spleen contains specialized vasculature that modifies circulating blood.

4.2. It provides the proper environment for final differentiation of reticulocytes, platelets, lymphocytes and monocytes.

4.3. The spleen monitors blood cells of the circulation. Imperfect, damaged or aged blood cells of all types are trapped by stave cells and destroyed by macrophages. In addition, particles or bacteria can be extruded from blood cells without damaging the cells as they pass through gaps between stave cells.

4.4. It sequesters monocytes from blood and facilitates their transformation into *macrophages*. These cells remove cell debris, effete red cells, leucocytes, platelets and microorganisms from blood. *Haemosiderin* granules from erythrocytes appear in the macrophage cytoplasm and is reutilized to form haemoglobin in new erythrocytes in marrow.

4.5. The spleen receives circulating T and B lymphocytes and sorts them into compartments where they interact with blood borne antigens or macrophages. T lymphocytes circulate through the spleen or through lymphatic sheaths where they remain for 4–6 hours. They carry out cytotoxic killing. B lymphocytes stay longer in nodules and germinal centers and transform into plasma cells. Under antigenic stimulation, macrophages and lymphocytes increase in number and the entire spleen may enlarge (*splenomegaly*).

4.6. From four months in utero, the spleen acts as a haemopoietic organ. In some anaemias and leukaemias, it can revert to this function.

4.7. The filling and emptying of venous sinusoids is controlled by sphincters at each end of sinusoids so that the spleen has a role in erythrocyte storage. In hypoxia, erythrocytes are discharged from the spleen.

5. Effects of Splenectomy

5.1. Although carrying out many important functions in filtering blood, the spleen is not essential to life. Partial removal of the spleen is followed by rapid regeneration.

SPLEEN

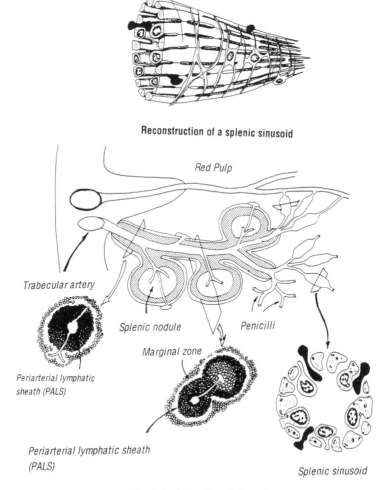

Reconstruction of a splenic sinusoid

Red Pulp

Trabecular artery

Splenic nodule

Penicilli

Marginal zone

Periarterial lymphatic sheath (PALS)

Periarterial lymphatic sheath (PALS)

Splenic sinusoid

Blood circulation through the spleen

5.2. *Splenectomy* in early life is accompanied by reduced immune capabilities and increased susceptibility to infection. Carried out later in life, splenectomy is accompanied by a transient leucocytosis. This is attributed to removal of humoral factors normally produced by the spleen which oppose the formation and release of cells from haematopoietic tissues.

CHAPTER 9

CARDIOVASCULAR SYSTEM

OBJECTIVES

After reading this chapter, you should be able to:
1. Describe the components of the cardiac impulse conducting system and give their functional significance.
2. Give an account of the histological structure of the heart wall, including the skeleton of the heart and structure of the heart valves.
3. Relate the function of arteries and arterioles to the structure of their walls.
4. Describe the structure and function of the microvasculature of metarterioles, capillaries, arteriovenous anastomoses and post capillary venules.
5. Describe the structure of components of the venous system.

CHAPTER OUTLINE

General functions and composition of the circulatory system.

Cardiac muscle.

Structure of the heart wall. Endocardium, Myocardium, Pericardium, Cardiac skeleton, Epicardium.

Valves of the heart. Development, Histology.

The cardiac cycle.

The impulse conducting system. Sinoatrial node, Atrioventricular node,

Atrioventricular bundle, Purkinje fibers.

Basic organization of blood vessels above precapillaries. Tunica intima, Tunica media, Tunica adventitia.

Tissue components of vascular wall. Endothelium, Smooth muscle, Vascular connective tissue, Vascular nerves.

Large elastic (Conducting) arteries.

Muscular (Distributing) arteries.

Arterioles.

Metarterioles.

Capillaries.

Arteriovenous anastomoses.

Post-capillary (Pericytic) venules.

Muscular venules.

Small and medium sized veins.

Large veins.

Vasa vasora.

Valves.

KEY WORDS, PHRASES, CONCEPTS

Arteries (Elastic, Muscular)

Capillaries (Continuous, Fenestrated)

Veins (Small, Medium sized, Large)

Impulse conducting system

Sinoatrial node

Atrioventricular bundle

Endocardium

Myocardium

Serous pericardium

Chordae tendineae

Tunica media

Vasa vasora

Arterioles

Venules (Post-capillary, Collecting, Muscular)

Cardiac cycle

Atrioventricular node

Pacemaker cells

Purkinje fibers

Epicardium

Fibrous pericardium

Cardiac skeleton

Tunica intima

Tunica adventitia

Venous valves

THE CIRCULATORY SYSTEM

1. General Functions and Composition of the Circulatory System

1.1. The circulatory system (or blood vascular system) is a closed system of tubes through which blood is forced by the pumping action of the four chambered contractile heart.

1.2. The tubular walls of the system are not impermeable. Exchange of materials takes place between the system of smaller vessels and their environment (cells, tissue spaces or a matrix of some kind) through formation of tissue fluids or special fluids (cerebrospinal fluid, aqueous humor or synovial fluid).

1.3. The lymphatic system collects fluids and colloids from tissue spaces and returns them to the bloodstream.

1.4. Materials are lost from blood, e.g., at the kidneys, lungs, skin, spleen, etc., while others are added, e.g., hormones, blood cells and antibodies, or replenished, e.g., by intake of foodstuffs, air and water.

1.5. The circulatory system is thus a chief integrator of the various systems of the body.

1.6. The circulatory system consists of:
   A. *The heart* is a blood vessel, but specialized for pumping.
   B. *Arteries* conduct blood away from the heart to the capillary bed. The quality of blood carried is not a factor in defining an artery — blood can be rich or poor in oxygen.
   C. *Arterioles.* 100 μm in diameter or less with a muscular wall control blood flow to capillaries.
   D. *Metarterioles or precapillary arterioles.* Terminal segments of arterioles where muscle in the wall is gradually replaced by pericytes. Of larger diameter than capillaries metarterioles give origin to capillaries, guarding them against damage from excessive pressure with *precapillary sphincters*. They may also provide a preferred channel by-passing the capillary bed.
   E. *Capillaries* form a meshwork of the smallest vessels.
   F. *Post-capillary or pericytic venules.* 8–30 μm in diameter, these segments receive blood from capillaries and are the important area of blood-interstitial fluid exchange. They are also the site of lymphocyte

entry into lymph organs from blood.

G. *Venules* have an increasingly complex wall structure. This segment is particularly important in the movement of cells (leukocytes) and fluid to tissue in inflammation.

H. *Veins* conduct blood to the heart from the capillary bed. The quality of blood carried is not a factor in defining a vein — blood can be rich in oxygen (in the pulmonary viens) or deficient in oxygen (in the vena cavae).

2. Cardiac Muscle

2.1. Striated cardiac muscle tissue (*myocardium*) comprises separate cellular units joined by intercalated discs. The discs are stepwise interdigitations at the Z band level with a horizontal part containing zonulae adherentes, desmosomes and gap junctions, and a longitudinal part which bears a gap junction. They permit mechanical and ionic coupling between cells. Z lines anchor thin filaments containing *alpha actinin* while adjacent Z bands are linked by intermediate filaments of *desmin*.

2.2. Contrasted with skeletal muscle:

2.2.1. Nuclei of cardiac muscle cells are situated in the interior (center) of the cell (fiber).

2.2.2 Cardiac muscle fibers contract spontaneously and although their activity is modified by nerve fibers, contraction is not under voluntary control. Additional output must be met by changes in function of the heart as a whole, not by recruitment of individual fibers.

2.2.3. There are more mitochondria in cardiac muscle (35% compared with 2% of cell volume in skeletal muscle), indicating more reliance of cardiac muscle on aerobic metabolism.

2.2.4. Sarcoplasmic reticulum is less abundant and less evenly distributed. This is associated with greater dependence of cardiac muscle on extracellular calcium in generation of action potentials.

2.2.5. T tubules in cardiac muscle contain *glycocalyx*, are wider and forms simpler associations (dyads) with sarcoplasmic reticulum.

2.3. Contractility is improved by hormones or drugs (positive inotropic effect).

2.4. Chronic excessive function of cardiac muscle results in cellular hypertrophy, i.e., an increase in the numbers of sarcomeres but not of fibers.

2.5. *Differences between atrial and ventricular muscle*:

2.5.1. Atrial muscle cells are smaller in diameter.

2.5.2. Atrial muscle cells are almost devoid of T system. Smaller cells equilibrate easier with extracellular calcium and transmit impulses faster than larger ventricular cells.

2.5.3. Atrial cells contain electron dense granules of *Atrial Natriuretic Factor (ANF)*, a peptide which exerts its effects on blood vessels, kidneys and suprarenal glands as well as regulatory regions in the brain. ANF regulates blood pressure and blood volume, excretion of sodium, potassium and water.

3. Structure of the Heart Wall

3.1. Endocardium, the innermost layer (cf. tunica intima of blood vessels), consists of three layers:

A. *Endothelium.* A single cell layer of squamous cells on a thin continuous basal lamina.

B. *Subendothelial layer.* The thickest layer in the endocardium contains loose connective tissue with a large number of elastic fibers, collagen and some smooth muscle cells.

C. The deepest layer (*myoelastic layer*) contains irregular connective tissue, fat cells and blood vessels as well as branches of the impulse conducting system.

3.2. *Myocardium*, the middle (muscular) layer comprises:

A. *Myocardium proper.* Layers and bundles of cardiac muscle.

In the atria, muscle cells intercalated with collagen and elastin form a lattice-work of ridges that resemble a comb (*pectinate muscles*).

In the ventricles, muscle cell bundles circumscribe chambers in complex, predominantly helical fashion. A *superficial group* encircle both ventricles while a *deep group* encircle each ventricle separately and forms the interventricular septum. Elastic fibers are scarce in ventricular myocardium.

Note that the myocardium has negligible regenerative capacity.

B. *Cardiac skeleton* is the fibrous base separating atrial from ventricular muscle on which cardiac valves and muscle insert. It comprises:

(i) A mass of dense fibrous tissue organized in rings (*annuli fibrosi*) surrounding the atrio-ventricular canals and origins of the aorta and pulmonary artery. Rings may contain elastic fibers and a few adipocytes. Annuli prevent the orifices from dilating in diastole and becoming incompetent.

(ii) The upper part of the interventricular septum forms a fibrous partition (*septum membranaceum*). The septum may contain islands of chondroid tissue which may calcify with age.

3.3. *Epicardium* (*visceral pericardium*) comprises:

A. *Mesothelium*. An outermost single layer of squamous epithelium.

B. *Subepicardial layer* contains loose connective tissue rich in elastic fibers and with a variable amount of adipose tissue. This layer contains blood vessels and nerve fibers.

4. Valves of the Heart

4.1. *Atrioventricular Valves*:

4.1.1. Between the 4 to 12 mm stages of human development, *endocardial cushions*, localized thickenings of mesenchyme covered by endocardium, divide the atrioventricular canal into right and left orifices.

4.1.2. Tissue located on the ventricular surface of these thickenings hollows out but newly formed valves remain attached to the ventricular wall by muscular cords.

4.1.3. Muscle tissue in the cords on the ventricular side degenerates and is partly replaced by dense connective tissue covered by endocardium. These cords (*chordae tendineae*) connect to the remaining (papillary) muscle.

4.1.4. The *left atrioventricular* (*mitral*) *valve* is bicuspid but the *right atrioventricular* (*tricuspid*) valve is tricuspid.

4.1.5. Histologically, atrioventricular valves are membranous flaps attached to annuli fibrosi with chordae tendineae attached to their free edges. Both surfaces are covered with endocardium while the subendocardial layer is thick on the atrial side, containing dense elastic fibers and scattered smooth muscle. A central flat sheet is very dense connective tissue continuous with the annulus. Blood vessels are absent from valves — nutrients for cells in the valves are obtained from circulating blood.

4.2. Semilunar Valves:

    4.2.1. Beginning at the 6 mm stage of development, *spiral ridges* of mesenchyme covered by endocardium, grow into the lee between two spiralling streams of blood as they leave the heart in the truncus and conus.

    4.2.2. The main spiral ridges fuse, separating the aorta from the pulmonary artery. Two minor ridges alternate in position with the major spiral ridges producing the anterior and posterior valves of the pulmonary and aortic valves respectively.

    4.2.3. Both pulmonary and aortic valves hollow out on their upper surfaces.

    4.2.4. Histologically, a central fibrous plate in semilunar valves forms a thickening (*nodule*) at the middle of its free border. There are no chordae tendineae.

5. The Cardiac Cycle

5.1. The *cardiac cycle* is a succession of events from the beginning of one heart beat to the beginning of the next.

5.2. Blood flows at first into relaxed atria.

5.3. Contraction begins in the right atrium initiated by cells of the *sinuatrial node* (*SAN*) near the opening of the superior vena cava.

5.4. A wave of depolarization spreads over muscle cells of both atria and the resulting contraction forces blood into the ventricles.

5.5. A brief delay at the atrioventricular junction allows the atria to complete contraction.

5.6. Ventricular contraction begins in the apex of the ventricles and spreads backwards toward the atrioventricular junction.

6. The Impulse Conducting System

6.1. The *impulse conducting system* is an elongated, branched collection of modified cardiac muscle cells that conducts impulses to parts of the myocardium. It insures a proper sequence and coordinated synchronous contraction of left and right hearts.

6.2. The impulse for contraction of the heart begins in the *sinuatrial node* (*SAN*). This is a group of specialized cardiac muscle cells located in fibroelastic connective tissue in the right hand wall of the superior vena cava at its junction with the right atrium.

6.3. *Nodal cells* are smaller than atrial cells. They lack a T system, contain glycogen, fewer and more poorly organized myofilaments than other atrial cells, and are connected by intercellular junctions but not intercalated discs. Parasympathetic nerve endings contact nodal cells but without forming specialized nerve endings.

6.4. Depolarization spreads through gap junctions between atrial cells to reach the *atrioventricular node* (*AVN*), a group of nodal cells situated at the lower end of the interatrial septum above the septal cusp of the tricuspid valve.

6.5. Nodal cells of the AVN depolarize spontaneously but at a slower rate than those of the SAN. Impulses are triggered by impulses from the faster SAN. The AVN slows conduction from the atria to ventricles (there is a delay between the contraction of the upper and lower chambers of the heart).

6.6. Impulses pass on to the *atrioventricular bundle* (*of His*). This is a collection of specialized conducting muscle fibers which extends from the AVN, penetrates the fibrous septum and divides into *right and left branches*. It travels distally in the deepest layer of endocardium.

6.7. Half-way down the septum, branches become bundles of large, rapidly conducting *Purkinje fibers* (*cells*). These are cells wider than ordinary cardiac muscle cells, contain few myofilaments, considerable stores of glycogen and have no T tubules. They are isolated from surrounding myocardium by connective tissue. Their role is to supply an impulse to papillary muscles, insuring that the papillary muscles take the strain on leaflets of the valves before the ventricles contract.

7. Basic Organization of Blood Vessels above Precapillaries

7.1. There is a common plan of histologic organization in blood vessels. Tissue components are arranged in concentric layers (tunics); however, some features are accentuated in particular local adaptations.

7.2. *Tunica Intima* (equivalent to endocardium) comprises:
Endothelium with basal lamina (and Pericytes).
Subendothelial connective tissue.
Internal elastic lamina.

7.3. *Tunica Media* (equivalent to myocardium) comprises:
Smooth muscle cells.
Elastic lamellae.
External elastic lamina.

7.4. *Tunica adventitia* (equivalent to epicardium or visceral pericardium) comprises connective tissue with its various components.

8. Tissue Components of Vascular Wall

8.1. *Endothelium*

8.1.1. *Endothelial cells* form a partially selective diffusion barrier which monitors bidirectional exchange of small molecules and restricted transport of macromolecules.

8.1.2. The cell membrane shows plasmalemmal vesicles and cells are joined by occluding (tight) junctions and communicating (gap) junctions.

8.1.3. The cytoplasm contains thick and thin filaments, indicating that they may contract.

8.1.4. Endothelial cells rarely divide and have a life span of 100–180 days. The source of new cells after damage may be from circulating blood cells, fibroblasts, smooth muscle cells, adjacent endothelial cells or undifferentiated subendothelial cells.

8.1.5. *Metabolic activities of endothelial cells*
A. Are actively engaged in *synthesis*, producing a wide range of products. They contribute to the metabolism of vasoactive substances, producing angiotensin converting enzyme, enzymes that inactivate norepinephrine, serotonin or bradykinin. They also synthesize prostaglandins which antagonise aggregation of platelets.

B. *Participate in hemostasis*, producing coagulant substances, tissue factor, plasminogen inhibitor as well as anticoagulant substances, plasminogen activator and prostacyclin.

      C. *Secrete blood group antigens A and B.*

      D. *Produce collagen* types IV and V for their own basal lamina, as well as elastin and glycosaminoglycans.

8.2. *Smooth muscle*:

  8.2.1. *Smooth muscle* is found in the walls of all vessels except capillaries and pericytic venules. Communicating (gap) junctions join smooth muscle cells, allowing conduction of impulses from one cell to another.

  8.2.2. Vascular smooth muscle cells behave like fibroblasts. They can produce most components of vessel walls — elastic fibers, collagen types I and III, glycosaminoglycans, as well as more muscle cells.

  8.2.3. Damage to the vessel wall stimulates migration of smooth muscle cells to the tunica intima. This migration is a feature of the formation of an atheromatous plaque. Cytoplasmic lysosomes may accumulate cholesterol in atheromatous lesions and cholesterol esters with aging.

  8.2.4. *Pericytes*, relatively undifferentiated cells encircling capillaries and postcapillary venules, can give rise to fibroblasts or smooth muscle cells.

8.3. *Vascular connective tissue*:

  8.3.1. *Elastic fibers* contain elastin and occur as microfibrils in isolated fibers or sheets. *Atherosclerosis* is associated with abnormal cross-linking of elastin.

  8.3.2. *Collagen fibers* concentrated between muscle cells. Aging is associated with increased cross-linking of collagen. *Arteriosclerosis* is associated with increased collagen synthesis with high proline — hydroxyproline activity.

  8.3.3. *Ground substance* is the extracellular matrix. It contains proteoglycans and controls the permeability of the vessel wall.

  8.3.4. Connective tissue cells include:

      A. *Mast cells* which produce, store and secrete histamine, heparin, chimase, beta glucuronidase and eosinophilic chemotactic factor of anaphylaxis (ECF-A). The cytoplasm of mast cells also contains leukotrienes, prostaglandins, platelet activating factor and hydrogen peroxide. These substances together regulate the viscosity of ground substance and insure optimum relationship between blood vessels and connective tissue.

B. *Macrophages* phagocytose material along blood vessel walls.

C. *Plasma cells* and *eosinophils* are responsible for local immunological reactions.

D. *Fibroblasts* secrete procollagen which is converted to collagen molecules in the extracellular space.

8.4. Vascular nerves

8.4.1. Bundles of postganglionic nerves from sympathetic ganglia form plexuses in the outermost layers of vessels. Some form knob-like endings near some, but not all, muscle cells. Arterioles have a particularly rich innervation.

8.4.2. Afferent nerves include those arising from pressure receptors (*baroreceptors*) and endings responding to the chemical composition of blood (*chemoreceptors*).

9. Arteries

9.1. The morphology of arteries is related to physical factors in various vessels of the system.

A. *Large elastic* (*conducting*) *arteries*. Blood delivered by the heart stretches elastic walls and recoil maintains pressure in this segment of the system.

B. *Muscular* (*distributing*) *arteries* regulate their diameter. Smooth muscle in the wall is under autonomic control and so the distribution of blood to areas depending on local needs is regulated.

C. *Arterioles and metarterioles* control the delivery of blood to capillary beds at low pressure and control the degree of pressure within the arterial system as a whole.

9.2. Large (*elastic*) Arteries

9.2.1. *Tunica intima* is thicker than other smaller arteries comprising 20% of the wall thickness (150 μm). It consists of:

A. Endothelium.

B. Subendothelial layer rich in interlacing collagen and elastin, small longitudinal smooth muscle bundles and fibroblast-like cells. There is no distinct internal elastic lamina.

9.2.2. *Tunica media* approximately 2 mm thick contains 50–70 concentric

2–3 μm fenestrated elastic laminae interconnected by elastic fibers and circumferential smooth muscle cells. Fibroblasts and a chondroitin sulphate ground substance are also present. There is no distinct external elastic lamina. Both tunica intima and tunica media in large arteries are nourished by diffusion.

9.2.3. *Tunica adventitia* is relatively very thin comprising a loose connective tissue containing vasa vasora, lymph vessels, myelinated and non-myelinated nerves.

9.3. Muscular (distributing) Arteries

9.3.1. Branches of major blood vessels have a larger potential volume than total blood volume so that helically arranged muscle cells in distributing arteries adjust the amount of blood delivered to local requirements.

9.3.2. *Tunica intima* comprises an endothelial layer, subendothelial layer of collagen and a few smooth muscle cells as well as an internal elastic lamina.

9.3.3. *Tunica media* contains 10–60 layers of helically arranged smooth muscle cells. Between muscle cells is a fine network of reticular, collagenous and elastic fibers.

9.3.4. *Tunica adventitia* comprises:

A. External elastic lamina.

B. Inner layer of dense connective tissue with longitudinal elastic fibers.

C. Outer layer of loose connective tissue with longitudinal collagen fibers and scattered smooth muscle cells.

D. Vasa vasora, lymph vessels and nerve fibers are present in this layer.

9.4. *Arterioles*

9.4.1. *Arterioles* have smooth muscle in their walls which respond to sympathetic nerve impulses and to metabolic stimuli reflecting local needs of tissues (autoregulation). They are the major regulators of blood flow.

9.4.2. *Tunica intima* comprises a simple non-fenestrated squamous endothelium and a thin internal elastic lamina. Gaps in the lamina allow formation of myoendothelial junctions.

9.4.3. *Tunica media* comprises 1–2 layers of helicoidally arranged smooth muscle cells.

9.4.4. *Tunica adventitia* is loose connective tissue containing macrophages, mast cells and non-myelinated nerves and is the same thickness as the media.

9.4.5. A relatively high hydrostatic pressure must be maintained to insure sufficient blood flow to tissues; however, blood must be delivered to capillary beds under low pressure to protect capillary walls. About half of the resistance to blood flow resides in arterioles.

9.5. *Metarterioles (precapillary arterioles)*

9.5.1. Metarterioles arise from terminal arterioles and are short segments 10–100 μm in length joined with a venule. Their diameter is larger than that of the capillaries to which they give rise. Smooth muscle cells in the wall form *precapillary sphincters* which control blood flow to the capillary bed.

9.5.2. *Tunica intima* is a single layer of endothelial cells with a thin subendothelial layer.

9.5.3. *Tunica media* is a single layer of smooth muscle cells replaced in some areas by pericytes.

9.5.4. *Tunica adventitia* is a loose connective tissue containing macrophages, mast cells and non-myelinated nerve fibers.

10. Capillaries

10.1. Capillaries are thin walled, 8–10 μm in diameter which form a semi-permeable partition between the vascular system and tissue space.

10.2. *Continuous capillaries* have an uninterrupted endothelium. Numerous micropinocytotic vesicles open at both basal and luminal cell surfaces as part of transendothelial channels. Zonulae occludentes and macula adherentes (desmosomes) join adjacent cells but gap junctions (nexuses) are rare. The basal lamina splits to enclose *pericytes*.

10.2.1. *Thick continuous capillaries* are found in muscular tissues, testis and ovaries.

10.2.2. *Thin continuous capillaries* have scarce pericytes and less micropinocytotic vesicles and are found in the CNS, lung, connective tissue, kidney, spleen, thymus, lymph nodes and bone.

10.3. *Fenestrated capillaries* have a very thin cytoplasmic wall perforated by pores. Cells are joined by zonulae occludentes and gap junctions in thicker areas while pericytes are rare. Fenestrated capillaries are found in endocrine glands, liver, spleen, bone marrow and kidney.

CARDIOVASCULAR SYSTEM

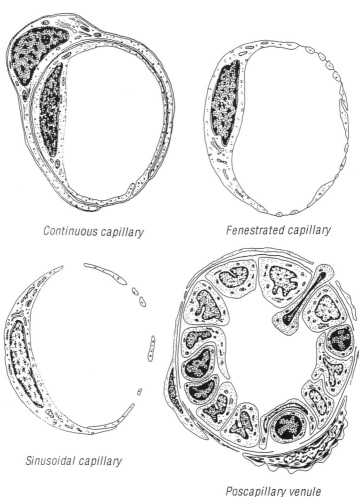

Continuous capillary   Fenestrated capillary

Sinusoidal capillary

Poscapillary venule

11. Arteriovenous Anastomoses

11.1. *Arteriovenous anastomoses* (*AVA's*) are coiled shunts between an arteriole and venule most commonly found in the distal parts of extremities, gastrointestinal tract, thyroid gland and in erectile tissue.

11.2. The walls are thick (12–15 μm) and muscular, of variable length (30–100 μm) and with a rich vasomotor innervation.

12. Post-Capillary (Pericytic) Venules

12.1. *Post capillary venules* are 10–50 μm in diameter and 50–700 μm long.

    12.1.1. *Tunica intima* comprises an endothelial layer 0.2–4 μm thick with overlapping and limited zonulae occludentes.

    12.1.2. *Tunica media* is a layer of flat pericytes.

    12.1.3. *Tunica adventitia* is thin and collagenous, containing some wandering cells.

12.2. Unlike capillaries, post capillary venules are:

    12.2.1. Easily affected by extreme temperature, inflammation and allergic reactions.

    12.2.2. Particularly labile and sensitive to histamine, serotonin, bradykinin and some prostaglandins which induce opening and leakage of their junctions.

13. Muscular Venules

13.1. Muscular venules are 50 μm–1 mm in diameter.

    13.1.1. *Tunica intima* is relatively thick comprising a continuous endothelium joined with occluding and gap junctions. Myoendothelial junctions occur with the tunica media.

    13.1.2. *Tunica media* comprises one or two layers of smooth muscle. The layer is incomplete in the spleen and kidney.

    13.1.3. *Tunica adventitia* is a relatively thick continuous layer of collagen fibrils containing non-myelinated nerve fibers. Muscular venules accompany arterioles.

14. Small and Medium Sized Veins

14.1. *Tunica intima* comprises an endothelium and basal lamina on a poorly defined internal elastic lamina or separated from the media by a small amount of subendothelial connective tissue.

14.2. *Tunica media* comprises circular smooth muscle. The layer is thinner than the same layer in an artery of the same diameter, contains more collagen and less elastin and is thinnest where the vein is protected by muscle.

14.3. *Tunica adventitia* is the thickest coat chiefly of collagen. In some veins, e.g., superficial veins of the leg, the tunica media is thick and muscular to counteract gravitational effects on venous return.

15. Large Veins

15.1. *Tunica intima* characteristically, the subendothelial layer thickens.

15.2. *Tunica media* is almost devoid of smooth muscle.

15.3. *Tunica adventitia* contains collagen and elastic fibers and is by far the thickest coat. In the inferior vena cava, there is a prominent layer of longitudinal muscle.

16. Vasa Vasora

16.1. These vessels are more plentiful in veins because they are supplied by poorly oxygenated blood.

16.2. With the low pressure in veins, they can approach the intima without collapse.

17. Valves

17.1. Leaflet type (flap) valves in veins are arranged to permit flow toward the heart only, especially in veins of the extremities.

17.2. The functions of valves are to:
A. Help overcome backflow from the force of gravity.
B. Enable veins squeezed by muscle to act as a pump by preventing backflow.

Chapter 10

RESPIRATORY SYSTEM
1. THE UPPER AIRWAY

OBJECTIVES

After reading this chapter, you should be able to:

1. Give an account of the development of the nasal cavities.
2. Describe in detail the epithelial lining of the vestibule, respiratory and olfactory regions of the nasal cavities.
3. Correlate histologic features of the nasal cavity with its functions in conditioning and filtering air.
4. Identify the particular histologic features of the epiglottis and larynx, relating them to the functions of these organs.
5. Give an account of the fine structure and function of laryngobronchial epithelium.
6. Identify the histologic features of the walls of the trachea, giving their functional significance.

CHAPTER OUTLINE

General. Conducting zone. Respiratory zone.

The nasal cavities. Vestibule. Respiratory region. Olfactory region.

Vascularization of respiratory mucosa.

Development of the nasal cavities.

Larynx. Functions of the larynx. Development of the larynx.
Trachea.

KEY WORDS, PHRASES, CONCEPTS

Conducting portion
Respiratory portion
Vestibule
Swell bodies
Lamina propria
Nasal conchae (turbinates)
Olfactory area:
  Olfactory receptor cells
  Olfactory vesicle
  Olfactory cilia
  Olfactory bulbs
  Sustentacular cells
  Basal cells
  Olfactory glands (of Bowman)
Paranasal sinuses
Nasal placodes
Trachealis muscle
Tracheal glands
Epiglottic glands

Oronasal membrane
Primitive choanae
Secondary palate
Epithelioid cells
Larynx:
  Vestibular folds
  Vocal folds
  Ventricles
  Saccule
  Cricovocal membrane
  Vocal ligaments
  Epiglottis
Tracheobronchial epithelium
Brush cells
Tracheal endocrine cells
Indifferent (intermediate) cells

Petiolus

1. General

1.1. The *respiratory system* conducts air through a series of conducting passages comprising the nasal cavity, nasopharynx, larynx, trachea, bronchi and bronchioles. This conducting zone represents 10% of total lung volume.

1.2. The respiratory system also provides for gaseous interchange in the lungs. This occurs in respiratory bronchioles, alveolar ducts together known as the *transitional zone* (30% of total lung volume) and terminal atria and alveolar sacs together known as the *respiratory zone* (60% of total lung volume).

1.3. The mature lung contains approximately 300 million terminal spaces (alveoli) with a surface area of 70–80 square meters.

2. Nasal Cavities

2.1. The paired nasal cavities are divided into three anatomical regions on the basis of the structure of the wall.

2.2. The *vestibule* is an antechamber with walls supported by cartilage. Covering epithelium is stratified squamous, gradually loosing its keratinized layer deeper into the nasal cavity. It contains coarse hairs, sebaceous and apocrine sweat glands.

2.3. The *respiratory region* covers most of the septum and lateral walls of the nasal cavity (160 cm^2).

2.3.1. Epithelium in this region is *pseudostratified ciliated with goblet cells* including intraepithelial glands. Mucus secreted by goblet cells traps particulate matter and cilia of the columnar cells beat toward the pharynx, expelling the mucus. The basal lamina varies from thin to thick.

2.3.2. The lamina propria is loose connective tissue infiltrated with lymphocytes and some eosinophils, plasma cells and macrophages.

2.3.3. Branched tubuloalveolar seromucous glands located in the lamina propria produce a secretion which also humidifies air and inactivates bacteria.

2.3.4. Arteries feed a subepithelial capillary plexus then large, thin-walled veins with enlargements (lacunae) resembling erectile tissue (*swell bodies*). Flow in these vessels is controlled by intimal cushions in their walls so that they contribute to warming of inspired air.

2.3.5. There is no submucosa, the lamina propria fusing with periosteum.

2.4. The *olfactory region* covers part of the roof of each nasal cavity extending onto small portions of the septum and superior conchae of each nasal cavity. Specialized epithelium is pseudostratified without goblet cells containing:

2.4.1. *Olfactory cells*. Long spindle-shaped bipolar neurones whose nucleus is situated in the lower half of the olfactory epithelium. A single dendritic process ends in a bulb-like swelling (the *olfactory vesicle or knob*) from which *olfactory cilia* project radially parallel to the epithelial surface. A single thin axon penetrates the basal lamina to join other non-myelinated axons of adjacent cells to form fascicles invested by Schwann cells. These penetrate the cribiform plate of the ethmoid bone and enter the paired *olfactory bulbs*.

2.4.2. *Supporting (sustentacular) cells* are tall columnar cells with apical microvilli joined to adjacent supporting cells by junctional complexes. Their cytoplasm contains lysosomes, granular ER and Golgi complex consistent with a role in metabolic exchange with olfactory cells.

2.4.3. *Basal cells* are small unspecialized cells adjacent to the basal lamina which can divide and differentiate into olfactory cells and perhaps supporting cells.

2.4.4. Branched tubuloalveolar *olfactory glands (of Bowman)* containing light (serous) and dark (mucous) cells continuously deliver a mixed secretion onto the surface of the olfactory epithelium to dissolve odoriferous substances, remove previous odors and moisten the olfactory mucosa.

3. Vascularization of Respiratory Mucosa

3.1. Muscular arteries supply a superficial capillary plexus beneath the epithelium.

3.2. Capillaries drain into venous lacunae whose walls contain smooth muscle that may form sphincters.

3.3. *Arteriovenous anastomoses (AVAs)* arising directly from the muscular arteries communicate directly with collecting veins. Their walls contain short, thick *epithelioid cells* in the tunica media but lack an internal elastic lamina.

3.4. Contraction of lacunar sphincters and AVAs promotes swelling of the venous plexuses (*swell bodies*), particularly over the middle and inferior conchae (turbinates).

4. Development of the Nasal Cavities

4.1. The site of formation of the nasal cavities is a localized thickening of surface ectoderm (*nasal or olfactory placodes*) on either side of the *frontonasal prominence* seen at 4 mm.

4.2. *Lateral and medial nasal prominences* surround the placodes, forming a central nasal pit. The lateral prominences form the alae of the nose while the medial prominences blend to form the nasal septum, upper lip, primary palate and maxilla.

4.3. The nasal pits deepen toward the forebrain where cells of the placodes become pseudostratified *olfactory epithelium*. The deepening pit also extends toward the stomodeum from which it is temporarily separated by an *oronasal membrane*.

4.4. The oronasal membrane ruptures at 7 weeks, establishing the *primitive choanae*.

4.5. *Lateral palatine processes* grow from each maxillary process medially and downward on either side of the tongue which at this time protrudes into the nasal cavity, reaching the nasal septum.

4.6. Rapid growth of the mandible in width and length allows the tongue to drop from the nasal cavity into the wider oral cavity.

4.7. Accentuated growth of mesoderm in the palatine processes causes them to adopt a horizontal position.

4.8. The palatine processes meet one another and with the nasal septum from in front posteriorly. Epithelium covering the processes breaks down by apoptosis and mesoderm penetrates, forming the definitive *secondary palate*, closing the primitive choanae posteriorly to the junction of the nasal cavity and pharynx.

4.9. *Conchae* (*turbinates*) develop as elevated folds from the lateral wall of the nasal cavity. The first develops from the maxilla (maxilloturbinal) then five appear sequentially from the ethmoid (ethmoturbinals). The inferior conchae originate from the maxilla, middle conchae from the first ethmoturbinal and superior conchae from the second and third ethmoturbinals.

4.10. Paranasal sinuses begin to appear at 4 months, expanding rapidly after birth.

5. Larynx (Larynx (Gk) A Throat)

5.1. Situated between the oro-pharynx and trachea, the larynx is a valve and sound producing organ. Its walls are kept patent during inspiration by cartilages interconnected by ligaments and intrinsic and extrinsic voluntary muscles.

5.2. Symmetrical mucosal folds project from the lateral walls:

   5.2.1. *Vestibular folds* are protective folds whose core is a lamina propria containing laryngeal glands, simple mixed tubulo-alveolar glands lacking intercalated and striated ducts. Their secretion moistens the laryngeal mucosa and vocal folds.

   5.2.2. The *saccule* is a diverticulum of the anterior end of the ventricle. It contains numerous mucous glands which can be squeezed by surrounding muscles. Their secretion also lubricates the vocal folds.

   5.2.3. *Vocal folds* (*cords*) are located below the vestibular folds and separated from them by the *laryngeal ventricles*. The vibrations of their cord-like free margins are required to produce sound.

5.3. The *cricovocal membranes* (*conus elasticus*) are paired triangular membranes of elastic fibers sweeping upwards and medially from the arch of the cricoid cartilage below to the inside of the thyroid cartilage near the point of fusion of its laminae (the thyroid angle).

5.4. The *vocal ligaments* are the thickened upper borders of the cricovocal membranes and extend from the thyroid angle in front to the vocal processes of the arytenoid cartilages behind. They form the core of the vocal folds while the *vocalis* (voluntary) *muscle* borders the ligaments laterally and runs parallel to them.

5.5. *Epithelium* lining the larynx is not uniform. Areas subjected to wear such as the vocal folds, aryepiglottic folds and the epiglottis are covered with *stratified squamous non-keratinizing epithelium*. Below the vocal folds, the epithelium is *pseudostratified columnar ciliated epithelium with goblet cells*. Cilia beat towards the pharynx.

5.6. The *basal lamina* is thin.

5.7. The *lamina propria* is rich in elastic fibers and unusually rich in mast cells. The secretion of *seromucous glands* protects the epithelium and mucus also reaches the larynx from the lower respiratory tract by coughing and ciliary action. Lymph nodules are present particularly in the ventricle and vestibular fold.

5.8. The *epiglottis* (epi (Gk) upon and glottis (Gk) larynx) is a flap-like leaf of elastic and fibrocartilage attached at the inner aspect of the thyroid angle and projecting upward from the top of the larynx. It has a passive role in keeping food/fluid out of the larynx. The larynx is drawn upwards and forwards in swallowing and the upper tubular part of the epiglottis is pressed against the laryngeal wall.

5.8.1. The core (*petiolus*) is a plate of fibrous and elastic cartilage whose perichondrium is continuous with the lamina propria of the mucous membrane.

5.8.2. *Epithelium* of the anterior and upper part of the posterior surface is stratified squamous non-keratinized. Epithelium of the lower posterior surface is pseudostratified columnar with goblet cells. Cilia move mucus towards the pharynx.

5.8.3. *Mucous* (*epiglottic*) *glands* occupy recesses in the epiglottic cartilage on the laryngeal side.

5.9. Functions of the larynx include:

A. *Phonation* (voice production).

B. *Protection of the lungs* during swallowing by preventing the ingress of foreign objects to lower respiratory structures. Stimulation of the sensitive aryepiglottic folds induces laryngeal spasm which stops the ingress of particles but can also cause asphyxia. The cough reflex expels foreign objects.

C. *In respiration*, the larynx not only controls the ingress of air but distributes the air by causing back pressure during expiration.

5.10. Development of the larynx:

5.10.1. The first indication of development of the respiratory system is the appearance at 3 mm (26 days) of a longitudinal epithelial (entodermal) lined evagination of the ventral wall of the foregut, the *laryngotracheal groove*.

5.10.2. The evagination grows caudally and is progressively separated from the esophagus by a longitudinal lateral pinching off which progresses from caudal to rostral.

5.10.3. The lower end of the laryngotracheal groove bifurcates at 4 mm so that at this stage, the respiratory organs comprise a

RESPIRATORY SYSTEM

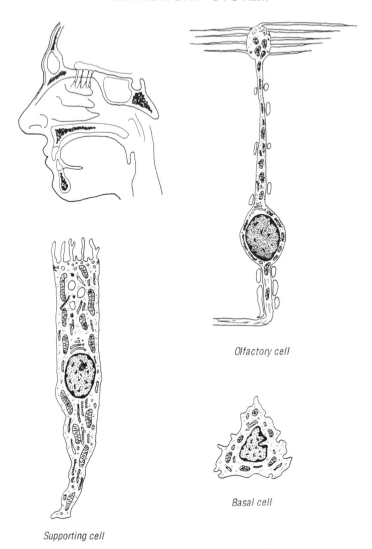

Olfactory cell

Basal cell

Supporting cell

laryngeal orifice between the fourth arches, a trachea and two primary bronchi.

5.10.4. *Laryngeal cartilages* are derivatives of pharyngeal arch cartilages: The *epiglottis* appears at the base of the third and fourth arches and differentiates internal cartilage at 4 months.

The *lesser horn and cranial part of the body of the hyoid* develop from the cartilage of the second (hyoid) arch.

The *greater horn and caudal part of the body of the hyoid* develop from the cartilage of the third arch.

Cartilages of the fourth, fifth and sixth arches fuse to form the *thyroid, cricoid and arytenoid cartilages.*

5.10.5. Laryngeal epithelium proliferates temporarily, occluding the lumen of the larynx; however, recanalization establishes the laryngeal ventricles.

5.10.6. Musculature of the larynx is derived from branchial arch muscles. Cricothyroid is a derivative of the fourth arch and supplied by the superior laryngeal branch of the vagus nerve. The remaining intrinsic muscles are derivatives of the sixth arches and are supplied by the recurrent laryngeal branch of the vagus nerve.

6. Trachea (from tracheia (Gk) rough, to distinguish it from smooth arteries. Both were thought in ancient times to carry "vital spirit").

6.1. The *trachea* is a flexible, extensible, airway tube with a constantly patent lumen. It extends from the cricoid cartilage to the carina (from carina (L) a keel) where the trachea divides into two primary bronchi.

6.2. Epithelial lining of bronchi is pseudostratified ciliated with goblet cells resting on a very thick basal lamina. Six cell types have been identified but squamous metaplasia from chronic irritation is common.

6.2.1. *Ciliated columnar cells* are most numerous. The cell surface is covered with 1–200 cilia which beat towards the larynx. The cytoplasm contains lysosomes, free and attached ribosomes and a large Golgi complex. Cells are interconnected by apical junctional complexes and mid-lateral desmosomes.

6.2.2. *Goblet cells.*

6.2.3. *Basal (Immature) cells* which can differentiate into ciliated or goblet cells.

6.2.4. *Brush cells*, tall cells with apical microvilli, are contacted by nerve fibers at their proximal (basal) pole and are considered to act as sensory receptors.

6.2.5. *Small granule cells (Tracheal endocrine cells)* are contacted by cholinergic nerve endings. These cells contain 1–300 nm

RESPIRATORY SYSTEM

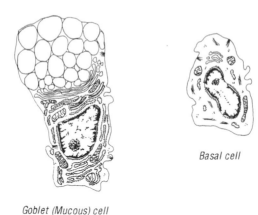

Goblet (Mucous) cell

Basal cell

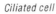

Ciliated cell

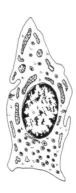

Endocrine cell

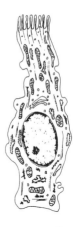

Brush cell

dense cored granules and some produce catecholamines while others produce polypeptide hormones.

6.2.6. *Indifferent* (*Intermediate*) cells are pyramidal cells with their base on the basal lamina but whose apical pole does not reach the tracheal lumen. These cells originate from basal cells and in turn divide and redifferentiate into mucous or ciliated cells.

6.2.7. *Migratory cells* are intraepithelial B lymphocytes and mast cells.

6.3. The *basal lamina* of the trachea is the thickest of any location in the body.

6.4. The *lamina propria* is a thin fibrous layer in which elastic fibers largely replace the muscularis mucosa. It contains lymphocytes, lymph nodules and fixed and wandering connective tissue cells.

6.5. The *submucosa* contains seromucous glands and extends into the adventitia between cartilages or penetrates the muscularis dorsally. *Tracheal glands* are mucous with serous crescents.

6.6. The *adventitia* contains 16–20 C or Y shaped hyaline cartilages which open posteriorly (facing the esophagus). They are bound together by a vertically arranged layer of dense fibroelastic tissue. Smooth muscle bundles (*Trachealis muscle*) stretch between the tips of tracheal cartilages and yield to expansion of the esophagus.

The adventitia holds the trachea open mechanically and provides extensibility and flexibility.

Chapter 11

RESPIRATORY SYSTEM
2. THE LUNGS

OBJECTIVES

After reading this chapter, you should be able to:
1. Describe a basis for lobulation and segmentation of the lungs.
2. Differentiate between the intrapulmonary conducting tubes and respiratory tubes of the lungs, identify their structural features and the functional significance of these features.
3. Describe the fine structure of alveolar walls.
4. Give an account of the blood and nerve supplies and lymphatic drainage of the lung.

CHAPTER OUTLINE

Lungs

General.

Bronchi.

Bronchioles.

Respiratory bronchioles.

Alveolar ducts.

Atria.

Alveoli. Cells of alveolar epithelium. Surfactant. Alveolar macrophages.

Air-blood interface.

Pulmonary circulation.

Nerve supply.

Development of the lungs.

KEY WORDS, PHRASES, CONCEPTS

Mediastinum

Lung buds

Pleura

Lobes

Secondary (Pulmonary) lobules

Primary lobules (Acini)

Main (Principal or Primary) bronchi

Lobar (Secondary) bronchi

(Tertiary) bronchi

Bronchopulmonary segments

Bronchial fluid

Respiratory bronchioles

Bronchial glands

Non ciliated bronchiolar (Clara)
    cells

Oncocytes

Alveolar ducts

Atria

Alveoli

Alveolar pores

Pulmonary epithelial cells

Type I pneumocytes

Type II pneumocytes

(Septal cells or Granular Segmental
    Pneumocytes)

Alveolar macrophages

Pulmonary arteries

Bronchial arteries

Pulmonary lymphatics

Ciliated bronchiolar
    cells

Neuroendocrine cells

1. General

1.1. Paired respiratory organs, the lungs are subdivided into nearly separate lobes.

1.2. Each lung is attached at the *hilum* where a main air conducting tube, the bronchus, enters and vessels enter and leave.

1.3. *Pleura* comprises a serous membrane (mesothelium) covering of the lungs and lining the pleural cavity and a densely innervated and vascular subserosal layer containing elastic fibers continuous with septa of the lung. At the hilum, the two portions of pleura become continuous — *parietal pleura* which lines the inner thoracic wall and *visceral pleura* reflected onto and enclosing the lung. Pleura is moistened by a friction-reducing fluid produced by mesothelial cells

1.4. Air conducting tubes in the lung include branches of *bronchi* and all ordinary *bronchioles* (cf. excretory ducts of a gland).

1.5. Respiratory tubes where gaseous exchange takes place with blood, include *respiratory bronchioles, alveolar ducts, atria and alveolar sacs* (cf. smaller ducts and alveoli of a gland). All respiratory tubes contain at least some air cells (*alveoli*) in their walls.

1.6. The smaller subdivisions of this system are closely crowded and displaced so that sections give a poor picture of true spatial relationships.

1.7. The lungs are divided into three lobes on the right side and two lobes on the left, all supplied by *secondary (lobar) bronchi*.

1.8. *Lobar bronchi* usually divide into 10 *tertiary (segmental) bronchi* in the right lung and 8 in the left lung. The area supplied by a tertiary bronchus is called a *bronchopulmonary segment*.

1.9. *Secondary (lung) lobules* are the area of lung supplied by bronchioles. The field supplied is shown at the lung surface as a polygonal area 10–20 mm in diameter bounded by interlobular septa. The boundary is often blackened by inhaled carbon particles contained in lymphatics.

1.10. *Primary lobules (lung units or acini)* are smaller units representing the area supplied by a respiratory bronchiole. They appear as polygonal areas on the lung surface approximately 1 mm in diameter.

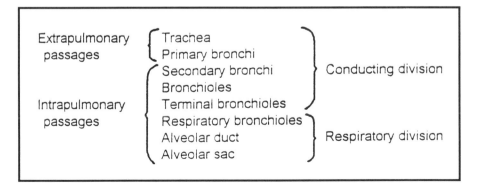

Pulmonary passages.

2. Bronchi

2.1. *Bronchi* conduct, moisten and warm inspired air and trap air-borne particles which are moved by ciliary action to the trachea and expelled by swallowing or coughing.

A. *Primary bronchi* are extrapulmonary extending from the tracheal bifurcation to the hilum.

B. *Secondary bronchi* are intrapulmonary extending between primary bronchi and bronchioles.

2.2. *Epithelium* lining bronchi is *pseudostratified ciliated with goblet cells* but reduced in thickness and layering compared with that of the trachea.

2.3. The *lamina propria* is loose connective tissue containing longitudinal elastic fibers and scattered lymphoid nodules.

2.4. The *muscularis mucosae* comprises interlacing spirals of smooth muscle whose contraction causes folding of the epithelial lining.

2.5. The *submucosa* is loose connective tissue containing a venous plexus and seromucous *bronchial glands*.

2.6. *Bronchial glands* are mixed, tubulo-alveolar glands which produce *bronchial fluid*. They are coextensive with the cartilaginous skeleton and as they disappear distally, surface goblet (mucous) cells increase.

2.6.1. Cells in bronchial glands include:

A. *Serous cells* which contain glycogen and small secretory granules. Their cell membranes have deep intercellular canaliculi and lateral interdigitations.

B. *Mucus cells*.

C. *Myoepitheliocytes* which send processes around alveoli and ducts.

2.6.2. Ducts of bronchial glands are lined with typical laryngobronchial epithelium but larger ducts contain single or groups of columnar acidophilic oncocytes. *Oncocytes* are rich in mitochondria and are considered to modify secretion of bronchial glands in a manner similar to striated duct cells in salivary glands.

2.6.3. *Bronchial fluid* produced by bronchial glands contains mucins, serum proteins filtered from blood, secretory immunoglobulin, some immunoglobulin M, muco and glycoprotein and lactoferrin, a bacteriostatic protein. The fluid protects and moistens the epithelium.

2.7. The *adventitia* contains separate cartilaginous plates which are hyaline but increasingly elastic.

3. Bronchioles

3.1. *Bronchioles* are conducting passages situated between bronchi and alveolar ducts. The largest is 1 mm in diameter and the smallest, 0.5 mm.

3.2. *Epithelium* lining bronchioles is simple columnar distally to the level of respiratory bronchioles where ciliated cells disappear and cells become low columnar to cuboidal.

Epithelial cells include:

A. *Non-ciliated bronchiolar (Clara)* cells are dome-shaped cells which contain dimorphic mitochondria, extensive RER and SER, indicating that they synthesize cholesterol and carbohydrates. Cytoplasmic granules contain proteolytic and mucolytic enzymes and non-enzymatic substances which modify the stickiness of secretions. In addition, they are considered to function in fluid absorption. These cells lie distal to the mucus-producing areas and keep the small airways dry.

B. *Ciliated bronchiolar* cells with apical cilia and long microvilli. These cells may be endocytic.

C. *Neuroendocrine (small granule) cells* containing amines (dopamine or serotonin) in small, dense core granules. They decarboxylate exogenous amine precursors so belong to the amine precursor uptake and decarboxylation (APUD) series. These cells are often found in clusters known as neuroepithelial bodies and are thought to be intrapulmonary chemoreceptors.

D. *Sensory brush cells.*

E. *Migratory cells* of the hematopoeitic series within the bronchiolar epithelium include lymphocytes, mononuclear leukocytes (which participate in immunological reactions), as well as neutrophils and eosinophils.

3.3. The *lamina propria* is a thin layer of loose connective tissue containing subepithelial elastic fibers.

3.4. The *muscularis mucosae* comprises spirally arranged smooth muscle proportionally thicker than elsewhere in the respiratory system. Activated by parasympathetic nerves, this muscle undergoes peristaltic movements and relaxes in inspiration and contracts at the end of expiration. It participates in the cough reflex and increases in tone in cold weather.

3.5. The *adventitia* is loose connective tissue containing small branches of bronchial arteries, veins and lymphatics and autonomic nerves.

3.6. In sections, bronchioles appear stellate-shaped because the mucosa folds with post-mortem shortening of muscle.

3.7. Bronchioles do not collapse during inspiration because stretching of surrounding respiratory tissue during inspiration causes them to expand.

4. Respiratory Bronchioles

4.1. *Respiratory bronchioles* are branches of terminal bronchioles 0.5 mm or less in diameter. The first alveoli or air sacs appear in the walls at this level.

4.2. *Epithelium* is low columnar and contains bronchiolar and ciliated cells. Goblet cells are absent.

4.3. The *lamina propria* is a thin layer of loose connective tissue with longitudinal elastic fibers.

4.4. *Muscularis* is a thin, discontinuous layer of interlacing smooth muscle cells which acts as a terminal sphincter. A few alveoli lying outside the muscular layer bud from the walls.

4.5. The *adventitia* is very reduced loose connective tissue. It contains branches of the pulmonary artery, fine lymphatics and autonomic nerves.

5. Alveolar Ducts

5.1. *Alveolar ducts* are branches of respiratory bronchioles in which the fraction of the wall taken up by alveoli increases until the wall is little more than a series of openings into alveoli.

5.2. Scattered spirals of smooth muscle appear in sections as knob-like enlargements at the mouth of alveoli. The muscle, in the form of rings, guards the openings of alveoli.

5.3. Many alveoli open into alveolar ducts.

6. Atria

6.1. Atria are 3–6 terminal branches of alveolar ducts representing antechambers to alveoli.

7. Alveoli

7.1. *Alveoli* are polyhedral sacs of uniform size (300 μm in diameter) where respiratory gas exchange occurs. One side, the aperture opening into an alveolar duct or respiratory bronchiole, is absent.

7.2. There are some 300 million alveoli in each mature human lung, representing a surface area of about 80 square meters. Two to five alveoli open off each atrium.

7.3. Interalveolar walls, the septa common to two adjacent alveoli, comprise an epithelium covering a highly vascularized connective tissue space. Connective tissue in interalveolar walls contains reticular and elastic fibers, fibroblasts, macrophages, occasional mast cells, lymphocytes and eosinophil leukocytes.

7.4. Anastomosing capillaries with an endothelial lining and basal lamina bulge into alveoli on both sides. This maximizes the surface area exposed to air. The capillary network in the lung is the richest in the body.

7.5. Alveolar pores are openings 7–9 μm in diameter between adjacent alveoli. They permit limited collateral air circulation so guard against collapse in the event of proximal blockage. Pores also represent a path for rapid spread of infection.

7.6. Alveolar epithelial lining is a continuous cuboidal entodermal lining in the embryo. It persists in the adult; however, the entodermal lining becomes squamous and the cytoplasm is greatly thinned.

    A. *Pulmonary epithelial cells* (*squamous alveolar cells, Type I pneumocytes*) have an attenuated cytoplasm (0.2 μm thick) in contact with air. Micropinocytotic vesicles indicate that small amounts of protein can be taken up from alveoli but the main role of pulmonary epithelial cells is to provide an intact, extremely thin surface which is permeable to gases.

    B. *Great alveolar cells* (*septal cells, Type II pneumocytes or granular pneumocytes*) are round or cuboidal cells resting on the common basal lamina shared with vascular endothelium deep to squamous epithelial cells. They may be found in the epithelium and joined to neighboring cells by continuous tight junctions. These cells contain well-developed cytoplasmic organelles associated with secretion. The cytoplasm also contains multilammellar bodies and cytosomes (0.2–1 μm, in diameter) with parallel or concentric lamellae. They contain phospholipid, mucopolysaccharide, proteins and lysosomal hydrolases. Great alveolar cells produce *surfactant* (*anti-atelectatic factor*), a detergent surface active phospholipid which coats the internal alveolar surface, reduces surface tension at the air – fluid surface and reduces the tendency of alveoli to collapse (atelectasis).

C. *Alveolar macrophages* (*alveolar phagocytes*, *dust cells*) are large, free phagocytes on the surface of alveolar cells which defend the respiratory region against contamination by microorganisms and inhaled particles. It is not known whether these cells arise from connective tissue in the lung or from circulating monocytes.

8. The Air-Blood Interface

8.1. The interface between air and blood in the alveoli comprises:
   A. A thin coat of *fluid* on the surface of alveolar cells.
   B. *Squamous alveolar cells*.
   C. *Great alveolar cells*.
   D. *Basal lamina* shared with:
   E. *Non-fenestrated endothelium* (of a blood vessel).
   F. *Elastic and reticular fibers* (excluded where capillary loops press against pulmonary epithelium).

9. Pulmonary Circulation

9.1. *Pulmonary arteries* deliver high volumes of deoxygenated blood at relatively low pressure to the lungs. The wall of pulmonary arteries contains relatively more smooth muscle and elastic tissue than pulmonary veins. The smallest vessels contain an inner elastic lamina.

9.2. *Pulmonary veins* are thin-walled vessels collecting oxygenated blood from lobules. For a short distance beyond their junction with the left atrium, pulmonary veins have an adventitial coat of cardiac muscle which acts as a valve and facilitates return of blood to the heart.

9.3. *Bronchial arteries* are small branches of the thoracic aorta supplying the walls of most airways.

9.4. *Bronchial veins* occur only near the hilum and provide accessory drainage from bronchial walls.

9.5. Anastomoses between branches of the bronchial arteries and pulmonary arteries occur at the level of respiratory bronchioles.

9.6. *Lymphatics* form plexuses superficially in the visceral pleura and deep within the walls of bronchi and pulmonary vessels. Both plexuses interconnect at the hilum. They also communicate near the origins of pulmonary veins and in interlobular septa arising from pleura. There are no lymphatic capillaries in interalveolar walls.

10. Nerve Supply

10.1. Autonomic nerves are abundant both superficial and deep to cartilages in conducting passages. A few unmyelinated fascicles can be traced to respiratory bronchioles.

10.2. Vagal stimulation causes transient vasoconstriction in the lung but sympathetic stimulation has no effect unless bronchial tone is first increased (it then produces bronchodilation). Sympathetic action thus appears to be inhibitory to parasympathetic fibers carried in the vagus.

10.3. Visceral afferent nerves poorly localize pain.

11. Development of the Lungs

11.1. The "lung bud" penetrates a median mass of mesenchyme (the mediastinum) and bifurcates at 4 mm. The stem will become the trachea while the branches are primary bronchi.

11.2. The *right primary bronchus* gives rise to two lateral bronchi and a stem bronchus. The *left primary bronchus* forms one lateral bronchus as well as its stem bronchus.

The right upper lateral bronchus (apical) supplies the upper lobe. The other lateral bronchus supplies the middle lobe and the stem bronchus supplies the lower lobe. The left lateral bronchus supplies the upper lobe and the stem bronchus supplies the lower lobe.

11.3. Right and left bronchial buds project into the narrow *pleural canals*, part of the intraembryonic coelom on either side of the foregut. Mesoderm covering the outside of the lung becomes the visceral pleura while the somatic layer becomes the parietal pleura.

11.4. The larger conducting tubes forming bronchi and bronchioles branch from 5 weeks to 4 months. At this stage (*the pseudoglandular stage*), the lung resembles an acinar gland. Acini of the lungs (the portion of the lung parenchyma supplied by a prospective terminal bronchiole) become delineated. Epithelium of the proximal airways contains ciliated, non-ciliated and goblet cells by week 13 while basal cells are found at 10 weeks. Pulmonary epithelium is high columnar.

11.5. Respiratory bronchioles form by further branching from 4–6 months. At this stage (*the canalicular stage*), acini are delineated and a typical air-blood barrier begins to form. The pulmonary epithelium differentiates (Type II cells give rise to Type I cells) and surfactant synthesis begins toward the end of the stage. Shortly before birth, the number of alveolar macrophages in air spaces increases sharply and the increase continues during the first post-natal month.

11.6. Alveolar ducts branch from 6 months to term (*the terminal sac stage*). Branching continues through the first eight years (*the alveolar stage*) for another 6 divisions until there are 24 generations of branches.

11.7. Primary septa between air spaces in the newborn are thick, three layered structures consisting of a central sheet of connective tissue with a layer of capillaries on both sides.

11.8. Alveolar formation begins at postnatal day 4. In addition, secondary septa arise from upfoldings of one of the capillary networks like crest-like protrusions from primary septa. These subdivide saccules into alveolar sacs and ducts. Two cell types in secondary septa are a dormant lipid containing cell and an active myofibroblast.

11.9. The appearance of elastic tissue is closely linked with alveolar formation.

11.10. Lung volume increases in the alveolar stage but tissue volume does not.

11.11. Septal reconstruction includes thinning of the interstitium, lengthening of the septum with expansion of the capillary meshwork and capillary fusion. There is also a dramatic appearance of *interalveolar pores*.

11.12. The number of alveoli increases from 20 million soon after birth to nearly 300 million in adulthood (alveoli also increase in diameter).

The air space surface increases from 2.8 square meters to 120 square meters.

LUNG

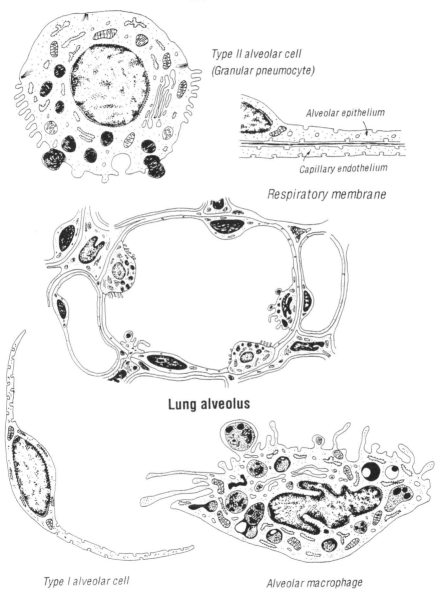

Type II alveolar cell
(Granular pneumocyte)

Alveolar epithelium

Capillary endothelium

Respiratory membrane

Lung alveolus

Type I alveolar cell
(Membranous pneumocyte)

Alveolar macrophage

Chapter 12

DIGESTIVE SYSTEM
1. ORAL CAVITY

OBJECTIVES

After reading this chapter, you should be able to:
1. Describe the regional specializations to the basic structural plan of the digestive tract exhibited in the walls of the oral cavity.
2. Give an account of the histologic structure of the lip and cheek.
3. Describe the regional differences in gingiva.
4. Describe the histologic structure of papillae of the tongue.
5. Give an account of the embryologic development of the tongue including a developmental explanation for its sensory and motor innervation.
6. Differentiate between the major salivary glands on the basis of histologic structure.
7. Describe the composition, functions and control of secretion of saliva.

CHAPTER OUTLINE

General. Structural plan of the mouth.

Lip.

Cheek.

Gingiva. Masticatory mucosa. Lining mucosa. Free gingiva. Attached gingiva. Interdental papillae.

Tongue. General. Detailed structure. Papillae: Filiform, Fungiform, Vallate, Foliate. Taste buds.

Hard Palate.

Soft Palate.

Salivary glands. General. Saliva: Functions of saliva.

Parotid gland.

Submandibular gland.

Sublingual gland.

Control of salivary gland function.

Development of the oral cavity.

Development of salivary glands.

KEY WORDS, PHRASES, CONCEPTS

Mucosa
Submucosa
Transitional zone of lip
Labial glands
Cheek
Free gingiva
Attached gingiva
Masticatory mucosa
Lining mucosa
Interdental papillae
Lingual papillae
Filiform papillae
Fungiform papillae
Vallate papillae
Stomodeum
Mandibular swelling
Maxillary swelling
Maxillary process
Second pharyngeal arch

Taste buds
Taste cells
Supporting cells
Taste chamber
Taste pore
Serous glands (of von Ebner)
Saliva
Parotid gland
Submandibular gland
Sublingual gland
Intercalated ducts
Striated ducts
Excretory ducts
Myoepitheliocytes
Maxillary swelling
Mandibular arch
Maxillary process
Meckel's cartilage
Lateral lingual swellings

Tuberculum impar
Terminal sulcus
Foramen caecum

Copula (Hypobranchial eminence)
Body of the tongue

THE ORAL CAVITY

1. General

1.1. The structural plan of the mouth and pharynx is:

    1.1.1. *Mucosa*.

        A. *Epithelium* is mostly stratified squamous and does not truly cornify in man. Cells desquamate into saliva. They can be examined histologically after scraping from the surface for carcinomatous changes or for indication of sex chromosome status. *Barr bodies* are heavily stained chromatin bodies first described in the nucleus of a much higher proportion of females than males. They comprise two X chromosomes attached to the inner nuclear membrane in the interphase nuclei.

        B. *Basal lamina*.

        C. *Lamina propria* forms tall vascular papillae that indent the epithelium.

        D. A *muscularis mucosa* is lacking in the mouth and pharynx.

    1.1.2. *Submucosa* is present in some regions as a lax layer which permits the mucosa to be lifted as a fold. In other regions, it attaches the mucosa to muscles or bone. It is absent from the hard palate, gingiva and dorsum of the tongue. Compound tubuloalveolar serous, mucous or seromucous glands may be in the submucosa or deeper but are not present in all regions.

    1.1.3. The *supporting wall* is skeletal muscle or bone to which superficial tissues attach.

    1.1.4. *Blood vessels, lymphatics and nerves* form a plexus in the submucosa. Branches pass into the mucosa, particularly into papillae which are also very sensitive.

2. Lip (Lippa (Anglo-saxon) Lip also Labium (L) a Lip)

2.1. The *outer surface* is typical thin skin containing hair follicles, sebaceous and sweat glands.

2.2. The *free margin* of the lip has a transitional zone (mucocutaneous junction) where relatively thin stratified squamous keratinized epithelium changes to thicker stratified non-keratinized epithelium (the *red border*).

    A. Tall, richly vascular papillae deeply indent the epithelium and blood in capillaries shows through, giving it a red color.

    B. Glands are virtually absent from the free margin rendering it susceptible to drying. This is normally overcome through moistening by saliva with the tongue.

2.3. The *inner surface* of the lip is a mucous membrane.

    A. *Epithelium* is thick, stratified non-keratinized epithelium.

    B. *Lamina propria* is thin, loose connective tissue with prominent papillae deeply indenting the epithelium.

    C. *Labial glands* are mixed seromucous (mostly mucous) glands in the submucosa with ducts opening into the vestibule.

3. Cheek

3.1. The *cheek* has an *outer surface* of thin skin with hairs, sweat and sebaceous glands and *hypodermis* rich in adipose tissue (particularly in newborns) adherent to the buccinator muscle.

3.2. The *inner surface* is a mucosa:

    A. *Epithelium* is stratified squamous non-keratinized with short papillae.

    B. *Lamina propria*, a compact layer rich in elastic fibers and bound to underlying muscle. This prevents folding and biting of the cheek during mastication.

    C. Mixed (mostly mucous) glands (*buccal glands*) open into the vestibule and may invade the muscular core (buccinator muscle) of the cheek.

4. Gingiva (Gingivae (L) Gums)

4.1. *Gingiva* is the part of oral mucosa that attaches to alveolar bone and surrounds the teeth.

4.2. Gingiva is divided structurally into:

A. *Masticatory mucosa* which bears the major forces of mastication, e.g., gingiva and the hard palate.

B. Lining mucosa which is not exposed to major forces, e.g., lining the vestibule lips and cheeks.

4.3. *Gingival epithelium* is stratified squamous with deep epithelial ridges. True keratinization (*orthokeratosis*) is replaced by cells progressing toward keratinization but superficial cells retain distinct nuclei (*parakeratosis*). In the gingival crevice surrounding teeth, epithelium is non-keratinized and devoid of epithelial ridges.

4.4. *Lamina propria* is poorly vascularized dense connective tissue firmly attached to periosteum or to the necks of teeth. It is rich in sensory Kraus' corpuscles.

4.5. Gingiva is normally coral pink in color but this depends on thickness of the keratinizing layers and pigmentation in colored races. Inflammation interferes with keratinization.

4.6. There are no glands or submucosa in gingiva.

4.7. Gingiva is divided topographically into:

A. *Free gingiva* parallel to the margin of teeth and separated from attached gingiva by a free gingival groove which is approximately opposite the base of the gingival sulcus. It is not always visible macroscopically.

B. *Attached gingiva* appears "stippled" because of the attachment of collagenous bundles of the periodontal ligament and of the alveolar crest into the superficial dermis. Stippling is a functional adaptation to mechanical impacts and varies in amount with age, sex and swelling (gingivitis).

C. *Interdental papillae* are the parts of gingiva filling the space between teeth. The buccal and lingual corners are high but the central part often dips below the contact point between teeth, forming a valley or col.

5. Tongue (Lingua (L) the Tongue also Glossa (Gk) the Tongue)

5.1. General:

5 1.1. The *tongue* is a mobile, mucosa covered muscular organ situated

in the floor of the mouth

5.1.2. It has a convex dorsum separated by a V-shaped groove, the *sulcus terminalis* into an anterior two thirds or *oral part* and posterior third or *pharyngeal part*. At the apex of the sulcus is the *foramen caecum* marking the site of developmental origin of the thyroid gland.

5.1.3. The oral part of the dorsum is covered by specializations of the mucosa known as *lingual papillae*. The pharyngeal part is marked by *lingual follicles*. Their *crypts* and *lenticular papillae* enclose lymphatic nodules of the *lingual tonsils*.

5.1.4. The ventral surface of the tongue is covered by oral mucosa but lacks specializations.

5.2. Detailed Structure:

5.2.1. *Mucosa* includes fairly thick stratified squamous epithelium which is partially keratinized and tightly bound down except on the ventral surface.

5.2.2. *Lamina propria* is compact and intimately bound to skeletal muscle bundles which form the core of the tongue.

5.2.3. *Lingual papillae* are vertical projections of the mucosa on the dorsal surface.

   A. *Filiform papillae* (filum (L) a thread), the predominant form of papilla, 0.5–3 mm long, are arranged in rows and constitute the "plush" of the tongue.

      (i) The papilla is a primary elevation of the lamina propria (*primary papilla*) which may be sub-divided into one or two *secondary papillae*.

      (ii) *Epithelium* covering filiform papillae ends in tapering points that point towards the pharynx. The epithelium is thinly keratinized and the papillae have an abrasive action in mastication.

   B. *Fungiform papillae* (fungus (L), a mushroom) are club-like projections with a narrow stalk. They are scattered singly and project above neighboring filiform papillae.

      (i) The largest is 1.8 mm high and 1 mm wide.

      (ii) The core is very vascular and because it is covered with translucent, non-keratinized stratified squamous epithelium, fungiform papillae appear red in color.

(iii) The primary connective tissue core bears secondary papillae which indent the epithelium but the free surface is smooth.

(iv) Some fungiform papillae bear one or more taste buds (vide infra).

C. *Vallate (circumvallate) papillae* (vallatus (L) walled or having a rim) form a V-shaped row in front of the sulcus terminalis at the division between the body and root of the tongue.

(i) There are 7–12 vallate papillae which are much larger than any other types of papillae measuring 0.5–1.5 mm. high and 1–3 mm wide.

(ii) The vallate papilla is the shape of an inverted, truncated cone with a flat top that does not project above the surface of the tongue (i.e., it is countersunk) and is surrounded by a deep trench.

(iii) The epithelial cover is exposed to abrasion and smooth but the deep layer is indented by many secondary connective tissue papillae.

(iv) Epithelium of the lateral wall contains some 200 taste buds and the wall facing the papilla also contains some 50 taste buds; however, numbers decrease with age.

(v) Serous glands (of von Ebner) open into the trench and are responsible for removing old taste stimuli.

D. *Foliate papillae* (folium (L) a leaf) are parallel mucosal folds on the dorsolateral margins of the tongue at the junction of the body and root.

(i) They are folds of the lamina propria covered by stratified squamous epithelium. Connective tissue cores form primary papillae and up to three secondary papillae.

(ii) In infants, foliate papillae are 4–8 well-defined, vertical folds but they are regressive or rudimentary in adult man.

(iii) Taste buds line the lateral aspects of folds.

(iv) Serous glands (of von Ebner) open into the base of trenches between folds.

5.2.4. *Taste buds* are barrel-shaped collections of chemoreceptor and supporting cells embedded in the surface epithelium. They are found in the lateral walls of circumvallate papillae and less frequently in the walls of foliate papillae, fungiform papillae, in the soft palate and laryngeal surface of the epiglottis.

A. *Taste buds* comprise groups of 20–30 fusiform cells 70 μm tall arranged like an onion. Microvilli of taste cells pierce the overlying epithelium at a taste pore (canal).

B. Cells identified in taste buds are:

   (i) *Supporting cells (Type 1 or dark cells)*. Tall columnar cells with dense cytoplasm containing secretory granules of glycosaminoglycans which are secreted into the taste chamber below the taste pore.

   (ii) Taste cells (Type 2 or clear cells). Spindle-shaped cells which extend from the basal lamina to the taste chamber. Here, the apical cytoplasm projects coarse microvilli (taste hairs). The base of these 4–20 cells is invaginated by unmyelinated nerve endings.

   (iii) *Taste cells (Type 3 or clear cells)* have densities near their base contacted by unmyelinated nerves.

   (iv) *Basal cells* (Type 4 cells) are undifferentiated progenitors of other cells in the taste bud.

   (v) *Peripheral cells* (Type 5 cells) at the periphery enclose nerve endings.

C. Cells of taste buds have a life span of about 10 days.

5.2.5. The *lingual tonsil* comprises lymphoid follicles grouped at the root of the tongue. They belong to the lymphatic ring of the pharynx.

A. *Lingual follicles* occupy the region between the sulcus terminalis and the epiglottis and comprise short crypts surrounded by lymphoid tissue and nodules.

B. *Crypts* are lined with stratified squamous non-keratinized epithelium.

C. Mucous *lingual glands* open into the base of crypts.

D. *Lenticular papillae* interspersed between lingual follicles do not possess crypts.

5.2.6. Bundles of skeletal muscle interlace at right angles in the core of the tongue. Intrinsic and extrinsic muscle groups run in vertical, longitudinal and transverse planes.

5.2.7. *Anterior lingual glands* are mixed serous and mucous glands opening onto the ventral anterior surface of the tongue.

6. Development of the Tongue

6.1. The tongue begins to form during the 4th week in the floor of the pharynx between the first, second and third pharyngeal arches.

6.2. Paired *lateral lingual swellings* and a median *tuberculum impar* (developing from the mandibular arches) are covered with ectoderm and contribute to the formation of the *body* of the tongue.

6.3. Caudally, another median swelling, the *copula* covered by entoderm, receives mesodermal contributions from the second, third and fourth pharyngeal arches and gives rise to the root of the tongue.

6.4. The line of junction between the body and root of the tongue is marked by a V-shaped depression, the *sulcus terminalis*.

6.5. Just behind the apex of the sulcus terminalis is a depression, the *foramen caecum* which marks the point of origin of the thyroglossal duct and thyroid gland.

6.6. *Intrinsic muscles* of the tongue originate from occipital somites rather than from local pharyngeal arches and are supplied by the hypoglossal nerve.

6.7. The *sensory innervation of the anterior two thirds of the tongue* is by way of the lingual branch of the trigeminal nerve (nerve of the first arch) while taste fibers are carried in a pretrematic nerve, the chorda tympani branch of the facial nerve (nerve of the second arch).

6.8. The *sensory innervation of the posterior third of the tongue* is by way of the glossopharyngeal nerve (nerve of the third arch) and the vagus nerve (nerve of the fourth arch). The area innervated by the glossopharyngeal nerve includes the vallate papillae and encroaches onto the territory of the chorda tympani.

6.9. The lateral lingual swellings enlarge while tuberculum impar lags, finally contributing little to the body of the tongue.

6.10. The root of the tongue is produced by the copula and adjacent parts of branchial arches. A small contribution is made by the epiglottic eminence to the back of the copula (the two together are known as the *hypobranchial eminence*).

ORAL CAVITY

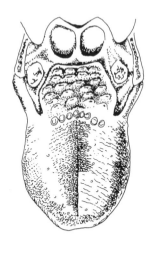

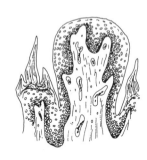

Filiform and fungiform papillae

Dorsal surface of the tongue

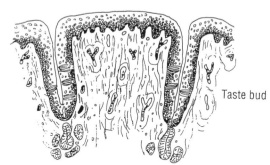

Taste bud

Gustatory (Ebner's) glands

Circumvallate papilla

7. The Hard Palate

7.1. The *hard palate* is the roof of the oral cavity (and floor of the nasal cavity) formed in its core by the palatine processes of the maxillae anteriorly and the horizontal plates of the palatine bones posteriorly.

7.2. It is covered on its *oral surface* by stratified squamous non-keratinizing epithelium (with thin keratinized patches) and a dense connective tissue lamina propria attached to the periosteum then called a mucoperiosteum.

7.3. The mucoperiosteum contains blood vessels and nerves and posteriorly mucous *palatine glands*. In the midline, it shows a sagittal ridge, the *raphe* (raphe (Gk) a seam) and several transverse palatine folds or *rugae* (ruga (L) a wrinkle).

7.4. Its *nasal surface* is covered by mucous membrane of the maxillary sinus and the floor of the nasal cavity.

7.5. The hard palate helps to grip food during mastication.

8. The Soft Palate (Velum Palatinum from Velum (L) a Curtain)

8.1. The *soft palate* is a fibromuscular fold suspended from the posterior border of the hard palate.

8.2. *Epithelium* covering the soft palate is mostly *stratified squamous non-keratinizing* on the oral side but this is replaced by *pseudostratified columnar ciliated epithelium* deep on its nasal side.

8.3. *Lamina propria* is a loose connective tissue containing mixed palatine or pharyngeal glands.

8.4. An *elastic layer* is situated deep to the epithelium on the oral side.

8.5. *Submucosa* exists only on the oral side where it contains mucous *palatine glands*.

8.6. A core of skeletal muscle consists of contributions from palatoglossus, palatopharyngeus, musculus uvulae, levator veli palatini and tensor veli palatini muscles. These all insert into an anterior *palatine aponeurosis* attached to the posterior border of the bony hard palate.

8.7. The soft palate contributes to closure of the nasopharynx in speech, swallowing and in phonation.

9. Salivary Glands

9.1. General

9.1.1. The major salivary glands are three large paired compound exocrine glands, the *parotid*, *submandibular* and *sublingual glands* located outside the oral cavity and provided with long ducts which open into the oral cavity.

9.1.2. *Saliva* is a moderately viscous, colorless fluid comprising the mixed secretions of all of the major salivary glands, the minor salivary glands of the palate and mucosa. In addition, it contains desquamated epithelial cells ("salivary corpuscles"), bacteria and leucocytes.

   A. Saliva is 99.5% water and 0.5% solids and has a pH of from 5.6–8.0 with an average value of 6.7.

   B. *Organic constituents* include proteoglycans, immunoglobulins, ptyalin (an enzyme active in the initial breakdown of carbohydrates) and kallikrein (a vasoconstrictive peptide produced by striated ducts of the major salivary glands).

   C. *Inorganic constituents* include sodium, calcium, potassium and small amounts of fluoride as well as bicarbonate and phosphate.

9.1.3. Saliva has a number of important functions:

   A. It *moistens and lubricates* food which facilitates swallowing.

   B. Saliva contributes to *digestion*. Ptyalin in saliva commences the digestion of starch.

   C. It has a *cleansing* action. The large volume of saliva (1.5 ltrs per day) cleans debris from the mouth and removes bacteria.

   D. Saliva *lubricates and protects soft tissues* from mechanical damage, excessive thermal change, chemicals and from dessication.

   E. *Teeth are protected* by physical washing and by saturation of elements in saliva required for mineralization.

   F. Saliva *protects against dissolution of tooth substance* by acid through its buffering action

   G. *Immunoglobulins and lysozyme* in saliva interfere with bacterial growth.

   H. Lubrication by saliva facilitates rapid movement of tongue and lips in *speech*.

   I. The volume produced depends on general level of body hydration so that saliva plays a *role in total body fluid balance*.

J. Certain heavy metals and drugs are *excreted* through the saliva.

9.2. Parotid Glands (para (Gk) near or beside and ous (Gk) an ear).

9.2.1. General:

    A. *Parotid glands*, the largest of the salivary glands, are situated below the zygomatic arch in front of the ear.

    B. Perforating septa from a fibrous capsule divide the gland into *lobes* and *lobules*. A finer connective tissue stroma often containing fat cells supports alveoli and smaller ducts.

9.2.2. Detailed Structure:

    A. *Alveoli* are elongated and branched. Cuboidal secretory cells contain an abundant basal and perinuclear RER and supranuclear Golgi complex, as well as membrane bound secretory granules.

    B. *Myoepitheliocytes* are located between alveolar cells and the basal lamina.

    C. *Intercalated ducts* are slender tubules attached to alveoli. They are lined with flat, low cuboidal cells and drain into:

    D. *Striated* (*secretory*) *ducts*, found only in salivary glands. These are intralobular channels lined with columnar epithelium. Duct cells contain apical secretory granules (of *kallikrein*). Rod shaped mitochondria are arranged vertically between basal infoldings form the basal striations of light microscopy. These cells can pump sodium out of the initial secretion and add lysozyme, kallikrein and potassium.

    E. *Excretory* (*interlobular*) *ducts* are lined with simple columnar epithelium becoming pseudostratified toward the outlet.

9.3. Submandibular Glands

9.3.1. General:

    A. These glands are paired, seromucous tubuloalveolar glands lying partly under the mandible and partly between the mandible and hyoid bone. They open through a long *submandibular duct* on the sublingual papilla at the side of the frenulum of the tongue.

    B. A connective tissue capsule gives septa that divide the glands into lobules.

9.3.2. Detailed Structure:

    A. Secretory end pieces are branched tubules which are either purely serous alveoli or mucous alveoli capped by serous cells (*"serous demilunes"*). Serous cells discharge their secretion into the lumen of tubules through narrow intercellular channels between mucus cells.

    B. *Myoepitheliocytes* are located between secretory epithelial cells and the basal lamina of alveoli.

    C. Short *intercalated ducts* continuous with alveoli are short.

    D. *Striated ducts* are longer than those of the parotid gland and are conspicuous in sections.

    E. The *excretory duct* (*of Wharton*) is lined with simple columnar epithelium initially but this becomes pseudostratified in its terminal portion.

9.4.   Sublingual Glands

  9.4.1. General:

    A. Sublingual glands are paired, mixed tubuloalveolar glands, actually a composite of one major and several minor glands.

    B. Each gland has an individual duct (there are some 20–30 ducts) which open into the floor of the mouth at separate papillae on the sublingual fold.

    C. An indistinct connective tissue capsule gives septa which divide the gland into lobules.

  9.4.2. Detailed Structure:

    A. The parenchyma comprises mucous tubules with and without serous demilunes. In man, mucous cells are much more numerous than serous cells.

    B. *Myoepitheliocytes* are present as in the other salivary glands.

    C. *Intercalated ducts* are mostly lacking and replaced by mucous tubules which are continuous with alveoli.

    D. *Striated ducts* are short and inconspicuous.

    E. *Excretory ducts* are formed at the junction of several interlobular ducts.

10. Control of Salivary Gland Function

10.1. Secretory autonomic nerve fibers (adrenergic and cholinergic) form plexuses beneath the epithelium. Nerve endings form close appositions with alveolar and duct cells.

10.2. Parasympathetic stimulation produces copious watery secretion through cholinergic stimulation of vasodilation, secretion and myoepithelial contraction.

10.3. Sympathetic stimulation causes secretion of smaller amounts of a more viscid saliva. While some alveolar cells have a dual sympathetic-parasympathetic innervation, the major effector of sympathetic nerves is smooth muscle of blood vessels.

10.4. Salivary gland function is also under local hormonal control. Vasodilation initiated by the nervous system is maintained by plasma kinins (*kallikrein*) released by secretory duct cells following sympathetic stimulation.

11. Development of the Oral Cavity

11.1. The *prochordal plate* is a thickening of entoderm in contact with ectoderm of the floor of the amnion at the cranial end of the embryo. With cranio-caudal folding of the embryo from approximately days 20–24, the prochordal plate swings beneath the forebrain in a depression, the *stomodeum*.

11.2. The prochordal plate (now known as the *buccopharyngeal or oropharyngeal membrane*) is surrounded by:
   A. Cranially, a proliferation of mesenchyme on the ventral surface of the developing brain, the *frontonasal process (frontal prominence)*.
   B. Caudally, the *mandibular processes* from the first pharyngeal arches.
   C. Laterally, the paired *maxillary processes* which have grown from the cranial edge of the mandibular process also form the lower border of the developing orbit.

11.3. The oropharyngeal membrane breaks down by the 4th week and the stomodeum then communicates with the foregut.

11.4. *Nasal placodes* (localized thickenings of surface ectoderm on each side of the lower part of the frontonasal prominences) form by the end of the 4th week.

11.5. *Medial and lateral nasal prominences (processes)* form as horseshoe-shaped swellings surrounding the nasal placodes. They result from mesenchymal proliferation at the margins of nasal placodes. The depressions in the placodes become the nasal pits.

11.6. The *maxillary prominences* grow medially and compress the medial nasal prominence.

11.7. The *medial nasal prominences* merge with each other and with the maxillary prominences to complete formation of the upper lip. The upper lip is thus formed by contributions from two maxillary prominences and two medial nasal prominences.

11.8. Merging medial nasal prominences form the *intermaxillary segment* of the upper jaw. This segment gives rise to:

  A. Middle portion of the upper lip (the philtrum).

  B. Middle part of the upper jaw and associated alveolus carrying four incisor teeth.

  C. The primary palate (premaxilla).

  D. Median portion of the nose.

11.9. The *labiogingival lamina,* a linear thickening of ectoderm medial to the site of formation of the lips and cheeks appears in each jaw. It grows into the underlying mesoderm and its central cells degenerate, forming a sulcus (the vestibule) which separates the lips and cheeks from the alveolar processes. A small part of the lamina persists in the midline as the *frenulum.*

11.10. *Maxillary prominences* give rise to:

  A. Lateral portions of the upper lip.

  B. Most of the upper jaw.

  C. The secondary palate.

11.11. *Lateral nasal prominences* remain separated from maxillary prominences by nasolacrimal grooves.

  A. Ectoderm in the floor of the grooves thickens into solid epithelial cords.

  B. The epithelial cords sink into underlying mesoderm and separate from surface ectoderm.

  C. Maxillary prominences and lateral nasal prominences fuse after detachment of epithelial cords.

  D. Cords become canalized, forming the nasolacrimal ducts.

11.12. *Palatine shelves* (*lateral palatine processes*) appear as horizontal mesoderm-filled projections from the oral side of each maxillary prominence.

    A. The shelves at first grow down on each side of the tongue.

    B. As the jaws grow, the tongue moves down and palatine shelves swing horizontally toward each other and fuse, forming the *secondary palate*.

    C. Palatine shelves also fuse with the primary palate and nasal septum, the process proceeding from anterior to posterior. The process of fusion occurs over the period of the 7th to 10th weeks.

    D. Membranous ossification occurs in the primary palate and anterior secondary palate which forms the hard palate. Mesodermal penetration of the posterior portion results in muscle formation in the soft palate.

    E. When the nasal pits first form, they deepen towards the forebrain and towards the oral cavity, remaining separated from the latter briefly by an *oronasal membrane*.

    F. The oronasal membrane ruptures and the primitive nasal cavity opens through *primitive choanae* behind the primary palate.

    G. Fusion of the secondary palate separates the oral and nasal cavities again and the *definitive choanae* are established where the nasal cavity opens into the nasopharynx.

12. Development of Salivary Glands

12.1. Salivary glands form from buds from the epithelial lining of the oral cavity.

12.2. The epithelial buds grow into the underlying mesoderm as a bush-like system of solid ducts

12.3. Secretory alveoli specialize at the tips of the branching ducts and continue to differentiate after birth.

12.4. The parotid glands are first to appear at 6 weeks, followed by the submandibular glands at 7 weeks and the sublingual glands at 8 weeks.

12.5. The duct system canalizes by 6 months.

ORAL CAVITY

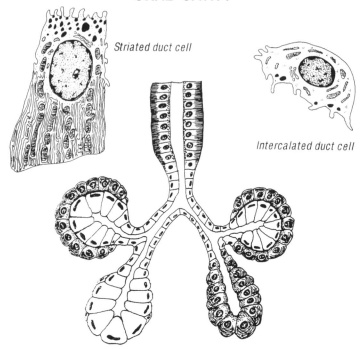

Striated duct cell

Intercalated duct cell

Organization of acini and ducts in salivary glands.

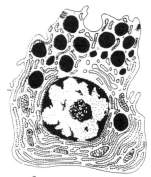

Serous cell

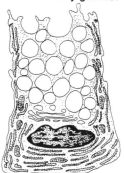

Mucous cell

Chapter 13

DIGESTIVE SYSTEM
2. TEETH

OBJECTIVES

After reading this chapter, you should be able to:
1. Identify the anatomical features of teeth and their supporting tissues.
2. Give an account of the composition of the primary and secondary dentition and differences between the two.
3. Describe the structure of dentine, its relationship to odontoblasts and its innervation.
4. Describe the structure and formation of enamel.
5. Describe the structure and function of cementum.
6. Describe the structure and functions of the periodontal ligament.
7. Describe the structure and functions of dental pulp.
8. Give an account of the development of teeth.
9. Give an account of the tissues involved in eruption and resorption of teeth.

CHAPTER OUTLINE

General. Dental nomenclature. Primary and secondary dentitions.

Detailed structure of teeth.

Enamel. Enamel rods, interrod enamel.

Dentine. Predentine, Odontoblasts, Innervation of dentine.

Cementum.

Pulp.

Periodontal ligament.

Alveolar bone.

Gingival (epithelial) attachment.

Development of teeth.

Dental lamina.

Enamel(dental) organ. Bud stage, Cap stage, Bell stage. Tome's processes, organic matrix, apposition, maturation, mineralization. Hertwig's epithelial root sheath.

Tooth eruption.

Exfoliation.

KEY WORDS, PHRASES, CONCEPTS:

Incisors
Canines
Premolars
Molars
Deciduous teeth
Permanent teeth
Apical foramen
Pulp canal (pulp chamber)
Anatomical crown
Root
Gingival (epithelial) attachment
Alveolar bone
Periodontal ligament
Dentinoenamel junction
Dentin
Predentin
Odontoblasts

Gingiva
Epithelial tooth buds
Dental lamina
Bud stage
Cap stage
Bell stage
Outer dental epithelium
Inner dental epithelium
Stellate reticulum
Ameloblasts
Tome's process
Enamel rods
Enamel matrix
Mineralisation of enamel
Maturation of enamel
Dentin formation
Dentinal matrix

Odontoblast processes
Cementum
Cementoblasts
Active eruption

Root formation
Hertwig's root sheath
Epithelial rests
Passive eruption

1. General

1.1. The adult human dentition comprises 32 permanent teeth embedded in an arch-shaped alveolar process. There are eight teeth in each half arch or dental quadrant.

1.2. Teeth are shaped and specialized to carry out some aspect of mastication or chewing. *Central and lateral incisors* are chisel-shaped for cutting and shearing. *Canines* are stout and pointed for grasping and tearing. *Premolars (or bicuspids)* and *molars* have a flattened occlusal surface for grinding.

1.3. There are 20 *deciduous or milk teeth* which begin to appear at 6 months and begin to be shed by 6–8 years. They are replaced over a 10–12 year period ending at 18 years. There are no deciduous forerunners of the permanent molars. The deciduous molars are replaced by premolars.

1.4. Parts of a tooth:

1.4.1. The *anatomical crown* is the part of the tooth covered by enamel. The *clinical crown* is the part of the tooth actually projecting into the oral cavity and may be more or less than the anatomical crown.

1.4.2. The *root* is the part covered by cementum and through its attachment to the periodontal ligament, responsible for anchoring the tooth in alveolar bone. There may be one or several roots of a tooth.

1.4.3. The *neck* or *cervix* is the constriction at the cementoenamel junction and is normally not seen as it is covered by gingiva.

1.4.4. The *pulp cavity* comprises a *pulp chamber* and one or more *root canals* which communicate with the periapical tissues through one or more *apical foraminae*. Blood vessels, nerves and lymphatics that supply the pulp enter and leave the pulp through apical foramina(e).

1.5. Dental nomenclature : Surfaces of teeth are identified by the structures they face.

    1.5.1. *Labial or buccal surface* faces the lips or cheeks.

    1.5.2. *Mesial surface* is closest to the midline.

    1.5.3. *Distal surface* is furthest from the midline.

    1.5.4. *Masticatory (occlusal) surface* comes into contact with a similar surface of an opposing tooth in the other jaw. This surface is a sharp edge in incisor teeth known as the incisal edge.

2. Enamel

2.1. *Enamel* is the most highly calcified substance in the body. It is very brittle, consisting of 96% inorganic material (mostly calcium hydroxyapatite) and a small amount of organic substance and water. The organic element differs in composition from keratin in that it has a very high content of proline, different ratios of histidine, lysine and arginine and minimal amounts of cystine.

2.2. Enamel is translucent and its color depends on its thickness and the color of underlying dentine.

2.3. It is permeable to some molecules and its mineral composition changes with age.

2.4. The structural unit of enamel is the *enamel rod* or prism which extends through the full thickness of enamel. To compensate for the difference in surface area, rods increase in diameter from 3 μm near the dentino enamel junction to 6 μm at the surface.

2.5. Rods are cylindrical, (fish-scale or keyhole cross section) and generally separated by an *interrod region* of similar nature but different crystal orientation from that of the core of the rod.

2.6. Each rod is surrounded by an organic, less calcified, 0.1 μm wide *rod sheath*. In cross section, the rod is U-shaped with the convexity directed towards the cusp while its open end is continuous with the interrod region.

2.7. Rods are perpendicular to the enamel surface but bend from side to side in a horizontal plane. When sectioned longitudinally, the side to side movement of rods gives rise to alternating light and dark bands seen in sections with a period of 1000 μm known as *Hunter-Schreger bands*.

2.8. *Gnarled enamel* occurs where rods are misaligned and irregularly intertwined.

2.9. *Cross striations* are thin transverse lines across enamel rods spaced every 4 μm. They contain more organic material and are less mineralized than the bulk of the rod. They represent the daily rhythm of enamel matrix formation by an enamel forming cell (*ameloblast*).

2.10. *Striae of Retzius* (*brown striae*) are accentuated imbrication lines with a period of 16–100 μm representing some systemic influence on enamel matrix formation. Striae may be hypo or hypermineralized.

    A. The *neonatal line* is an accentuated stria caused by an abrupt change in nutrition from prenatal to postnatal sources.

    B. At the surface of the tooth, striae form curved ridges parallel to the gingival margin called *perikymata*. These wear from the surface with time after eruption.

2.11. An organic layer covers the surface of newly erupted teeth. This is formed by remnants of the enamel organ (the *reduced enamel epithelium*) which covered developing enamel and a product of ameloblasts (the *primary enamel cuticle*). Together, these two layers are known as *Nasmyth's membrane*. The layer is worn off post eruptively except in protected areas.

2.12. *Lamellae* are leaf-like vertical sheets of organic or hypomineralized enamel matrix extending occlusally from the cementoenamel junction. They are thought to develop along lines of tension during enamel formation which then leads to faulty mineralization. They may also represent clefts in crowded areas of matrix formation. Lamellae become filled with cells of the enamel organ or secondarily with organic material from saliva.

2.13. *Tufts* are ribbon-like hypomineralized structures which extend from the dentino-enamel junction for about one third of the width of enamel. They correspond to widened rod sheaths associated with contractions of matrix during calcification.

2.14. The *dentino-enamel junction* comprises scalloped depressions of dentine which fit into projections of enamel and increase the bonding between the two.

3. Dentin

3.1. *Dentine* forms the bulk of the crown and roots of the tooth. It is harder than bone, light yellow in color and highly elastic. It consists of a mineralized matrix but unlike bone, contains only the processes of its formative cells (*odontoblasts*).

3.2. *Odontoblasts* form an irregular layer on the pulpal surface of dentine. They send a single, branched process in a tubule through about one quarter of the thickness of dentine toward the dentinoenamel junction. The perikaryon contains RER and secretion granules of procollagen and is connected to adjacent odontoblasts by junctional complexes. Odontoblasts synthesize and secrete collagen and ground substance of dentinal matrix.

3.3. *Dentinal tubules* follow a curved path through dentine and are more spaced in the peripheral layers. Odontoblast processes fill the entire tubule only in recently formed teeth. In older teeth, the outer tubules are filled with proteinaceous material which calcifies.

3.4. *Dentine* is about 70% by weight crystalline hydroxyapatite and amorphous calcium phosphate and 30% by weight water and collagen. It varies in composition and structure:

A. *Peritubular dentine* immediately surrounding dentinal tubules is highly mineralized.

B. *Intertubular dentine* constituting the remainder of dentine between tubules is less mineralized than peritubular dentine.

C. *Mantle dentine* is the outermost and first formed layer of dentine situated beneath enamel and cementum. It is rich in ground substance and poor in collagen.

D. *Interglobular dentine*, most frequently found beneath the dentino-enamel junction contains areas of deficient mineralization of matrix. The structure represents interstices between calcospherites which have failed to fuse completely.

E. *Primary dentine* is dentine which has formed prior to the completion of root formation.

F. *Secondary dentine* is added posteruptively to the entire pulpal surface of dentine and may be deposited at an irregular rate through life.

G. *Tertiary or reparative dentine* is formed beneath areas of erosion, caries or operative procedures as a defense mechanism to protect the pulp. The course of tubules in this dentine is twisted or tubules may be sparse or absent.

H. *Transparent or sclerotic dentine* appears when odontoblastic processes degenerate and tubules (*dead tracts*) are obliterated by calcium salts. This gives a homogeneous, transparent appearance in ground (undemineralized) sections.

I. *Predentine* is the unmineralized matrix first formed by odontoblasts which is subsequently mineralized by linear and globular calcification. A layer of predentine always lines the pulpal surface of dentin, separating odontoblasts from the mineralized matrix.

J. *Tomes granular layer* is a layer adjacent to cementum. It represents the cut ends of branched, looping and bending dentinal tubules in the first formed root dentine.

3.5. *Incremental lines* (*of von Ebner*) are fine hypomineralized lines perpendicular to dentinal tubules spaced 4–8 μm apart, representing daily deposition of dentinal matrix by odontoblasts. *Contour lines* (*of Owen*) are accentuated incremental lines of which the *neonatal line* found in deciduous teeth and the first permanent molar teeth is most marked.

3.6. *Innervation of dentine* is poorly understood. Fine unmyelinated nerve fibers approach the cell body of odontoblasts and form a plexus (of Raschkow) on their pulpal side. Fine branches loop into predentin and others pass into dentinal tubules for about one third of the thickness of the dentine. It is not clear whether stimulation of nerves results from movement of fluid through dentine, whether nerves are stimulated directly or whether the odontoblast processes themselves conduct impulses to nerve fibers ending on odontoblast cell bodies.

4. Cementum

4.1. *Cementum* is the hard tissue covering the anatomical root of teeth. It extends from the cementoenamel junction to the apex and attaches the periodontal ligament.

4.2. Cementum is yellowish in color, permeable and not as hard as dentine. The inorganic phase (45–50% by weight) is mostly calcium hydroxyapatite and the organic phase is collagen and proteoglycan ground substance as well as water.

4.3. *Cementoblasts* are stellate cells of mesenchymal origin which form cementum. In mature cementum, they form a layer on the surface of newly deposited cementum matrix (cementoid). When they become trapped in the matrix, they occupy lacunae and canaliculi and become known as *cementocytes*. Although resembling osteocytes, the processes of cementocytes are less numerous and directed primarily toward the source of nutrition, the periodontal ligament.

4.4. *Cementoid* is recently formed, unmineralized cementum matrix (intrinsic matrix) like osteoid and predentin. Periodontal ligament fibers (extrinsic collagen fibers) pass between cementoblasts into cementoid and cementum (cemental fibers or Sharpey's fibers) but attachment of the tooth is confined to the superficial layers.

4.5. Continuous appositional growth of cementum occurs throughout life so that the width of the periodontal ligament remains constant. This process is essential for continuous eruptive movements of teeth and to compensate for occlusal wear.

4.6. Cementum occurs in two forms:

A. *Cellular cementum*, like bone, comprises a mineralized matrix, a system of lamellae and cementocytes in lacunae.

B. *Acellular cementum* comprises only matrix without enclosed cells. It is located adjacent to root dentine from the cementoenamel junction to the apex and at the bifurcation of multirooted teeth. It is thinnest at the cementoenamel junction (20–50 μm) and thickest toward the apex (150–200 μm) surrounding the apical foramen and it may extend to the inner dentine wall.

4.7. The *cementoenamel junction* may be a sharp line (in 30%) or cementum may overlap enamel (in 60%) or it may not reach the cervical edge of enamel (in 10%).

4.8. The *cementodentinal junction* is smooth in permanent teeth but scalloped in deciduous teeth.

4.9. The functions of cementum are to:

A. Anchor the tooth to the alveolus.

B. Compensate by growth for loss of tooth substance resulting from occlusal wear.

C. Contribute by growth to continuous mesio-occlusal eruption.

5. Pulp

5.1. *Pulp* is a gelatinous connective tissue filling the pulp chamber and pulp horns (*coronal pulp*) and root canals (*radicular pulp*). Pulp tissue is continuous with the periapical tissues through the apical foramen.

5.2. In the young, the pulp chamber is large and its outline follows that of the outer surface of dentine. Because of continuous formation of dentine, the size of the pulp chamber and amount of pulp tissue decreases with age.

5.3. Root canals may be multiple or branched. The *root canal* has a wide open apex early. The opening narrows as cementum is laid down on the inner surface of the root dentine.

5.4. The *apical foramen* varies in shape, size and location — a regular, direct opening is rare. It may be on the lateral side of the root or there may be multiple distinct apical foraminae. Its location and shape may change from functional influences on teeth.

5.5. Cells of the pulp include:

A. *Fibroblasts* which decrease in relative numbers with age as the amount of fibers increases.

B. *Odontoblasts* form a layer of varying thickness along the inner or pulpal surface of predentin. Postnatally, fibroblasts are capable of differentiating into odontoblasts

C. *Defense cells* include macrophages, undifferentiated mesenchymal cells and wandering lymphocytes. The number of undifferentiated cells decreases with age.

5.6. The *cell free (subodontoblastic) zone (of Weil)* is a region of the pulp situated immediately beneath odontoblast cell bodies. It contains nerve fibers in a plexus, collagen fibers, capillaries and ground substance but no cells.

5.7. Fibers in the pulp are reticular and some are collagenous but elastic fibers are lacking. *Korff's fibers* are reticular fibers originating within the pulp that thicken into bundles and pass between odontoblasts and attach to predentin.

5.8. Intercellular substance of the pulp is a gelatinous *proteoglycan*.

5.9. *Blood vessels* are arteries, arterioles and fenestrated, pericytic capillaries which drain into venous vessels that begin beneath odontoblasts. Arteriovenous anastomoses also occur.

5.10. *Nerves* follow blood vessels into the pulp and myelinated sensory nerves branch joining the subodontoblastic plexus. They interpret all forms of stimulation as poorly localized pain. Unmyelinated autonomic nerves supply smooth muscle of blood vessels which controls their diameter.

5.11. *Regressive changes* occur in the pulp with age:

A. *Pulp stones* (*denticles*) are either *true denticles* which contain dentine and arise from remnants of Hertwig's root sheath or *false denticles* which arise from concentric layers of calcified tissue around a nidus usually of necrotic cells. Pulp stones may be free within pulp, attached to dentine or embedded in dentine. They increase in incidence with age.

B. *Diffuse calcifications* are irregular calcific deposits in the pulp usually following collagen bundles.

6. Periodontal Ligament

6.1. The *periodontal ligament* surrounding a tooth is a connective tissue suspensory ligament which attaches the tooth to its bony alveolar socket. It is continuous with the connective tissue of the gingiva.

6.2. Component white collagenous fibers follow a wavy course from alveolus to cementum and allow limited movement of the tooth.

6.3. Collagen bundles form distinctive groups:

A. The *gingival ligament* fibers run from cementum near the neck of the tooth, breaking up into a meshwork in the gingiva. This group is responsible for stippling of the gingiva and binds the gingiva firmly to the tooth so that it resists stripping by masticatory forces.

B. *Transeptal* (*interdental*) *fibers* run between adjacent teeth over the alveolar crest.

C. *Alveolodental fibers* run from the tooth to bone and are divided into:

D. *Alveolar crest group* runs from the cervical cementum to the crest of the alveolus.

E. *Horizontal group* runs from cementum of the root to alveolar bone at right angles to the long axis of the tooth.

F. *Oblique group* runs from cementum coronally to alveolar bone. This group forms the bulk of periodontal ligament fibers and is disposed like a sling to oppose forces of mastication.

G. *Apical group* is an irregular group radiating from the apex of the tooth.

H. *Interradicular fibers* pass from the bifurcation of multirooted teeth to the crest of the interradicular septum.

Forces of mastication are resisted by periodontal ligament fibers but primarily dissipated by compression and emptying of veins in the periodontal space. As a result, osteoclasts are not stimulated.

6.4. Cells in the periodontal ligament include:

A. *Fibroblasts* which form and maintain fibers of the ligament. They may differentiate into cementoblasts or osteoblasts.

B. *Osteoblasts* secure fibers of the ligament to alveolar bone.

C. *Cementoblasts* are active in the formation and maintenance of cementum.

D. *Osteoclasts* are involved in remodelling of the alveolus. They are present in large numbers on the resorbing roots of deciduous teeth.

6.5. Loose connective tissue is located between collagen fiber bundles in the periodontal ligament. It contains blood vessels, lymphatics and nerve fibers.

6.6. The *blood supply* of periodontal tissues is from three major sources:

A. Blood vessels to the pulp which also supply the periapical area.

B. Interalveolar arteries which enter the periodontal ligament through openings in the alveolar wall and provide the major blood supply.

C. Gingival arteries supply the alveolar crest area.

6.7. The major sensory nerve endings are free nerve endings, knob-like swellings and loops around ligament fiber bundles. They respond to painful stimuli and can inhibit the jaw closing reflex. Proprioceptors are direction sensitive to forces applied to teeth.

6.8. Epithelial structures (*epithelial rests of Malassez*) are groups of epithelial cells found close to cementum. They are remnants of Hertwig's epithelial root sheath which is part of the enamel organ involved in root formation (vide infra).

6.9.   *Cementicles* are calcifications formed around groups of degenerated cells. They are found in the periodontal ligament of older persons and may be free or joined to cementum.

6.10. Functions of the periodontal ligament include:

A. *Formative*.   Cementoblasts, osteoblasts and fibroblasts produce their characteristic fibers or matrices.

TEETH

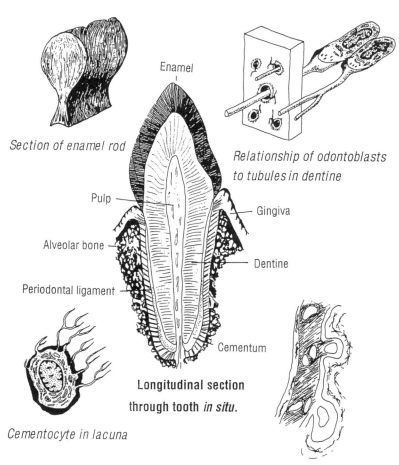

Section of enamel rod

Relationship of odontoblasts
to tubules in dentine

Enamel

Pulp

Gingiva

Alveolar bone

Dentine

Periodontal ligament

Cementum

**Longitudinal section
through tooth *in situ*.**

Cementocyte in lacuna

Longitudinal section through
periodontal ligament

B. *Supportive*. The ligament maintains a constant relation between teeth and hard and soft tissues.

C. *Protective*. By limiting the movement of teeth in mastication, the supporting tissues and blood supply to the tooth is protected.

D. *Sensory*. Nerve endings provide feedback in masticatory movements and pain receptors protect the tooth and supporting tissues.

E. *Nutritive*. Blood vessels of the ligament also supply neighboring supporting tissues.

7. Development of Teeth

7.1. At 6 weeks, the basal cells of the oral ectoderm thicken in a band along the future dental arches, forming the *dental lamina*.

7.2. At ten points along the dental lamina in each jaw, local round or oval swellings of the epithelium (*tooth buds*) arise. These will give rise to the deciduous teeth and the stage of development is known as the *bud stage*.

7.3. Unequal growth of the epithelial tooth bud (the *enamel organ*) leads to apparent invagination of the deep surface of the bud and formation of a cap-shaped structure. This is the cap stage of development.

7.4. Another thickening of epithelium (the vestibular lamina) develops at the same time in front of the dental lamina and parallel to it. Its central cells will degenerate, forming the vestibule which separates the lips and cheeks from the alveolar arches.

7.5. Histodifferentiation of tooth forming cells begins. The enamel organ gives rise to epithelial layers related to enamel formation and indirectly to dentine formation.

7.5.1. The *outer enamel epithelium* is a convex outer single layer of cells continuous at the edge of the cap (at the cervical loop) with the inner enamel epithelium.

7.5.2. The *inner enamel epithelium* is the concave layer of cells lining the invaginated cup. It will form enamel of the tooth.

7.5.3. *Stellate reticulum* is the name given to cells in the core of the enamel organ. These cells produce hydrophilic acid proteoglycans and push away from one another but they remain in contact through long slender processes. Stellate reticulum provides mechanical support and protection as well as nutrition to enamel forming cells.

7.5.4. The *enamel knot* is a swollen mass of cells in the center of the inner enamel epithelium with a cellular condensation (*enamel cord*) linking the dental lamina and inner enamel epithelium. The knot contributes cells to the stellate reticulum.

7.5.5. The *succedanous lamina* is an additional epithelial downgrowth from the dental lamina that will give rise to the enamel organ of the permanent tooth which will replace the deciduous tooth.

7.6. The *dental papilla* derived from ectomesoderm, fills the concavity of the enamel organ and will be responsible for the formation of dentine.

7.7. The *dental sac* is a condensation of mesenchyme surrounding the enamel organ and dental papilla. It gives rise to the periodontal ligament, alveolus and cementum.

7.8. Mitotic activity in the enamel organ enlarges the cap and changes its shape to that of a bell. This is known as the *bell stage* of development.

7.8.1. The outer enamel epithelium is cuboidal and ridged by a capillary network.

7.8.2. The inner enamel epithelium becomes a row of enamel matrix secreting *ameloblasts*. This cell layer apposes the site of formation of dentine by cells of the dental papilla so the stage establishes the future dentinoenamel junction. Establishment of the shape of the tooth is known as morphodifferentiation.

7.8.3. *Stratum intermedium* is an additional layer of cells that appears at this time in close apposition with the ameloblasts. These cells are thought to nourish ameloblasts and provide calcium during mineralization.

7.8.4. Stellate reticulum increases in volume by further synthesis of acid proteoglycans.

7.8.5. Ameloblasts, prior to matrix secretion, become tall, columnar cells with organelles polarizing sequentially from the tip of cusps towards the cervical loop.

7.8.6. In response to ameloblasts, cells of the dental papilla become tall *odontoblasts* which form dentine.

7.8.7. The *dental lamina* connecting the enamel organ to the oral cavity begins to disintegrate. Note that in addition to initiating formation of the entire deciduous dentition, the dental lamina has two additional important functions:

A. *Initiation of the permanent successor teeth* from a lingual growth of the enamel organ of deciduous teeth (from 5 miu to 10 months postnatal).

B. *Initiation of formation of permanent molars* by distal extension of the dental lamina (4 miu to 5 years postnatal).

7.9. *Apposition* refers to the deposition of enamel and dentine matrix. It is characterized by:

A. Collapse of the stellate reticulum which brings the outer enamel epithelium in contact with the stratum intermedium.

B. The outer enamel epithelium being thrown into folds which are occupied by blood vessels.

C. Odontoblasts beginning to form *mantle dentine*.

D. Ameloblasts beginning to secrete enamel matrix. The thickness of enamel and or dentine in various regions of the tooth will be a function of the length of time that cells of that region have spent in hard tissue formation.

7.10. Dentine formation (*dentinogenesis*) is characterized by the production of collagen and ground substance by odontoblasts. They secrete and retreat toward the center of the papilla away from the dentinoenamel junction.

A. Odontoblasts begin with several (collateral) processes accommodated in tubules of the matrix. As they retreat from the enamel matrix, processes become longer and merge into a single process.

B. Odontoblasts retreat and deposit matrix at a daily rate of 4–8 μm per day.

C. Mineralization of dentine is accompanied by budding from odontoblasts of small vesicles (matrix vesicles) that carry a high concentration of calcium and act as nidi of crystallization.

D. The layer of dentinal matrix most recently formed by odontoblasts (*predentin*) remains unmineralized.

7.11. *Enamel formation* (*amelogenesis*) is characterized by formation of aprismatic enamel matrix and the retreat of ameloblasts in a direction away from dentine.

A. Ameloblasts develop short blunt cytoplasmic processes (*Tome's process*) at their distal end. These segments of the cell contain no organelles but secretory and pinocytotic vesicles. Enamel matrix is secreted around the process.

B. The ameloblast retreats away from the dentinoenamel junction, leaving a rod space filled in by enamel matrix. The block of matrix formed is a rod segment formed by four ameloblasts at the rate of 4 μm daily.

7.12. *Mineralization* of enamel occurs in two stages:

A. The first enamel formed is partly mineralized (20–30%).

B. Subsequently matrix is fully mineralized (to 96%) in a process known as *maturation*.

7.13. Ameloblasts pass through several morphologic and functional stages:

A. *Organizing stage*. the cells elongate and organelles polarize.

B. *Formative stage*. cells secrete matrix.

C. *Maturative stage*. A process in which matrix is mineralized and protein and water withdrawn.

D. *Protective stage*. Ameloblasts, stratum intermedium and outer enamel epithelium form a cellular sheath, the *reduced enamel epithelium* which protects newly formed enamel, participates in formation of the dentogingival junction and assists in eruption of the tooth by desmolysis.

7.14. *Root formation* begins when the cells of the entire cervical loop undergo mitotic activity forming an epithelial cylinder, *Hertwig's epithelial root sheath*.

A. The stratum intermedium and stellate reticulum are absent from the enamel organ in the sheath which will not form enamel. The sheath will however induce the dental papilla to form odontoblasts.

B. Hertwig's sheath elongates and the inferior rim is folded medially to form an epithelial diaphragm which tapers the root.

C. The diaphragm shows differential areas of mitotic activity in multirooted teeth. As a result, the sheath shows local expansions which coalesce, dividing the original pulp tissue. This results in two or more separated openings in dentinal tissue in the apical region.

D. The root sheath shows partial degeneration resulting in *cell rests* (*of Malassez*).

TEETH

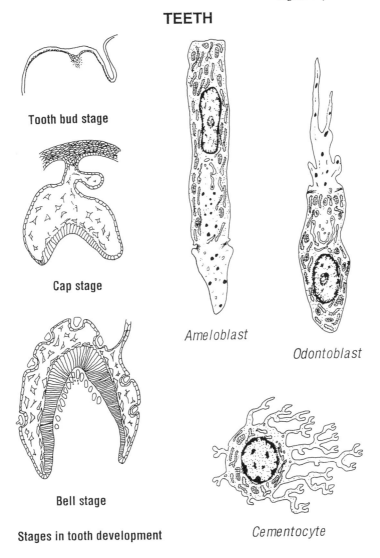

Tooth bud stage

Cap stage

Ameloblast

Odontoblast

Bell stage

Stages in tooth development

Cementocyte

E. Dental follicle cells (ectomesenchymal) penetrate gaps in the broken sheath, reach dentine and differentiate into cementoblasts.

8. Tooth Eruption

8.1. *Eruption* of teeth includes the processes involved in the tooth reaching the oral cavity, entering it and reaching and maintaining occlusion.

8.2. The *preeruptive stage* refers to motion of the entire tooth germ prior to root formation. This stage is accompanied by remodelling of developing alveolar bone.

In this stage:

A. The *gubernacular cord* is an epithelial remnant of the dental lamina of the permanent tooth germ which joins the permanent tooth germ to the oral epithelium through an opening in the alveolar bone (the gubernacular canal). The cord may assist in eruption by guiding the tooth.

B. The *reduced enamel epithelium* fuses with the oral epithelium, forming the primary attached epithelium.

8.3. The *eruptive stage* occurs during, but probably not as a consequence of, root formation. The tooth moves axially.

A. The first signs of the eruptive stage are when there is apical movement of Hertwig's sheath and deepening of the bony socket.

B. Horizontal trabeculae of bone form in the base of the bony crypt.

C. Oral epithelium fuses with the reduced enamel epithelium and replaces it. There is no bleeding as the connective tissue is not exposed. The epithelium is however permeable and there may be an inflammatory response.

8.4. The *posteruptive stage* refers to the period subsequent to the time when the tooth reaches occlusion in response to growth at the temporomandibular joint and interproximal wear of tooth substance.

A. Additional deposition of cementum occurs at the root apex as a result rather than a cause of posteruptive movements.

B. Interproximal wear is responsible for mesial drift of teeth (*active eruption*).

C. The dentogingival junction moves apically (*passive eruption*).

8.5. There are several theories concerning the source and nature of eruptive force:

A. The *cushion hammock ligament* is a condensation of collagen fibers separating the periodontium from the pulp. It was considered to protect the alveolar bone from forces generated within the pulp which then forced the tooth into occlusion. This ligament has been shown not to be attached to the socket wall.

B. Differential pressures between those of tissue above the tooth and those generated within the pulp. These may not be enough to account for the entire movement.

C. The periodontal ligament containing contractile *fibroblasts* may provide the force necessary for eruption.

8.6. There is no bleeding during eruption as the tooth erupts through an epithelial cord and the surrounding connective tissue is not exposed.

9. Exfoliation

9.1. The locus of resorption of the deciduous tooth depends on the location of the succeeding tooth (the lingual surface of incisors or interradicular region of molars).

9.2. *Odontoclasts* (cf. osteoclasts) appear in Howship's lacunae in cementum and dentine of the root.

9.3. Resorption and repair may appear to alternate but eventually resorption predominates.

9.4. It is thought that the chief cause of resorption is the inability of deciduous teeth to withstand the increased forces of mastication.

Chapter 14

DIGESTIVE SYSTEM
3. ESOPHAGUS AND STOMACH

OBJECTIVES

After reading this chapter, you should be able to:

1. Describe components of the four concentric layers comprising the general structure of the gastrointestinal tract viz. mucosa, submucosa, muscularis externa and serosa (or adventitia) as they appear in the esophagus and stomach.
2. Give an account of the development of the caudal part of the foregut.
3. Describe the development of the stomach, giving implications of differential growth of its walls to anatomical features of the adult stomach, its nerve supply and mesenteries.
4. Give the particular features of the histological structure of the wall of the esophagus.
5. Describe the histological features and functional correlates of cells of the gastric glands.
6. Describe the functions of the stomach.
7. Indicate how sections of the pyloric region differ from the fundic region of the stomach.

CHAPTER OUTLINE

Esophagus.

General.

Detailed structure. Mucosa. Submucosa. Tunica muscularis. Tunica adventitia.

Blood supply.

Nerve supply.

Development.

Stomach.

General. Anatomical regions, Histological regions.

Detailed structure. Tunica mucosa. Gastric glands. Tunica submucosa. Tunica muscularis. Tunica serosa.

Functions of the stomach.

Development of the stomach.

KEY WORDS, PHRASES, CONCEPTS

Esophagus
Submucosal glands
Cardiac region of stomach
Body (Fundic region) of stomach
Pyloric region
Gastrin
Pepsinogen
Pepsin
Rennin (Chymosin)
Lipase
Rugae
Gastric pits (foveolae)
Mucous columnar cells
Gastric (zymogenic) glands
    Base
    Isthmus

Primitive yolk sac
Definitive yolk sac
Foregut
Midgut
Buccopharyngeal membrane
Pharyngeal pouches
Mucosa (mucous membrane)
Lamina propria
Muscularis mucosae
Submucosa
Submucosal plexus
Muscularis externa
Myenteric plexus
Serosa
Blood supply to digestive tube

Neck
Mucous neck cells
Parietal (oxyntic) cells
Chief (zymogenic) cells
Enteroendocrine cells (GEP cells)

Adventitia
Lymphatics of digestive tube
Gastric epithelial renewal
Pyloric region
Pyloric sphincter

THE ESOPHAGUS

1. General

1.1. The *esophagus* (Oiso (Gk), future of phero, I carry and phagein (Gk) to eat) is a muscular passageway 25 cm long extending from the pharynx to the stomach.

2. Detailed Structure

2.1. In color, the *mucosa* (tunica mucosa or mucous membrane) comprising an epithelial layer, lamina propria and muscularis mucosae is reddish above but pale below. Because of the tonus of circular muscular fibers in the wall, the lining is thrown into temporary longitudinal folds (*plicae or rugae*) which disappear with distension.

    2.1.1. The *epithelium* lining the esophagus is stratified, non-keratinized squamous which is very thick (300 μm). In the human, keratinization is rare unless there is unusual trauma. At the cardioesophageal junction, there is an abrupt change to simple columnar epithelium.

    2.1.2. The *lamina propria* is a loose connective tissue (less cellular than in the lower digestive tube) sending papillae into the epithelium. It contains occasional lymphoid nodules.

    2.1.3. The *muscularis mucosae* comprises a thick (2–400 μm) layer of smooth muscle which is sparse at the beginning, longitudinal in the middle and plexiform below. This layer replaces an elastic layer of the pharynx.

2.2. The submucosa (tunica submucosa) is a thick (3–700 μm) layer containing coarse elastic fibers, accumulations of lymphoid tissue, large blood vessels, nerves and mucous glands. The layer allows for distension in swallowing.

2.2.1. *Submucosal (esophageal) glands* are scattered tubular down growths or tubular racemose (racemus (L) a bunch of grapes) mucous glands most common in the upper half of the esophagus.

2.2.2. The glands have long ducts, the smallest of which are lined with columnar epithelium while larger ducts are lined with stratified to squamous epithelium.

2.3. *The muscularis (tunica muscularis)* is 0.5–2 mm thick, comprising inner circular and outer longitudinal layers. At the upper end of the longitudinal fibers do not form a complete layer. They divide posteriorly to form two bands that pass around to the front and unite to form a tendinous attachment to the posterior surface of the cricoid cartilage.

2.3.1. In the upper third of the esophagus, the muscularis is entirely skeletal muscle. In the intermediate part, it is a mixture of skeletal and smooth muscle fibers while in the lower third, the muscularis is entirely smooth muscle.

2.3.2. At the upper extremity, there is a *superior esophageal (pharyngoesophageal) sphincter*.

2.3.3. At the lower extremity, the muscular layer remains unthickened but there is a physiologic *inferior esophageal sphincter* contributed to by:

A. The split right crus of the diaphragm.

B. The phrenicoesophageal ligament comprising connective tissue from the inferior surface of the diaphragm which blends with the submucosa of the terminal esophagus.

C. Obliquity of the gastroesophageal junction.

D. Contraction of the muscularis mucosae which produces mucosal folds and contributed to by the difference between intra-thoracic and intra-abdominal pressures.

The exact functional mechanism of the inferior sphincter remains uncertain.

2.3.4. In the third stage of swallowing, food is propelled toward the stomach by peristaltic movements in the esophageal wall.

2.4. *Tunica adventitia* (instead of a serosa), the outermost layer, contains loose connective tissue rich in elastin to allow for distension during swallowing and contains longitudinally oriented blood vessels, lymphatics and nerves.

3. Blood Supply of the Esophagus

3.1. The arterial supply of the esophagus is from several sources including:
  A. Inferior thyroid branch of the thyrocervical trunk.
  B. Descending aorta.
  C. Bronchial arteries.
  D. Left gastric branch of the coeliac trunk.
  E. Left inferior phrenic branch of the abdominal aorta.
      Branches run longitudinally in the submucosa and smaller branches rise to the serosa.
3.2. Venous drainage of the esophagus is to several destinations:
  A. The cervical esophagus drains to the inferior thyroid vein.
  B. The thoracic esophagus drains to azygos, hemiazygos and accessory hemiazygos veins.
  C. The abdominal esophagus drains to the left gastric vein.
  3.2.1. Venules in the mucosa anastomose in the submucosa.
  3.2.2. The left gastric vein is part of the portal system. With portal obstruction or hypertension (e.g., with liver cirrhosis) the site of anastomoses with systemic veins within the submucosa of the esophagus may become varicosed (esophageal varices) and be subjected to damage.
  3.2.3. Lymphatics run long distances in the esophageal walls and there is no constant localized pattern to drainage to phrenic, posterior mediastinal and tracheal lymph nodes.

4. Nerve Supply

4.1. The vagus (parasympathetic) and sympathetic nerves supply autonomic and sensory nerves to the esophagus.
4.2. Neurones of intramural parasympathetic ganglia are located:
  A. In nodes of a *submucosal plexus* (*of Meissner*) located deep in the submucosa and whose fibers supply the muscularis.
  B. Between two layers of the muscularis (the *myenteric plexus of Auerbach*) which innervates blood vessels and the muscularis.
      Nerve cells of these intramural plexuses contain acetyl choline as well as VIP, somatostatin, gastrin, CCK and SP.
4.3. Parasympathetic activity increases muscular activity, circulation and secretion.

4.4. Sympathetic vasoconstrictive activity is reinforced by catecholamine release from the suprarenal medulla.

5. Development

5.1. Folding of the embryo between the presomite and 22 somite stages leads to formation of the *intraembryonic coelom* divided by a median partition, the primitive mesentery. The mesentery is divided into a *dorsal* and *ventral mesentery* by the central gut.

5.2. In the region of the middle part of the esophagus, the mesentery (mesoesophagus) gives rise to the mediastinum.

5.3. The *dorsal mesentery* (*mesoesophagus*) is short and broad but longer like a typical mesentery only near its attachment to the stomach. This portion contributes to the formation of the diaphragm.

5.4. Up to 4 weeks, the esophagus is very short, but it elongates rapidly thereafter.

5.5. The epithelial lining is ciliated up to 10 weeks but this is replaced by stratified squamous epithelium by 5 months.

THE STOMACH

1. General

1.1. The *stomach* (stomachos (Gk) stomachus (L) gullet or esophagus from stoma (Gk) mouth and cheo (Gk) I pour. Greeks also used the word gaster, stomach) is a piriform-shaped dilated part of the alimentary canal located between the esophagus and duodenum predominantly in the upper left abdomen.

1.2. Five anatomical regions of the stomach include:

A. The *cardia* (kardia (Gk) a heart) which adjoins the esophagus and is separated from the fundus by the cardiac notch.

B. The *fundus* (fundus (L) bottom or base) or rounded upper end above the level of the esophageal opening.

C. The *body* or *corpus* comprises two thirds of the remainder of the stomach from the fundus to the pyloric antrum and separated from the pyloric antrum by the angular notch.

D. The *pyloric antrum* (pyle (Gk) a gate) is the slightly dilated part of the stomach below the body.

E. The *pyloric canal* is the cylindric portion between the antrum and the pyloric sphincter.

1.3. Three histologically distinct regions are:

A. The *cardiac region* which surrounds the cardiac orifice and contains cardiac glands in its mucosa.

B. The *body* or *fundic region* includes the anatomical body and fundus which both have the same histologic structure.

C. The *pyloric region* (pylorus) includes the pyloric antrum, canal and sphincter.

1.4. The empty (contracted) stomach shows folds or *rugae* in the mucous membrane which contain cores of submucosa. They are flattened out when the stomach is distended.

2. Detailed Structure

2.1. The *mucosa* comprises epithelium, lamina propria and muscularis mucosae (smooth muscle) and contains gastric pits and simple tubular glands, the gastric glands.

2.1.1. *Epithelium* is simple columnar (*mucous columnar or surface mucous cells*) covering the surface and extending into *gastric pits or foveolae* (foveola (L) diminutive for a pit). Cells contain mucigen droplets and continuously secrete a glycoprotein which stains with the PAS method.

2.1.2. *Gastric pits* (*foveolae*) open onto the surface lining of the stomach and descend into the lamina propria. They become continuous with the upper ends of gastric glands. Two or three glands deliver their secretion (*gastric juice*) into each pit.

2.1.3. *Gastric glands* are simple branched tubular glands located in the tunica mucosa. They differ in composition in different regions of the stomach where they are known as *cardiac glands, fundic glands* or *pyloric glands*.

A. Parts of *gastric* (*zymogenic*) *glands* are:

(i) A deepest part or *fundus* (*base or body*).

(ii) A middle part or *neck*.

(iii) An upper part or *isthmus*.
Gastric pits into which glands open are not part of gastric glands.
B. Cells of gastric glands include:

 (i) *Neck mucous cells* located in the middle and upper parts
  of gastric glands are pyramidal-shaped cells containing
  large glycosaminoglycan granules which stain with PAS.
  Their function is unknown but they are thought to be
  non-differentiated cells which replace surface mucous
  cells or they may be precursor cells of parietal and chief
  cells.

 (ii) *Parietal (Oxyntic) cells* are located in the middle and
  upper part of glands but are less common in pyloric
  glands. These cells are large pyramidal- or spheroidal-
  shaped cells bulging on their outer surface. They have
  an acidophilic cytoplasm which contains many mitochondria,
  a well-developed SER and distinctive intracellular (secretory)
  canaliculi lined with microvilli. At rest, canaliculi are
  relatively inconspicuous and reduced to tubulo-vesicles.
  The basal cell membrane contains receptors for histamine,
  gastrin and acetylcholine. These substances stimulate
  the secretion of HCl into the gastric lumen and bicarbonate
  into the interstitium of the wall. Parietal cells synthesize
  and secrete hydrochloric acid (0.1 N) and a glycoprotein
  (*intrinsic factor*) essential for normal erythropoesis.

 (iii) *Chief (peptic or zymogenic)* cells located mostly in the
  basal half of gastric glands are cuboidal basophilic cells
  which contain a rich basal RER and large supranuclear
  secretory granules (not preserved in routine preparations).
  Chief cells synthesize *pepsinogens* (a mixture of at least
  seven proteases) and precursors of *pepsin* which hydrolyses
  proteins to smaller molecules in an acid environment.

 (iv) *Enteroendocrine (gastroenteropancreatic or GEP cells)*
  resemble peptide synthesizing cells in endocrine glands
  and are characterized by a clear cytoplasm which contains
  unit membrane bound, dense cored secretory granules.
  Enteroendocrine cells belong to the APUD cell group.

Some produce true peptide hormones which are secreted into the blood stream (e.g., *gastrin*, *secretin* and *cholecystokinin*) and influence the activity of target organs. Others, such as those that produce *somatostatin*, release their product into the subepithelial connective tissue from long cytoplasmic processes and modify the action of cells in the vicinity (*paracrine secretion*). Some enteroendocrine cells produce both a peptide and a biogenic amine which interact with neural elements to modify the function of organs.

In the stomach, the following *enteroendocrine cells* have been identified by immunocytochemical means:

A. *EC cells* found throughout the mucosa produce serotonin.

B. *A cells*, occurring only in the upper third of the stomach, produce glucagon and may be involved with carbohydrate metabolism.

C. *D cells* occur in the middle part of the stomach, producing somatostatin.

D. *G cells* secrete gastrin in response to elevated pH and to autonomic stimulation.

On the basis of staining for light microscopy, enteroendocrine cells include:

A. *Enterochromaffin cells* (also known as *Argentaffin cells, EC cells, Kulchitsky's cells or pheochrome cells*), many of which stained with potassium dichromate.

B. *Argentaffin cells* (sometimes used interchangeably with enterochromaffin cells) precipitate silver from ammoniacal silver nitrate.

C. *Argyrophilic cells* precipitate silver only when a chemical reducing agent is present.

2.1.4. Epithelium is renewed from stem cells in the isthmus of gastric glands. These cells give rise to surface epithelial cells, mucous neck cells, parietal cells and enterochromaffin cells. Epithelial cells are replaced very rapidly (inside one hour) following injury. In addition, cells migrate from the base of glands to cover areas denuded of epithelium.

    2.1.5. In the *pyloric region*:
- A. Pits are deeper and glands shorter.
- B. Most cells in glands are mucus and pepsinogen secreting.
- C. Enteroendocrine cells present in pyloric glands include, EC cells, D cells and G cells.

2.2. The *submucosa* has no glands except in the pyloric part near the duodenum.

2.3. The *muscularis externa* has three smooth muscle layers instead of two as in the remainder of the gastro-intestinal tract. Layers are *innermost oblique, middle circular* and *outermost longitudinal*.

    2.3.1. The function of the muscularis is to churn stomach contents (chyme) and pass fluid digested food periodically into the duodenum through a thickening of the muscularis (*pyloric sphincter*) while retaining solid, undigested food.

    2.3.2. Patterns of activity in the muscularis include non-propulsive peristalsis, segmentation, pendular movements and propulsive peristalsis. Peristaltic movements spread from the upper part of the body ("pace-maker") towards the pylorus.

2.4. The *serosa* comprises loose connective tissue which carries blood vessels and is covered by mesothelium.

3. Functions of the Stomach

3.1. As an exocrine organ, the stomach produces, after each meal, a large volume of a mixed acidic secretion (*gastric juice*) which contains the protease, *pepsin* (secreted as pepsinogen and converted to pepsin in an acid environment).

    3.1.1. The stomach also produces rennin (chymosin), which curdles milk, and lipase, to a small extent, which splits fats.

    3.1.2. Gastric juice secretion is controlled by:
- (i) Conditional reflexes which initiate gastric secretion (the "Cephalic Phase"). Vagal nerve (cholinergic) action causes release of *gastrin* from G cells and *histamine* from enteroendocrine cells.
- (ii) Vagal nerve action, local cholinergic reflexes, histamine and gastrin release are triggered by products of digestion within

STOMACH

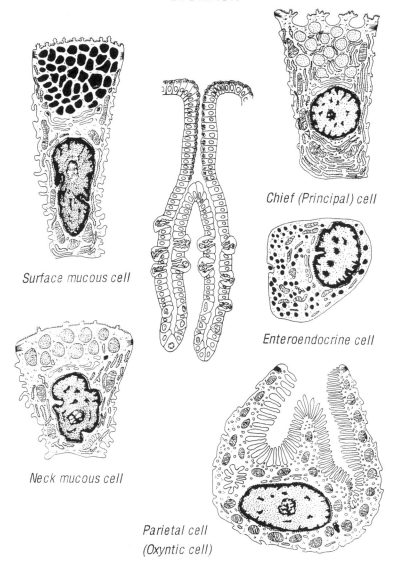

Surface mucous cell

Chief (Principal) cell

Enteroendocrine cell

Neck mucous cell

Parietal cell
(Oxyntic cell)

the stomach (the "gastric phase" of secretion) and this action may continue for some time.

(iii) Chyme release into the duodenum causes gastrin release from G cells in the duodenal wall which stimulates gastric

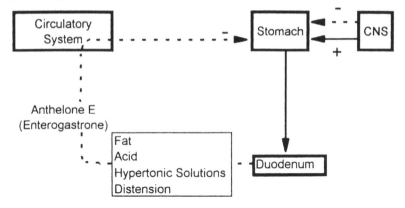

Control of gastric motility.

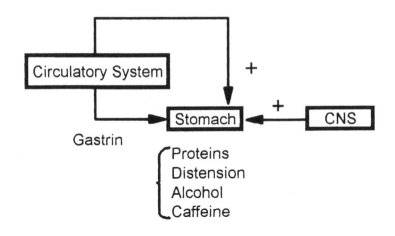

Control of acid secretion in the stomach.

secretion (the "intestinal phase" of secretion). This is followed by inhibition of secretion by release of gastric inhibitory peptide (GIP) release by K cells and *cholecystokinin-pancreozymin (CCK-PZ)* release by I cells in the duodenal wall.

3.2. The mucosa is protected from desiccation by acid contents by a thin layer of mucus produced by surface epithelial cells.

3.3. The stomach produces *"intrinsic factor"*, a glycoprotein which combines with vitamin B_{12} to form a complex. The complex passes to the ileum where it is necessary for the absorption of vitamin B_{12}.

3.4. As an endocrine organ, the stomach produces several hormones, including *gastrin* which influences gland function, muscle function, activity of pancreas and small intestine.

3.5. Stomach walls are distensible so that it acts as a *reservoir* whose outlet is guarded by a prominent muscular thickening, the pyloric sphincter. The smooth muscle of the wall relaxes and rugae in the wall flatten. There is also vagally mediated receptive relaxation.

3.6. Stomach walls, particularly in the pyloric part, contract rhythmically, mixing food. The contents are diluted with gastric juice produced in the body and the admixture is known as chyme.

3.7. Vigorous antral peristalsis releases chyme into the duodenal bulb. When this occurs, the antrum is nearly closed off from the body and there is longitudinal shortening of the pyloric canal.

3.8. Gastric emptying is controlled by an *enterogastric reflex* mediated by the Vagus nerve in which emptying is inhibited by filling of the duodenal bulb. Gastric emptying is also inhibited by secretin, GIP, and CCK release from S, K and I cells in the duodenal wall following the entry of fat or hydrochloric acid into the duodenum.

3.9. As an absorptive organ, the stomach absorbs some water, salts, alcohol and some drugs.

4. Development

4.1. The stomach is first discernible at 4 mm as a spindle-shaped enlargement of the gut tube. It is attached to the dorsal and ventral body walls by folds of mesentery, the *dorsal and ventral mesogastria*.

4.2. At 4–7 weeks the stomach changes shape and orientation:

A. It increases in length.

B. The dorsal border grows faster than the ventral border to produce the *greater curvature*.

C. The *fundus* bulges near the cranial end.

D. The stomach undergoes a 90° rotation until the greater curvature (dorsal border) lies to the left while the lesser curvature (ventral border) lies to the right.   As a result, the right vagus nerve is carried dorsally and the left vagus nerve, ventrally.

E. The cranial end of the stomach is displaced to the left by the liver while the caudal end is anchored by a ventral mesentery.

4.3.   Gastric pits are observed at 7 weeks and glands develop from them by 14 weeks.

Chapter 15

DIGESTIVE SYSTEM
4. INTESTINES

OBJECTIVES

After reading this chapter, you should be able to:

1. Differentiate between the histological features of duodenum, jejunum, ileum, colon and rectum based on the distinctive features in the layers of their walls.
2. Describe the structure and functions of cells found in the mucosa of the intestines.
3. Give an account of the structure and function of villi, adding notes on additional devices by which the surface area of the intestines is increased for absorption.
4. Describe the distribution and function of nerve plexuses in the wall of the intestine.
5. Give an account of the blood supply and lymphatic drainage of the gut wall.
6. Describe the development of the midgut with particular reference to its extent, physiological herniation and retraction and origin and fate of the mesenteries.

CHAPTER OUTLINE

Intestines

General structural plan of the gastrointestinal tract. Mucosa (mucous membrane), Submucosa, Muscularis, Adventitia or Serosa.

Development. Foregut, Midgut, Hindgut.

Small Intestines

General features of the small intestine.

Detailed structure and function.

Mucosa. Plicae, Villi, Intestinal crypts.

Epithelial lining of the small intestine. Absorptive (Villous) columnar cells. Goblet cells. Paneth cells. Enteroendocrine cells. Undifferentiated crypt base cells.

Changes in the small intestine along its length.

Immune defence mechanisms.

Absorption. Lipids, Proteins, Carbohydrates.

Development of the midgut. Extent of the midgut. Physiologic herniation. Rotation. Re-entry. Completion.

Large Intestines

General features.

Regional details.

Mucosa. Crypt base columnar cells. Columnar absorptive cells. Goblet cells. Enteroendocrine cells.

Nerve supply of the large intestine.

Development of the hindgut. Functions of the large intestine. Production of faeces. Motility of the large intestine.

KEY WORDS, PHRASES, CONCEPTS

Villi

Intestinal crypts (of Lieberkuhn)

Absorptive columnar cells

Faeces

Taeniae coli

Haustra

Goblet cells
Undifferentiated crypt base
  columnar cells
Enteroendocrine cells
Epithelial cell renewal
Plicae circulares
Microvilli
Gut Associated Lymphoid
  Tissue (GALT)
M cells
Chylomicrons

Anal columns
Anorectal junction
Myenteric plexus
Submucous plexus
Vitelline duct
  Primary intestinal loop
  Physiological herniation
    and retraction
  Dorsal mesentery
Peyer's patches

INTESTINES

1. General Structural Plan of the Gastrointestinal Tract

1.1. The gastrointestinal tube is constructed of four concentric layers. From the lumen outwards, these are:

1.2. Mucosa (Mucous membrane) which has three components:

A. Epithelium. The type of epithelium depends on functions of the particular part of the tract. Stratified squamous epithelium is protective in the esophagus and anus. Columnar epithelium is absorptive and secretory in the intestine.

Secretory cells along the length of the gastrointestinal tract may be located as:

(i) Individual secretory cells.

(ii) Secretory cells which invaginate the lamina propria (mucosal glands) or submucosa (e.g., in the esophagus and duodenum).

(iii) Glands which develop from lining cells but are located outside of the tract (e.g., salivary glands, liver and pancreas). They retain their contact through ducts which open into the lumen of the tract.

B. *Lamina Propria* comprises loose, vascularized connective tissue rich in immunocompetent cells (*Gut Associated Lymphoid Tissue or GALT*) and containing fenestrated capillaries and lymph capillaries. Lymphocytes, both isolated and in unencapsulated nodules, form a major source of IgA which is transported to the gut lumen.

C. *Muscularis Mucosae* comprises two layers of smooth muscle, a thin inner circular or helical layer and an outer longitudinal layer. This layer allows movement (folding) of mucosa independent of the remainder of the gut wall. Smooth muscle fibers from this layer extends into villi which can change their shape and the relationship of the villus to gut contents for absorption.

1.3. *Submucosa* comprises a layer of loose connective tissue which conveys larger blood vessels. The submucosa may contain mucus-secreting glands (in esophagus and duodenum) and accumulations of lymphoid tissue.

1.3.1. The deep *submucosal (Meissner's)* plexus, comprising autonomic (parasympathetic) ganglion cells and nerve fibers, post-ganglionic sympathetic nerves and interneurons, supplies smooth muscle cells of the gut wall and of blood vessels, as well as secretory cells of mucosal glands.

1.4. *Muscularis (Externa)* comprises substantial inner circular and outer longitudinal (helical) layers of smooth muscle. Tonus of the inner layer determines the overall shape of the lumen of the gut.

1.4.1. There are two main movements of the gut, a churning movement and peristaltic movements which propel gut contents. These movements are coordinated by autonomic impulses in a second nerve plexus, the *myenteric (Auerbach's) plexus* located between the circular and longitudinal muscle layers. The plexus contains parasympathetic post-ganglionic (to the vagus) nerve cells.

1.5. *Adventitia (or Serosa)* comprises a layer of loose alternately collagenous and elastic connective tissue which contains blood vessels and nerves. Where suspended in a peritoneal fold, the gut is covered by a squamous mesothelium and the layer is termed a *serosa*. Where the segment of the gut is attached to surrounding body wall, the layer blends with surrounding fascia and is termed an *adventitia*.

A. Arteries within the mesentery divide into ascending and descending branches which anastomose with branches above and below, thus forming primary arcades. Arteriae rectae pass to each side of the intestine. Radial branches reach and course longitudinally in a plexus in the submucosa. From these vessels, two sets of capillaries branch perpendicularly one to the mucosa and the other to the muscularis.

B. Veins arising in the mucosa anastomose in the submucosa and pass out of the gut alongside arteries.

C. Lymphatic vessels begin as blind tubes (*lacteals*) in the mucosa which extend into villi. Lymphatic capillary endothelial cells lack pores but contain many micropinocytotic vesicles. Large lymphatic branches in the submucosa have valves. Vessels in the mesentery have muscular walls which can propel the contents towards the venous system.

2. Development

2.1. At 8 days, the entodermal layer is a sheet of flat epithelial cells immediately under the ectodermal embryonic disc.

2.2. Entodermal cells extend along the wall of the primitive yolk sac by the 15th day, forming the inner lining of the primitive yolk sac.

2.3. Head and tail fold formation occurs between 21 and 30 days. The entodermal-lined yolk sac is thus sub-divided into:

A. An intraembryonic *primitive gut*.

B. An extraembryonic *yolk sac* and *allantois* (allas (Gk) a sausage and oeides (Gk) shape) which extends within the body stalk.

2.4. The primitive gut is a blind ended tube comprising:

A. A cephalic part, the *foregut*.

B. A middle part, the *midgut* opposite and remaining connected with the yolk sac by the *vitelline* (*omphalomesenteric*) *duct*.

C. A caudal part, the *hindgut*.

2.5. The cranial part of the foregut (or *pharyngeal gut*) extending from the buccopharyngeal membrane to the respiratory diverticulum is closely associated in its development with that of the pharyngeal pouches.

2.6. The caudal part of the foregut extends from the respiratory diverticulum to the duodenum (origin of the hepatic diverticulum) and gives rise to the esophagus, stomach, part of the duodenum and derivatives of the tract (liver, gall bladder and pancreas).

2.7. Up to 4 weeks, the esophagus is short but lengthens rapidly with development of the neck, the heart and lungs.

INTESTINES

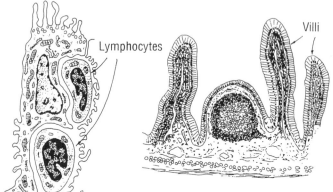

Lymphocytes

Villi

Section of ileum showing Peyer's patch (Aggregated lymphoid follicle).

M Cell
(Follical associated
epithelial (FAE) cell)

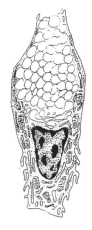

Goblet cell
(Mucous cell)

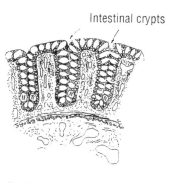

Intestinal crypts

Section of large intestine

2.8. The stomach is discernible at 4 mm as a spindle-shaped enlargement of the caudal foregut. It is attached to the dorsal and ventral body walls by folds of peritoneum — the *dorsal and ventral mesenteries*.

2.9. The *midgut* forms the duodenum beyond the hepatopancreatic ampulla, the jejunum, ileum, caecum, appendix and proximal two thirds of the large intestine.

2.10. The *hindgut* forms the distal third of the large intestine and upper part of the anal canal (as well as some urogenital organs).

2.11. The gut is supplied by a series of ventral branches of the dorsal aorta which originally supplied the yolk sac. Progressive fusion reduces these to three major vessels, the celiac trunk (to the caudal foregut), the superior mesenteric artery (to the midgut) and the inferior mesenteric artery (to the hindgut).

SMALL INTESTINE

1. General Features of the Small Intestine

1.1. The *small intestine* is about 2.8 meters long, presenting a large internal surface area for absorption.

1.2. It is divided anatomically and histologically into three distinguishable segments — the *duodenum* (from duodenarius (L) containing twelve, i.e., twelve finger breadths in length), jejunum (from jejunus (L) fasting, i.e., a segment that appeared empty at post mortem) and *ileum* (eilein (Gk) to twist).

1.3. It is suspended by a *mesentery*, two apposed sheets of peritoneum which carries blood vessels and nerves to and from the gut wall. Lymph vessels pass from the intestine and the mesentery contains interposed lymph vessels and nodes.

2. Detailed Structure and Function

2.1. The small intestine has a serous coat except for part of the duodenum and terminal ileum which are fixed to the posterior abdominal wall.

2.2. It has a *muscularis* comprising two complete inner circular and outer longitudinal layers of smooth muscle.

2.2.1. Products of digestion are moved through the intestine by propulsive *peristalsis*, a contraction of the circular muscle layer that progresses as a wave along the tube usually preceded by a wave of relaxation.

2.2.2. Food is mixed by:

    A. *Non-propulsive peristalsis.* Peristalsis propagated over only short distances;

    B. *Segmentation.* The simultaneous contraction of circular muscle at closely adjacent alternating points; and

    C. *Pendular movements.* Contractions of the longitudinal muscle over a distance causing the mucosa to slide over the intestinal contents.

2.3. A *submucosa* comprises areolar tissue occupied by compound tubular mucous glands (of Brunner) only in the duodenum.

2.4. There are two nerve plexuses with aggregations of ganglion cells throughout the length of the intestines. They are:

    A. The *myenteric (Auerbach's)* plexus situated between the two outer muscle layers. This plexus primarily influences intestinal motility.

    B. The *submucosal (Meissner's) plexus* between the circular muscle and submucosal layers. This plexus influences motility and secretion. Both plexuses comprise aggregations of autonomic ganglion cells, most of which receive synaptic input from fibers of the vagus nerve and post-ganglionic sympathetic fibers from the coeliac ganglia and which terminate chiefly on smooth muscle fibers and the smooth muscle of blood vessels walls.

2.5. The *mucosa* includes:

2.5.1. A *muscularis mucosae* comprising inner circular and outer longitudinal layers of smooth muscle.

2.5.2. *Plicae circulares* are permanent, transverse, semilunar folds involving the mucosa and submucosa in the wall of the small intestine. They are most prevalent in the distal duodenum but decrease in height and frequency distally in the ileum. Plicae increase the surface area of the mucosa for absorption by some three times.

2.5.3. *Villi* (villus (L) a hair) are small finger or leaf-like projections of the mucosa up to 1 mm long and 3–500 μm in diameter.

They are broadest and leaf-shaped in the duodenum, tongue-shaped in the jejunum and finger-shaped in the ileum.

A. The core of a villus contains:

(i) A basal lamina beneath the surface epithelium.

(ii) A central lymphatic capillary (Lacteal).

(iii) Blood vessels.

(iv) Smooth muscle strands connecting with the muscularis mucosae.

(v) Loose stroma comprising reticular and elastic fibers infiltrated with white blood cells.

B. Movements of villi are controlled by:

(i) *Vagal fibers* via the submucosal plexus affecting contraction of smooth muscle in the core of villi.

(ii) *Villikinin*, a factor released from intestinal mucosa in response to acid chyme entry into the duodenum.

C. Villi increase the surface area for absorption by some thirty times.

2.5.4. The surface area of the lining of the intestine is further increased some six hundred times by microvilli on the surface of absorptive epithelial cells (see below) so that the total area of the intestinal lining for absorption is increased to some 200 square meters.

2.5.5. Products of digestion are moved in relation to absorptive cells by contraction of smooth muscle in the villi, contractions of the muscularis mucosae and of the main muscle coats.

2.5.6. *Intestinal crypts* (*of Lieberkuhn*) are short (0.1–0.3 mm), simple tubular glands which descend into the mucosa from the general surface of the intestine. They open into the gut lumen between the bases of villi.

2.5.7. The *lamina propria* forms the core of villi and also extends between the tubules of glands.

2.5.8. The epithelial lining of the small intestine includes:

A. *Absorptive columnar* (*villous columnar*) *cells or enterocytes* cover the general lining surface of the small intestine, the villi and extend into crypts. They are held together by apical junctional complexes and lateral interdigitations.

(i) These cells have a prominent striated or brush border

which in electron micrographs comprises microvilli and a fuzzy coat or glycocalyx. The glycocalyx is a filamentous layer rich in glycolipids, sialic acid and proteoglycans in which enzymes produced by absorptive cells are embedded and which protects the cell from digestion. Also adsorptively embedded in the glycocalyx are enzymes of pancreatic juice and membrane-bound enzymes which are released when the membrane is destroyed. Carrier molecules for active transport are embedded in the cell membrane.

(ii) *Absorptive cells* also have a secretory function producing new components of cell membranes, ATPase, alkaline phosphatase and enterokinase (which cleaves and activates trypsinogen to trypsin).

(iii) The basolateral plasma membrane contains ATPase for pumping sodium (with water) into the intercellular space from the intestine.

B. *Goblet cells* contain membrane-bound mucus droplets which coalesce. The number of goblet cells increases distally along the length of the small intestine.

C. *Paneth cells* are pyramidal-shaped cells located at the base of crypts. They are held together laterally by tight junctions and have a few apical microvilli. The supranuclear cytoplasm contains acidophil, refractile secretory granules which contain glycosaminoglycans and anti-bacterial lysozyme. Paneth cells have a longer life span than absorptive cells, ~16 days.

D. *Enteroendocrine cells* produce *somatostatin, gastrin, secretin, CCK-PZ* and *glucagon*. *Enterochromaffin cells* produce *serotonin* and *endorphin*. Hormones produced by cells of the intestinal wall alter its motility and secretion.

(i) *G cells* in the epithelium particularly of the pylorus and duodenum produce the polypeptides *gastrin I* and *II*. Gastrin increases hydrochloric acid production by parietal cells of gastric glands, promotes motility of the antrum and delays gastric emptying.

(ii) *S cells* in the crypts of Lieberkuhn in the duodenum produce the polypeptide *secretin* which increases secretion of pancreatic juice and increases bicarbonate production by cells of pancreatic ducts. Secretin also antagonizes gastrin action.

(iii) *I cells* of the duodenum, jejunum and ileum produce the polypeptide *Cholecystokinin-Pancreozymin* (CCK-PZ) which promotes the contraction of the gallbladder and secretion of enzyme rich pancreatic juice by pancreatic acinar cells.

E. *Undifferentiated crypt base columnar cells* have few surface microvilli and have smooth lateral borders. They are capable of division, migration and differentiation into either or all of the cell types described above. Undifferentiated cells divide in crypts to produce another stem cell and a differentiating daughter cell. The latter is displaced towards the tip of a villus and lost from the tip of the villus to the lumen within 3 days.

3. Changes in the Small Intestine along Its Length

3.1. Only the upper third of the duodenum contains compound tubulo-alveolar *duodenal (Brunner's) glands*. These glands secrete a very viscous mucous fluid with high bicarbonate content.

3.2. *Plicae circulares* are best developed in the jejunum and decrease in number and size distally.

3.3. The *shape and number of villi changes* distally along the intestine. Villi are tallest and most numerous in the jejunum.

3.4. *Goblet cells increase* in numbers from duodenum to the ileo-caecal valve.

3.5. *Lymphoid tissue increases* in amount in the intestine wall from proximal to distal.

4. Immune Defense Mechanisms

4.1. *Gut associated lymphoid tissue (GALT)* comprises aggregates of unencapsulated lymphatic nodules and solitary nodules distributed throughout the length of the intestines. It is part of a generalized mucosal immune system which includes dispersed lymphocytes and plasma cells in the lamina propria and wandering intra-epithelial lymphocytes.

4.2. Most intra-epithelial lymphocytes are T lymphocytes which contact a pseudopod of a macrophage in the underlying lamina propria.

4.3. *M cells* are specialized absorptive cells scattered in the epithelium covering Peyer's patches. They sample antigens by endocytosis of macromolecules and transport them in small vesicles to intra-epithelial lymphocytes which invaginate their basal surface.

4.4. *Plasma cells* in the lamina propria either:
   A. Secrete *IgG and IgE* which is taken up by lymphatic capillaries; or
   B. Secrete *IgA* which is taken up by epithelial cells, linked to a glycoprotein and secreted into the gut lumen (*Secretory IgA*).

5. Absorption

5.1. *Lipids*

   5.1.1. Cholesterol esters, phospholipids and triglycerides are split within the intestinal lumen by hydrolase, phospholipase A and lipase in pancreatic juice.

   5.1.2. Lipid droplets are emulsified by bile salts, forming micelles, which enter the space between microvilli, are broken down by pancreatic lipase and enter the absorptive cell without energy consumption.

   5.1.3. Free fatty acids and monoglycerides diffuse across the surface membrane of absorptive cells to accumulate in the apical cytoplasm.

   5.1.4. In the SER, resynthesized triglycerides combined with cholesterol esters and phospholipid appear as droplets.

   5.1.5. Cholesterol, phospholipid and apoprotein are added to form chylomicrons, which are transported in membrane-bound vesicles.

   5.1.6. Chylomicrons are released by exocytosis at the basolateral cell membrane into lymphatics and reach the blood through the thoracic duct.

5.2. *Proteins*

   5.2.1. Proteins are split by pepsins, trypsin and chymotrypsin and absorbed as amino acids by active transport systems in the luminal membrane of the absorptive cells.

   5.2.2. Amino acids leave the lateral and basal cell membranes by passive diffusion and active transport.

5.3. *Carbohydrates*

5.3.1. Carbohydrates are split by alpha amylase in saliva and pancreatic juice and by glucosidase in the brush border.

5.3.2. Monosaccharides attach to a carrier and diffuse to the interior of the absorptive cell. Sugars are extruded from the lateral and basal cell membrane.

6. Further Development of the Midgut

6.1. At 4 weeks (5 mm), the intestine is a simple tube extending from the stomach to the cloaca and suspended from the dorsal body wall in the midline by a dorsal mesentery. A ventral mesentery exists only in the region of the duodenum.

6.2. The midgut retains a connection with the yolk sac and elongates to form a simple loop. The cranial limb of the intestinal loop above the yolk sac connection (vitelline duct) will form the duodenum, jejunum and much of the ileum. The caudal limb will form the remainder of the ileum, colon and rectum.

6.3. In the fifth week, the intestinal loop elongates rapidly and cannot be accommodated in the small abdominal cavity. As a result, it undergoes several changes:

A. *Herniation* and coiling as it protrudes ventrally into the extra-embryonic coelom (where it remains for 4 weeks before returning).

B. *Rotation* in an anti-clockwise direction (viewed from in front) as the loop elongates and is displaced around the axis of the superior Mesenteric artery by the developing liver.

C. *Re-entry* into the abdominal cavity beginning at the end of the third month when growth of the liver declines relatively and the trunk enlarges.

The proximal part of the jejunum returns first to the left side and more caudal parts re-enter progressively to the right. The caecum is last to re-enter and is temporarily located in the upper right quadrant.

D. *Completion* which involves:

(i) Fixation of the duodenum against the dorsal body wall with loss of its mesentery.

(ii) Relative lack of growth of the caecal swelling resulting in formation of the vermiform appendix.

SMALL INTESTINE

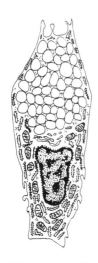

Mucous cell

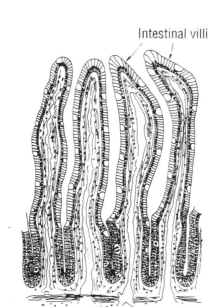

Intestinal villi

Small intestine showing intestinal villi and crypts.

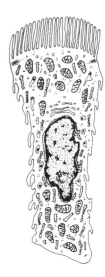

Enterocyte

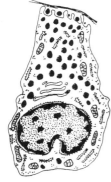

Enteroendocrine cell

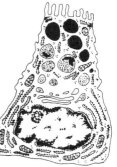

Paneth cell

   (iii) Loss (in all but 2–4% of people) of attachment of the vitelline duct.

   (iv) Establishment of the hepatic flexure of the colon as the liver decreases relatively in size. Both the ascending and descending colons are applied to the dorsal body wall, losing their mesenteries.

6.4. Proliferation of epithelium lining the intestine leads to occlusion of the lumen from 6–7 weeks but coalescence of intercellular vacuoles soon restores the lumen.

6.5. Villi appear at 8 weeks, intestinal glands at the end of the third month, and duodenal glands soon after. Peristalsis has been observed at 11 weeks.

LARGE INTESTINE

1. General Features

1.1. The *colon* begins at the caecum and is divided anatomically but not histologically into four parts, ascending, transverse, descending and pelvic or sigmoid colon. The caecum has the blind *vermiform appendix* extending from its posteromedial wall.

1.2. The transverse and sigmoid parts of the colon are intraperitonal structures and are completely invested with a serosa (*peritoneum*) and each has its own mesentery (*mesocolon*).

1.3. The terminal part of the large intestine descends into the pelvis as the rectum (rectus (L) straight from Galen who observed the straight terminal bowel in some animals). This segment is characterized by three transverse *rectal folds* involving the mucosa, submucosa and circular and longitudinal muscle layers. The folds help to support rectal contents.

1.4. The *anal canal* is the portion of the tract caudal to the *pectinate line* (mucocutaneous junction) although the boundary is considered by some to be at the level of the pelvic floor and upper border of the voluntary sphincter.

2. Regional Details

2.1. The ileum joins the caecum medially or posteromedially and the ostium is guarded by the *ileocaecal valve*. The valve comprises two transverse folds (*frenula*) of mucosa, submucosa and the circular smooth muscle layer of the ileum.

2.1.1. The *ileocaecal valve* retains ileal contents partly by tonic muscle contraction and partly by mechanical stretch of the frenula with caecal distension. The valve opens with a peristaltic wave from the ileum.

2.1.2. The sphincter is inhibited by distension of the caecum through a *caeco-ileal* reflex which prevents overfilling of the caecum and inhibits contractions of the terminal ileum. The functional competence of the ileo-caecal valve is low.

2.2. The *appendix* has continuous muscle coats in its wall. It has few crypts and the mucosa is mainly occupied by lymphoid tissue. The muscularis mucosae may be deficient and lymphoid tissue then extends into the submucosa.

2.3. In the *colon* and *caecum*, the outer longitudinal smooth muscle coat is divided into three bands or *taenia coli* (taenia (L) a band). Tonus in the taeniae causes puckering or sacculation of the walls of the tube, forming *haustra* (haustra (L) a pouch). *Appendices epiploicae* are fat-filled, finger-like projections of peritoneum which project from the external surface of the colon.

2.4. The *rectum* has a continuous outer longitudinal smooth muscle sheet.

2.5. The mucosa of the *anal canal* or terminal part of the rectum is thrown into longitudinal *anal columns* (of Morgagni). These are joined at their lower ends by transverse folds completing *anal valves* enclosing pocket like *anal sinuses*.

2.5.1. The epithelial lining changes near the beginning of the anal valves from simple columnar to stratified squamous at the *anorectal junction* (or *pectinate line*).

2.5.2. The submucosa of the anal canal is very vascular and contains many sensory nerves. Veins form the large *internal haemorrhoidal plexus* beneath the anal valves.

2.5.3. The circular layer of the (involuntary) muscularis is thickened to form the *internal anal sphincter* supplied by the hypogastric plexus. More distally skeletal muscle surrounds the external orifice, forming the *external anal sphincter* supplied by the inferior rectal nerves (S2,3).

2.5.4. In the submucosa of anal columns are large *arteriovenous anastomoses* communicating with rectal veins together forming the internal hemorrhoidal plexus. These communicate through small openings in the rectal walls with the superior hemorrhoidal veins of the portal system. Since this system has no valves to support pressure of the portal system and the connections are constricted by standing or straining, they may varicose producing, *internal hemorrhoids*.

2.5.5. The end of the anal canal is the poorly defined *anal verge* (ano-cutaneous junction). Skin surrounding the external orifice is hairy, lacking in sweat glands and contains simple tubular *apocrine (circumanal) glands* which secrete an oily material.

2.5.6. Veins of the internal hemorrhoidal plexus communicate with branches of the subcutaneous inferior hemorrhoidal veins via an *external rectal (hemorrhoidal)* plexus situated in the subcutaneous tissue surrounding the lower anal canal. These drain into the systemic system via the inferior rectal vein. Spasms of the anal sphincter shut off the venous outflow, causing *external hemorrhoids*.

3. Mucosa

3.1. There are no villi or plicae circulares, only crypts in the mucosa of the large intestine.

3.2. *Epithelium* of the large intestine is simple columnar containing:
  A. *Crypt base columnar cells* which are immature (undifferentiated) stem cells located in the base of crypts.
  B. *Goblet cells* more numerous than in the small intestine. Dehydrated faeces are lubricated by goblet cell mucus.
  C. *Columnar absorptive cells* which develop in crypts from stem cells and at first contain a glycoprotein which they secrete into the intestinal lumen as well as glycocalyx material. Upon reaching the lumen surface, absorptive cells loose their vesicles and become simple epithelium with microvilli and a rapidly renewed glycocalyx. These cells absorb water, vitamins, sodium and chloride.
  D. *Enteroendocrine cells*.

4. Nerve Supply of the Large Intestine

4.1. Preganglionic nerve fibers to the intestine arise from cell bodies in the dorsal motor nucleus of the vagus nerve (parasympathetic) and intermediolateral column of the second to fourth sacral spinal cord segments (parasympathetic) and from the intermediolateral column of the thoracic and lumbar spinal cord segments (sympathetic).

4.2. The *myenteric plexus* (*of Auerbach*) comprises groups of perikarya of postganglionic parasympathetic neurons, fibers and synapses between the layers of the muscularis externa. Postganglionic fibers supply smooth muscle of the external muscles. Congenital absence of the myenteric plexus causes constriction from lack of neural inhibition (relaxation). Above the constriction, the colon is greatly distended (congenital megacolon or Hirschsprung's disease).

4.3. The *submucosal plexus* (*of Meissner*) also contains groups of postganglionic parasympathetic neurons, fibers and synapses situated deep in the submucosa. It supplies postganglionic fibers to the muscularis mucosae, smooth muscle in vessel walls and secretory epithelium.

4.4. Sympathetic post-ganglionic nerves from extramural ganglia supply nerve endings to smooth muscle of the intestinal wall and of blood vessels. Their action in the intestine is inhibitory, opposing that of the parasympathetic system.

5. Development of the Hindgut

5.1. The *hindgut* arises from the caudal limb of the intestinal loop which gives rise to the distal third of the transverse colon, the sigmoid colon, rectum and upper part of the anal canal in the adult.

5.2. With cephalo-caudal folding of the embryo, a wedge of mesenchyme (the *urorectal septum*, cf. septum transversum) fills the interval between the hindgut and allantois and begins to push caudally. By the seventh week, it separates the cloaca into a ventral *bladder* and *urogenital sinus* and a dorsal ano-rectal canal.

5.3. The urorectal septum reaches the *cloacal membrane*, dividing it into an *anal membrane* and urogenital membrane and establishes the intervening *perineum*. Both membranes rupture by the ninth week.

5.4. The anal membrane is surrounded by mesenchymal swellings covered by ectoderm and form a central pit, the *proctodeum* (proktos (Gk) anus and odaios (Gk) a way).

5.5. The upper part of the anal canal is lined with entoderm, is relatively insensitive and is supplied by the inferior mesenteric artery.

5.6. The lower part of the anal canal below the pectinate line is lined with ectoderm, is very sensitive and supplied by the internal pudendal artery.

6. Functions of the Large Intestine

6.1. *Production of faeces*:

6.1.1. Products of digestion are concentrated in the colon by reabsorption of water. Electrolytes and water soluble vitamins are also reabsorbed.

6.1.2. The colon is populated soon after birth by saphrophytic *bacteria* which further degrade carbohydrate by fermentation and protein by putrifaction.

6.1.3. *Faeces* contains cellulose and other insoluble components, bacteria, insoluble calcium and iron salts, some fat and shed epithelium. Its color results from the breakdown of bile pigments.

6.2. *Motility of the large intestine*:

6.2.1. The movements of the colon are rhythmic segmental and non-propulsive peristalsis. Several times a day, mass contractions sweep from the caecum toward the rectum (*peristaltic rushes*).

6.2.2. Filling of the rectum stimulates stretch receptors in the wall and afferent impulses are conveyed to a reflex center in the spinal cord. Efferent impulses in parasympathetic nerves reduce the tone in smooth muscle of the internal sphincter. The striated muscle of the external sphincter is voluntarily relaxed and *defecation* (expulsion) is aided by contraction of the abdominal muscles which increase intra-abdominal pressure.

6.2.3. The defecation reflex can be voluntarily suppressed to some extent but frequent suppression leads to constipation. The fecal mass dries and the threshold of receptors is raised, requiring greater filling of the rectum to initiate the "call to stool".

Enzymes in protein digestion.

Site of Production	Enzyme	Substrate and Action
Gastric Glands (Chief Cells)	Pepsinogen (Pepsin)	Splits peptide bonds (pH optimum 1.3–3.5)
Exocrine Pancreas	Trypsinogen (Trysin)	Splits proteins between COOH groups of lysine and arginine and NH2 of other amino acids.
	Chymotrypsinogen (Chymotrypsin)	Splits proteins between COOH groups of aromatic amino acids except glutamic acid and asparagine (pH optimum 7.5–8.5)
	Carboxypeptidase A and B	A splits aromatic non-polar amino acids at terminal end and from polypeptides. B splits basic amino acids from same position of polypeptides.
Duodenal mucosa	Enterokinase	Splits trypsinogen between isoleucine and lysine.
Enterocytes (Brush border)	Tripeptidase	Splits N terminal or C terminal amino acids from proteins and polypeptides.
	Aminopolypeptidase	An exopeptidase splitting di and tri peptides.
	Aminopeptidase	Splits amino bonds from di and tri peptides.

Gastrointestinal Hormones.

Secretion	Location	Major actions
Gastrin I and II	Gastrin antrum and duodenum. (G Cells)	Increased gastric secretion, antrum motility and delayed gastric emptying.
Secretin (Oxykrinin)	Duodenum (S Cells)	Increased secretion and bicarbonate concentration of pancreatic juice and bile. Decreases gastric secretion.
Cholecystokinin (CCK) -Pancreozymin	Duodenum (I Cells)	Stimulates secretion of enzyme rich pancreatic juice. Empties gall bladder.
Motilin	Duodenum, Jejunum (EC2 cells)	Increases gastric motility.
Gastric Inhibitory Peptide (GIP)	Duodenum (K Cells)	Inhibits gastric secretion and motility.
Vasoactive Intestinal Polypeptide (VIP)	Entire length of GIT (D1 Cells)	Increases blood circulation of GIT.
Enteroglucagon	Intestines (Glucagon like immuno-reactive cells (GLI cells)	Stimulates glycogenolysis.
Substance P	Entire length of GIT (EC1 cells)	Stimulates smooth muscle contraction directly and indirectly through enteric neurons.
Somatostatin	Entire length of GIT (D cells)	Inhibition of exocrine secretion, neuroendocrine secretion, motility and intestinal transport.
Bombesin	Stomach and small intestines (P cells)	Promotes gastrin release and acid secretion
Neurotensin	Small intestines (N cells)	Stimulates smooth muscle, intestinal motility, gastric acid secretion, increases GIT blood flow, increases bicarbonate secretion from exocrine pancreas and insulin and glucagon from endocrine pancreas.

Chapter 16
Digestive System
5. Digestive Glands

OBJECTIVES

After reading this chapter, you should be able to:
1. Identify the major histologic features of liver.
2. Give the anatomical and functional bases for division of the liver parenchyma into hepatic lobules, portal lobules or acini.
3. Describe the lining of hepatic sinusoids and the anatomy and function of the Space of Disse.
4. Give an account of the functions of the liver relating these functions to particular cells.
5. Trace the path taken by bile from its formation to its injection into the duodenum. Add notes on the factors which control bile flow into the duodenum.
6. Give an account of the development of the liver and of the venous system from the yolk sac and placenta.
7. Identify histologic features of the exocrine pancreas.
8. Describe the origin, function and composition of pancreatic juice and factors which regulate its secretion.
9. Describe the development of the pancreas and its ducts.

CHAPTER OUTLINE

Liver

General.

General structure. Lobes, lobules, hilum, capsule. Hepatocytes, bile canaliculi.

Detailed structure. Hepatocytes, Sinusoids, Endothelial cells, Kupffer cells, Space of Disse. Bile ducts.

Structural units of the liver. Hepatic (Classic) lobule. Portal lobule. Liver acinus.

Functions of the liver. Secretion. Steroid hormone circulation. Glycogen synthesis and glucose secretion. Blood protein synthesis. Lipoprotein synthesis. IgA secretion. Transformation and conjugation.

Development of the liver. Hepatic diverticulum. Fate of the vitelline and umbilical veins.

Gall Bladder

General.

Detailed structure.

Functions of the gall bladder.

The Exocrine Pancreas

General.

Detailed structure. Acini. Acinar cells, Pancreatic juice.

Regulation of secretion.

Development of the duct system.

Structure of the duct system. Centroacinar cells, Intercalated ducts, Intralobular ducts, Interlobular ducts, Pancreatic and Accessory Pancreatic ducts. Sphincter of the hepatopancreatic ampulla.

KEY WORDS, PHRASES, CONCEPTS

Lobes
Lobules
Porta Hepatis

Bile preductules
(Canals of Hering)
Bile ductules

Capsule
Hepatocytes
Sinusoids
Portal area (tract or radicle)
Hepatic artery
Portal vein
Bile duct
Bile
Hepatic (Classic) lobule
Bile canaliculi
Portal lobule
Liver acinus
Endothelial cells
Kupffer cells
Pancreatic duct
Accessory Pancreatic duct

Hepatic ducts
Gall bladder
Cholecystokinin-
Pancreozymin (CCK-PZ)
Vitelline veins
Umbilical veins
Hepatic diverticulum
Pancreatic acini
Acinar cells
Pancreatic juice
Secretin
Centroacinar cells
Intercalated ducts
Intralobular ducts
Choledochal sphincter
Sphincter of the hepato-pancreatic
    ampulla

THE LIVER

1. General

1.1. The *liver* (from lifer (Anglo-Saxon) liver, also hepar (Gk) liver, thus the adjective, hepatic) is the largest gland in the body accounting for one twentieth of the body weight of a neonate and one fiftieth of the body weight of an adult.

1.2. The liver is basically a compound tubular serous gland but is highly modified in mammals. Anastomosing and branching cellular plates replace tubules and the pattern of lobulation is related to the interposed blood vessels rather than the duct system.

1.3. *Bile*, the exocrine secretion of the liver, empties into the duodenum through the bile duct. Bile is secreted by parenchymal cells (*hepatocytes*) into tiny intercellular passageways (*bile canaliculi*) between parenchymal cells.

1.4. Internal (endocrine) secretions of hepatocytes including glucose, plasma proteins and lipoproteins are liberated directly into the bloodstream.

1.5. The liver is thus described as partly an endocrine and partly an exocrine organ.

2. General Structure

2.1. The liver is divided into four incompletely separated *lobes*.

2.2. A thin, strong *capsule* (of Glisson) is covered by peritoneal mesothelium except for a large area, the *bare area*, where the liver rests directly against the diaphragm.

2.3. The *hilum* (porta hepatis) is the area on the inferior surface where vessels and ducts enter or leave.

2.4. The parenchyma is subdivided into approximately one million small (*hepatic*) *lobules* shaped like irregular prisms 1–2 mm in diameter and incompletely isolated by connective tissue.

2.5. Lobules comprise polyhedral glandular, epithelial cells of entodermal origin (*hepatocytes*) arranged in anastomosing trabeculae or curved perforatedplates which radiate from an axis, a central venule. *Hepatocytes* are separated by *hepatic sinusoids*. In most places the trabeculae (plates) are one cell thick with one cell having two surfaces bordering on sinusoids.

2.6. Hepatocytes have microscopic channels or *bile canaliculi* between their lateral borders. The exocrine secretion (*bile*) is liberated into these canaliculi.

2.7. Bile flows in the canaliculi towards the periphery of a lobule to *portal tracts*. Blood flows from the periphery of the lobule from portal tracts to the central venule, i.e., in the opposite direction to the flow of bile.

2.8. Hepatic sinusoids converge radially between cellular plates to the *central venule* and connect vessels at the periphery of the lobule (branches of the *portal vein*) with the central vein. These vessels converge to the suprahepatic part of the inferior vena cava via hepatic veins.

2.9. Connective tissue at the edges of lobules constitutes a *portal area* (or *portal tract*). It contains branches of the Hepatic artery, Portal vein and bile duct.

2.10. The liver has a dual blood supply:

A. The *portal vein* from the intestine brings venous blood containing products of digestion to the liver and supplies 75% of its blood supply.

B. The hepatic artery (from the coeliac trunk) provides oxygenated blood (25%) to the tissue in portal areas but this blood eventually mixes with portal blood passing through liver lobules.

3. Detailed Structure

3.1. *Hepatocytes* are polyhedral cells making up trabeculae of hepatic lobules.

   3.1.1. The cytoplasm is rich in organelles reflecting diverse functions. There is a rich RER, SER and multiple Golgi complexes, as well as glycogen granules, mitochondria, lysosomes (especially near bile canaliculi) and microbodies (peroxisomes) with crystalline nucleoids.

   3.1.2. Some cells contain two to four nuclei.

   3.1.3. The cell surface facing the Space of Disse toward the sinusoid is covered with microvilli. This presents a large surface area for exchange.

   3.1.4. The lateral cell surfaces contact apposed hepatocytes and form half of a *bile canaliculus* (0.5–1.5 μm in total diameter). Microvilli protrude into the bile canaliculus which is closed by junctional complexes. The immediately subjacent cytoplasm contains microfilaments, which insert into attachment plaques of desmosomes.

4. Sinusoids

4.1. *Endothelial cells* line sinusoids. These cells have large fenestrae through their cytoplasm and smaller pores closed by sieve plates. They are separated by large intercellular openings that do not present a barrier to the fluid phase of blood.

4.2. *Kupffer cells* are large, stellate macrophages, some found in the wall of sinusoids and some beneath the wall lining. These cells guard against blockage of endothelial pores joining sinusoids and the Space of Disse and phagocytose debris and effete red blood cells from blood.

4.3. The *Space of Disse* is the narrow space between the endothelial-Kupffer cell lining of sinusoids and hepatocytes. The space contains:

A. *Plasma*, but not blood cells and platelets, which are excluded.

B. *Collagen bundles* and *laminin* (a non-collagenous glycoprotein product of fibroblasts); and

C. *Lipocytes*, which support the Space of Disse and also store fat and vitamin A.

5. Bile Ducts

5.1. *Bile canaliculi* begin blindly between hepatocytes near central veins.

5.2. They empty into short *terminal bile ductules* bordered partly by hepatocytes and partly by duct cells (*Canals of Hering*) at the periphery of the liver lobule.

5.3. Bile then passes into *bile ductules* in the portal areas. These are lined with low cuboidal duct cells.

5.4. Bile ductules then empty into *interlobular bile ducts*. These ductules are lined with cuboidal cells characterized by microvilli on their free surface, apical junctional complexes and lateral surface interdigitations.

5.5. Larger bile ducts (*right and left hepatic ducts, common hepatic duct and cystic duct*) are lined with columnar epithelium.

6. Structural Units of the Liver

6.1. The Hepatic (Classic) Lobule

    6.1.1. The *hepatic lobule* is demarcated by interlobular connective tissue septa (unclear in the human but clear in the pig). The hepatic lobule is hexagonal in cross section.

    6.1.2. Connective tissue in at least some corners of the lobule is known as the *portal tract, area or radicle*. It contains branches of the portal vein, hepatic artery and bile duct, together with one or more lymphatics.

    6.1.3. Blood arrives from the portal vein and hepatic artery enters the periphery of wide anastomosing hepatic sinusoids and percolates to the central vein.

6.2. The Portal Lobule

    6.2.1. This subdivision represents a group of hepatocytes which discharge their exocrine secretion (bile) into the same intralobular bile duct.

6.2.2. The portal lobule is triangular in shape and the central axis is a bile duct in a portal tract. It therefore comprises parts of three adjoining classic lobules.

6.2.3. The direction of bile flow is toward the center of the portal lobule (the portal tract).

6.3. The Liver Acinus

6.3.1. The liver acinus is a grouping of hepatocytes according to their proximity to the afferent blood supply. It is not a secretory unit equivalent to the acinus of an exocrine gland.

6.3.2. This structural unit is like two wedge-shaped pieces sharing a common base and incorporating contiguous parts of two neighboring lobules. Peripheral landmarks of an acinus are two neighboring central veins.

6.3.3. Blood is delivered to sinusoids by small branches of portal and hepatic vessels conveyed in portal tracts. Side branches of portal tract vessels occur at intervals in any of three directions to contiguous classical lobules.

6.3.4. Acini are divided into zones depending on the proximity of hepatocytes to the blood supply, i.e., branches of interlobular arteries and veins.

A. *Zone 1* cells are closest to the blood supply (closest to the base of the wedge), obtain excellent supply of oxygen and nutriments, and synthesize glycogen and plasma proteins.

B. *Zone 2* cells are in an intermediate position.

C. *Zone 3* cells are near central veins and most distant from the source of blood supply. They are the last cells to receive nutrients, most vulnerable to hypoxia, susceptible to damage by toxic metabolites and the main site of alcohol and drug detoxification.

7. Functions of the Liver

7.1. *Secretion*:

7.1.1. *Bile* contains bilirubin, a pigmented waste product of haemoglobin breakdown by macrophages, cholesterol, lecithin, fatty acids, bile salts, calcium, chloride, sodium, potassium and bicarbonate ions and water.

7.1.2. *Bile salts* facilitate digestion of fats by forming complexes (micelles). They also have surfactant or detergent properties and are reabsorbed by the intestine and reused.

7.1.3. *Steroid hormones* of the suprarenal cortex and sex glands are absorbed by hepatocytes, secreted into bile and reabsorbed in the intestines. This process is known as the *enterohepatic circulation of steroid hormones*.

7.1.4. Bile secretion by the liver is continuous but can double during digestion.

7.2. *Glycogen synthesis and glucose secretion*:

7.2.1. Hepatocytes absorb excess glucose from blood under the influence of insulin and convert glucose to glycogen.

7.2.2. Cortisol leads to glycogen formation in hepatocytes from protein catabolism.

7.3. *Blood protein synthesis*:

7.3.1. Hepatocytes secrete albumins, fibrinogen and most of the globulins of blood plasma.

7.4. *Lipoprotein synthesis*:

7.4.1. Most plasma lipids are complexed triglycerides and cholesterol esters combined with protein and hence hydrophilic. The remainder are a complex of fatty acids and albumin.

7.4.2. Hepatocytes remove chylomicrons from blood following a fatty meal.

7.5. *Immunoglobulin A and Secretory Component (SC) production*:

7.5.1. IgA is captured by hepatocytes from blood by secretory component, a glycoprotein surface receptor. The complex is secreted in bile and thus reaches the lumen of the small intestine.

7.6. *Transformation and conjugation*:

7.6.1. Hepatocytes play a role in the detoxification of endogenous and exogenous compounds, e.g., of ammonia to urea.

8. Development of the Liver

8.1. The development of the liver is associated not only with growth of its parenchyma (from gut entoderm), but with the influence of parenchymal development on the fate of veins approaching the heart from the placenta (*umbilical veins*) and yolk sac (*vitelline veins*).

8.2. A ventral outgrowth of gut entoderm near the entry of the vitelline duct (*the hepatic diverticulum*) appears between the pericardial cavity and the attaching yolk sac at 2.5 mm.

8.3. The diverticulum grows into splanchnic mesoderm of the septum transversum and splits into:

   A. A cranial part giving rise to glandular tissue, the liver parenchyma, and biliary duct system.

   B. A caudal part giving rise to the gallbladder and cystic duct.

8.4. Epithelial cords bud from the tip of the cranial part of the hepatic diverticulum.

8.5. The cords become closely associated at first with the vitelline veins and are thus separated from one another by *sinusoids*. These sinusoids link supplying (portal) and draining (hepatic) vessels. Regularity of branching of the vitelline network is responsible for the creation of hepatic lobules.

8.6. The *vitelline veins* form an anastomosis around the duodenum before entering the septum transversum on their way to the heart. The proximal parts of the vitelline veins enter the right and left horns of the sinus venosus.

8.7. Of the distal parts of the vitelline veins:

   A. The anastomosis around the duodenum forms a single vessel, the *portal vein*.

   B. The superior mesenteric vein is the remainder of the right vitelline vein.

   C. The distal part of the left vitelline vein disappears.

8.8. Of the proximal parts of the vitelline veins draining into the sinus venosus:

   A. The left sinus horn disappears and the left side of the liver rechannels to the right vitelline vein. This segment becomes the suprahepatic part of the inferior vena cava.

   B. The proximal part of the left vitelline vein disappears.

8.9. *Umbilical veins* enter the embryo via the connecting stalk and septum transversum to end in the right and left horns of the sinus venosus.

8.10. Liver cord growth interrupts the umbilical veins, which become connected to liver sinusoids.

A. The proximal part of both umbilical veins (to the developing liver) disappear as does the remainder of the right umbilical vein.

B. The left umbilical vein is the only vessel remaining to carry blood from the placenta to the liver.

C. Increased placental circulation forms a channel from the left umbilical vein to the right hepatocardiac channel, the *ductus venosus*. This channel largely by-passes the liver sinusoidal plexus.

D. At birth, the left umbilical vein and the ductus venosus are obliterated, forming the *ligamentum teres* and the *ligamentum venosum* respectively.

8.11. From 2–7 months, red and white blood cells differentiate between hepatocytes and the endothelial-Kupffer lining of sinusoids. These haematopoietic cells in the liver are seeded from primary centers in the yolk sac wall. The potential of the liver to be a site of haematopoeisis remains latent throughout life.

GALL BLADDER

1. General

1.1. The gall bladder is an elongated, pear-shaped, thin-walled reservoir for the storage and concentration of bile.

1.2. The lining tunica mucosa is thrown into primary and secondary folds.

2. Detailed Structure

2.1. The gallbladder is lined by a simple, high columnar absorptive epithelium with surface microvilli, sealed with junctional complexes and bordered with interdigitating lateral surfaces. Cells concentrate bile by pumping sodium and water into the intercellular spaces and through the basal lamina into vessels of the lamina propria.

2.2. The *lamina propria* is loose, vascular connective tissue.

2.3. There is no *muscularis mucosae*.

2.4. *Tunica muscularis* comprises irregular spirally arranged bundles of smooth muscle intermingled with collagen and elastic fibers. External spiral and internal longitudinal bundles are described. Near the entry into the cystic duct, spiral bundles become more longitudinally arranged, throwing the duct into a series of spiral folds (*the spiral valve*).

2.5. *Tunica adventitia* is a layer of loose connective tissue containing blood vessels, lymphatics and nerves where the gall bladder contacts the liver. In some areas, the gallbladder is covered by peritoneum (serosa).

3. Functions of the Gall Bladder

3.1. The gall bladder stores and concentrates bile ($\times 10$).

3.2. Contractions of gall bladder wall and relaxation of the sphincter choledochus, located in the bile duct at its junction with the pancreatic duct, are initiated by *cholecystokinin-pancreozymin* (*CCK-PZ*) produced by *I cells* in the walls of the duodenum, jejunum and ileum in response to contact with chyme.

3.3. Absence or removal of the gallbladder results in compensatory dilation of bile passages.

THE EXOCRINE PANCREAS

1. General

1.1. The exocrine pancreas comprises acini, pear-shaped secretory end pieces attached to short excretory tubules.

1.2. Acini are surrounded by a basal lamina but differ from salivary glands in lacking subjacent myoepitheliocytes.

2. Detailed Structure

2.1. *Acinar cells* are pyramidal-shaped cells making up the major part of pancreatic acini.

    2.1.1. They contain a conspicuous Golgi complex, numerous mitochondria, and extensive RER (responsible for basal basophilia). Supranuclear dense secretion granules are acidophilic *zymogen granules*.

    2.1.2. Cells have apical microvilli and tight junctions and interdigitations with adjoining acinar cells.

    2.1.3. Cholinergic and adrenergic axon terminals contact the basal surface of some cells.

2.2. *Pancreatic juice*, the secretion of acinar cells, is an alkaline digestive juice containing the following enzymes:

Trypsin	Chymotrypsin	Esterase
Deoxyribonuclease	Ribonuclease	Amylase
Phospholipase A	Carboxypeptidases A&B	Elastase
Lipase		

These enzymes are activated after reaching the alkaline intestine.

3. Regulation of Secretion

3.1. *Nervous regulation* of secretion is by parasympathetic stimulation through the Vagus nerve (or parasympatheticomimetic drugs like pilocarpine).

3.2. *Hormonal regulation* is by two gastrointestinal hormones released by enteroendocrine cells of intestinal mucosa following stimulation by acid stomach contents.

    A. *Secretin* (secreted by S cells in the intestinal crypts) which stimulates release of bicarbonate ions by duct cells of the pancreas.

    B. *Cholecystokinin-pancreozymin* (*CCK-PZ*) produced by I cells of the small intestine wall. CCK-PZ stimulates release of enzymes from acinar cells.

4. Development of the Duct System

4.1. Both ventral and dorsal pancreatic buds have axial *ducts*.

4.2. The duct of the *dorsal pancreas* enters the duodenal wall directly.

4.3. The duct of the *ventral pancreas* enters the common bile duct.

4.4. Duodenal torsion brings the two pancreatic primordia side by side with the ventral pancreas below the dorsal pancreas. The short ventral duct taps the dorsal duct.

4.5. The definitive *pancreatic duct* is formed from:

    A. A long distal segment, the axial duct of the dorsal pancreas.

    B. A short anastomosis between the axial ducts resulting from fusion of the two primordia.

    C. The proximal part of the duct of the ventral pancreas.

4.6. Secretory alveoli of the exocrine part of the pancreas appear as terminal and side buds of the branching ducts at 3 months.

5. Structure of the Duct System

5.1. *Centroacinar cells* are small, flattened cells containing abundant mitochondria which incompletely border the lumen of pancreatic acini. They may be responsible for producing bicarbonate-rich fluid and have a role in solubilizing zymogen granules. Centroacinar cells are continuous with:

5.2. *Intercalated ducts* which are lined with cuboidal epithelium. This duct segment is more extensive than in any other digestive gland.

5.3. *Intralobular ducts* lined with simple cuboidal or low columnar epithelium.

5.4. *Interlobular ducts* between lobules are lined with low columnar epithelium.

5.5. The *pancreatic duct* and *accessory pancreatic duct* are lined with simple cuboidal to columnar epithelium with outpocketings which may be mucous type glands. Smooth muscle surrounds the junction of the pancreatic duct with the ductus choledochus.

5.6. The *sphincter muscle of the hepatopancreatic ampulla* is a complex of smooth muscle guarding the opening of the ductus choledochus and pancreatic duct at the pancreatic ampulla. It comprises:

   A. A circular group of fibers surrounding the ampulla;
   B. A longitudinal bundle passing from the points of entry of choledochus and pancreatic ducts;
   C. The sphincter of the pancreatic duct; and
   D. The sphincter of the choledochus duct.

LIVER

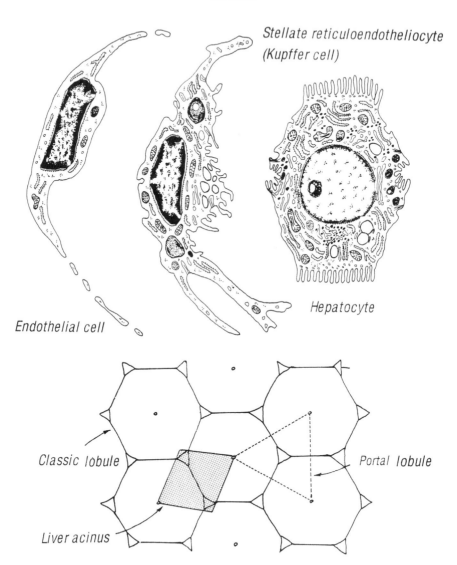

Stellate reticuloendotheliocyte
(Kupffer cell)

Hepatocyte

Endothelial cell

Classic lobule

Portal lobule

Liver acinus

Structural and functional organization of the liver.

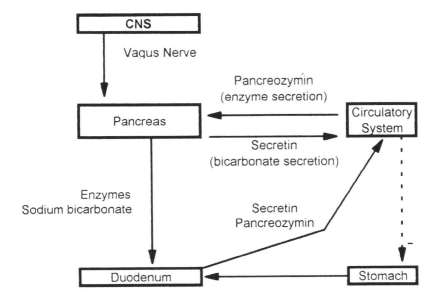

Control of pancreatic exocrine secretion.

EXOCRINE PANCREAS

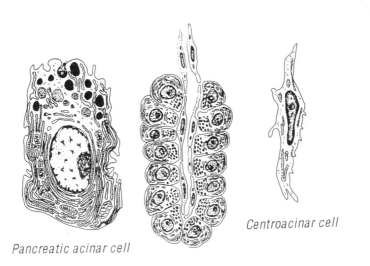

Pancreatic acinar cell

Centroacinar cell

Pancreatic acinus

Chapter 17

URINARY SYSTEM
1. KIDNEY

OBJECTIVES

After reading this chapter, you should be able to:

1. Give an account of the functions of the kidney.
2. Identify the histological features of the parts of a uriniferous tubule and explain their distribution in the kidney lobules.
3. Give an account of the developmental origin of the secretory and excretory parts of the kidney and how the pronephros, mesonephros and metanephros differ from and contribute to the development of one another.
4. Describe the detailed structure of a glomerulus with particular emphasis on the nature of the glomerular filtration barrier.
5. Give a detailed histologic account of the structure of the walls of the secretory and excretory portions of the nephron.
6. Describe the structure and function of the juxtaglomerular apparatus, relating it to the secretion of aldosterone by the suprarenal cortex.

CHAPTER OUTLINE

General. Components of the urinary system. Functions of the urinary system.

General structure of the kidney.

Development. Intermediate mesoderm. Pronephros. Mesonephros. Metanephros.

Detailed structure. Renal (Malphigian) corpuscle. Glomerulus, Glomerular capsule, Podocytes, Glomerular filtration barrier. Renal tubule. Proximal convoluted tubule, Loop of Henle, Distal convoluted tubule. Juxtaglomerular apparatus, Mesangial cells, Juxtaglomerular cells, Macula densa. Arched collecting tubule. Straight collecting tubule, Papillary ducts.

Blood supply of the kidney.

Further functions of the kidney. Counter current multiplier and counter current exchangers. Anti-diuretic hormone (ADH). Aldosterone. Atrial natriuretic factor (ANF).

KEY WORDS, PHRASES, CONCEPTS

Uriniferous tubules
Nephron
Collecting tubule
Secretory portion of the
Uriniferous tubule
Excretory portion of the
   uriniferous tubule
Cortex
Renal columns (of Bertin)
Pars radiata (Medullary Rays)
Pars convoluta (Labyrinth)
Medulla
Pyramids
Lobes
Lobules
Intermediate mesoderm
Pronephros
Nephrostome
Pronephric duct
Mesonephros
Angiotensinogen
Angiotensin II

Metanephros
Ureteric bud
Metanephric blastema
Calyces (major, minor)
Renal (Malphigian) Corpuscle
Glomerulus
Vascular pole
Urinary pole
Glomerular capsule
   Parietal layer
   Visceral layer
Podocytes
   Pedicles
   Filtration slits
   Glomerular filtration barrier
Mesangial cells
Proximal tubule
Loop of Henle
Distal tubule
Juxtaglomerular apparatus
Macula densa
Juxtaglomerular cells

1. General

1.1. The *urinary system* comprises two *kidneys* (renes (L) kidney thus renal and nephros (Gk) kidney thus nephron), two *ureters* (oron (Gk) urine and tereo (Gk) to preserve), a bladder (blaedre (Old English) a blister) and a *urethra*.

1.2. The paired kidneys are compound tubular glands which elaborate urine, a filtrate of wastes from blood.

1.3. The ureters are fibromuscular tubes conducting urine to a single urinary bladder where fluid accumulates for periodic evacuation via the urethra.

1.4. The functions of the kidneys include:

A. *Excretion* of waste products of metabolism.

B. *Elimination of foreign substances* and their breakdown products from blood.

C. *Regulation of total body fluid.*

D. *Maintenance of extracellular fluid volume.*

E. *Regulation of various salts* to be excreted or retained.

F. Control of *acid-base balance*.

G. Kidneys produce *erythropoietin*, a glycoprotein hormone which stimulates proliferation and differentiation of responsive cells to differentiate through CFU-E's to proerythroblasts. Erythropoietin also stimulates haemoglobin synthesis in erythroblasts.

2. General Structure

2.1. The kidney is covered by a thin, fibrous and elastic *capsule*.

2.2. The medially placed *hilum* expands inside the kidney into a large cavity, the *renal sinus*, which accommodates the expanded upper end of the ureter, the *renal pelvis*. The renal sinus also contains fat, vessels and nerves.

2.3. The renal pelvis divides within the sinus into 2–3 *major calyces* each ramifying into 4 to 13 *minor calyces*. These are cup-shaped ducts that receive the *renal papillae*.

2.4. The basic functional unit of the kidney is the *nephron*, a blind tubule invaginated at its distal end by an anastomosing capillary tuft or *glomerulus* (glomerare (L) to roll up, from glomus (L) a ball). There are more than a million nephrons in each kidney.

2.4.1. The nephron or *secretory portion* of the uriniferous tubule is divided into segments: Glomerular capsule, proximal tubule (convoluted portion, straight portion), thin segment of Henle's loop, distal tubule (straight portion, convoluted portion).

2.4.2. The nephron joins a collecting tubule, *excretory or duct portion* of the uriniferous tubule whose segments include: Arched collecting tubule, straight collecting tubule, papillary duct.

2.4.3. The nephron (or secretory portion) and the collecting duct (or excretory portion) together constitute a *uriniferous tubule*. Portions of the uriniferous tubules are concentrated in such a way as to give the kidney its characteristic gross subdivisions seen in a sliced section.

2.5. The *medulla* comprises 10–15 conical renal pyramids whose apices converge toward the renal sinus.

2.5.1. Two or three pyramids commonly fuse at their apices to end on a common renal papilla (there are 8–18 papillae) which project into minor calyces.

2.5.2. The medulla is also divided into *outer and inner zones* containing particular segments of ducts and tubules.

2.6. The *cortex* arches over the base of pyramids as cortical arches or lobules and extends between pyramids as *renal columns (of Bertin)*.

2.6.1. The cortex is divided into *outer and inner (juxtamedullary)* zones in which the structure of nephrons differ (vide infra).

2.6.2. The cortex is also divided into alternate radially oriented areas:

A. *Medullary rays (pars radiata)* contain concentrations of proximal tubules, arched tubules and collecting ducts.

B. *Convoluted parts (the pars convoluta or labyrinth)* which contain a high proportion of renal corpuscles, proximal and distal convoluted tubules.

These divisions can be observed with a hand lens in a cut specimen.

3. Development

3.1. In the third week, intraembryonic mesoderm differentiates into three distinct parts:

    A. The medially placed *paraxial mesoderm* which forms the somites.

    B. Laterally placed *lateral plate mesoderm* which splits into *somatic and splanchnic layers* lining the intra-embryonic coelom.

    C. *Intermediate mesoderm* which temporarily connects the paraxial and lateral plate mesoderm.

3.2. Intermediate mesoderm is segmented in the cervical region but caudally forms an unsegmented mass, the *nephrogenic cord*. This caudal mass forms the excretory units of the urinary system.

3.3. In the cervical and thoracic regions, intermediate mesoderm cell clusters (*the nephrotome*) elongate and canalize to form a tubule.

    3.3.1. Medially, the nephrotome opens into the intra-embryonic coelom. Laterally, it grows caudally, uniting with other segments, canalizes, and forms a longitudinal duct, the *pronephric duct*.

    3.3.2. Serial branches of the dorsal aorta ending in capillary tufts (*glomeruli*) grow toward the nephrotome and wastes are filtered through them via the nephrotome to the coelom.

3.4. In phylogeny (and repeated in a rostro-caudal sequence in human development), three types of kidney have developed, the *pronephros* (pro (Gk) before and nephros (Gk) kidney), *mesonephros* (mesos (Gk) middle) and *metanephros* (meta (Gk) after).

3.5. The *pronephros* is vestigial in man, appearing as about 7 pairs of rudimentary tubules which disappear by the end of the forth week.

    3.5.1. One end of the pronephric tubule opens into the coelom. The other end joins with adjacent segments, forming a longitudinal cellular cord which reaches the cloaca caudally, fuses with its lateral wall, and canalizes to complete the longitudinal pronephric duct.

    3.5.2. Nearby but separate from each tubule, an arterial tuft projects into the coelom, forming an external glomerulus filtering wastes into the coelom.

    3.5.3. A mixture of urine and coelomic fluid is taken up by the tubules and carried by currents created by cilia on epithelial cells lining the tubules to the main excretory ducts.

3.6. The *mesonephros* first appears while the pronephros is beginning to degenerate.

    3.6.1. The mesonephros differs from the pronephros in that:

     A. It contains more tubules than the pronephros.

     B. Tubules are longer and more complicated.

     C. It only differentiates into tubules which secondarily connect with the pronephric duct (which now becomes known as the mesonephric duct). The mesonephros thus has a double origin comprising a secretory system and a collecting system.

     D. The glomerulus is internal indenting the blind end of the tubule and passing wastes directly into the tubule.

     E. The nephrostome is transitory, never serving as a functional opening into the coelom.

3.6.2. The mesonephros is most highly developed by the mid second month; degenerating by the end of the same month.

3.6.3. The mesonephric duct is used in the male as the ductus deferens but disappears in the female.

3.7. The *metanephros* forms the definitive kidney.

    3.7.1. It has a double origin, as does the mesonephros:

     A. Secretory units develop from intermediate mesoderm in the caudal solid mass of intermediate mesoderm, the metanephric blastema.

     B. Collecting ducts develop from a branching bud from the mesonephric duct.

    3.7.2. The collecting system arises in the forth week as a dorsomedial bud, the ureteric bud, from the mesonephric duct near its entrance to the cloaca.

    3.7.3. The ureteric bud penetrates the metanephric blastema where it splits into cranial and caudal parts, the major calyces. These continue to divide in 13 or more generations.

    3.7.4. Major calyces absorb the proximal ducts up to the third or forth generations, establishing the minor calyces.

    3.7.5. The fifth and later generations form definitive collecting tubules.

    3.7.6. The secretory system arises from tissue of the metanephric blastema.

    3.7.7. The distal part of each newly formed tubule is covered with a tissue cap. Parts of the cap separate from the main tissue mass, forming cell clusters on each side of the tubule.

    3.7.8. The cell clusters develop a vesicle (renal vesicle) which gives rise to the excretory tubule or nephron. The proximal end of the nephron becomes invaginated, forming the glomerular (Bowman's) capsule. The distal end of the nephron connects with, and then opens into, one of the collecting tubules.

3.7.9. Glomeruli develop as a solid sphere of mesodermal cells in which vessels develop by canalization. They mature by 6–12 years.

3.8.10. Secretory tubules lengthen, forming the loop of Henle.

4. Detailed Structure

4.1. *Renal (Malpighian) corpuscles* are 0.2 mm in diameter and comprise:

   A. A *glomerulus*, a lobulated tuft of capillaries. An afferent arteriole enters the glomerulus and an efferent arteriole emerges close by. The glomerulus invaginates the capsule at a point opposite to the point of continuity of the capsule with the tubule and is known as the vascular pole of the capsule.

   B. The *glomerular capsule (of Bowman)* is the expanded end of a renal tubule which is deeply invaginated by the glomerulus.

     (i) Squamous cells line the outer wall of the capsule forming the *parietal epithelium of Bowman's capsule*.

     (ii) Specialized epithelial cells (Podocytes) cover the glomerulus (*visceral epithelium of Bowman's capsule*).

Between the layers of the capsule is the *urinary (Bowman's)* space.

4.2. *Podocytes* are flattened, stellate cells with dendrite-like processes which interdigitate with processes of other podocytes and cover the basal lamina of glomerular endothelium.

   4.2.1. *Primary (major) processes or trabeculae* extend from the cell body and bear smaller secondary and tertiary processes. These branch to thin interdigitating pedicles or podocyte feet which are separated from pedicles of other podocytes by filtration slits.

   4.2.2. *Filtration slits* are 20–30 nm gaps between pedicles. They are spanned by shelf-like filtration (glomerular) slit diaphragms.

4.3. The glomerular basal lamina has pale staining inner and outer layers (laminae rara) and a dense, fibrous central layer (lamina densa). It contains type IV collagen, sialic acid and glycosaminoglycan (rich in heparin sulphate) and is the principal filter of macromolecules. The lamina is constantly being renewed mainly on its epithelial side.

4.4. The vascular endothelium of the glomerulus is simple squamous epithelium with a fenestrated cytoplasm. Only a few fenestrae have diaphragms.

4.5. The total *glomerular filtration barrier* through which blood borne molecules must pass to reach the urinary space comprises:

    A. Capillary endothelium.

    B. Glomerular basal lamina.

    C. Filtration slits between podocyte end feet.

    The barrier favors passage of molecules no larger than 100 nm in diameter and without a high negative charge.

4.6. *Mesangial cells* are phagocytic and contractile cells found around the base of glomerular capillary tufts, that is, in the intraglomerular mesangial region. They clear the glomerular filter of cloggng substances and can contract when stimulated by angiotensin to decrease capillary blood flow.

4.7. The tubular portion of the uriniferous tubule comprises the following parts in sequence:

    A. *Proximal tubule* connected to the capsule at the neck has an initial convoluted part and more distal straight part.

        (i) It is lined with cuboidal cells (*nephrocytes*) with tall apical microvilli but whose shape depends on the degree of distension of the tubule (they are tall post-mortem). Cells are strongly eosinophilic with a base highly folded into complex mitochondria containing pleats. They are also attached to adjacent cells by a tight, belt-like band of junctions adjacent to the lumen and complex interdigitations of lateral cell membranes. Endocytic channels and lysosomes indicate some uptake and hydrolysis of proteins.

       (ii) *Nephrocytes* present a large surface area of membrane contacting tubular and extra tubular space. They transport ions and small molecules against steep concentration gradients actively transporting sodium into the intercellular space or basal labyrinth. Water and other ions also follow between cells passively, thereby reducing the volume of filtrate by 80% of its original volume.

    B. *Loop of Henle* is a sharp recurving part of the nephron comprising a thick descending limb or straight portion of the proximal tubule, thin segment and thick ascending segment or straight portion of the distal tubule.

(i) The component of the tubule actually making the *apex* of the loop varies. If the loop dips deeply into the medulla, a long thin segment makes the loop. If the loop is high in the medulla, the thick ascending segment forms the apex. Nephrons with glomeruli near the corticomedullary border (*juxtamedullary nephrons*) have a longer loop of Henle that extends farther into the medulla than the loop of nephrons situated in the outer region of the cortex.

(ii) The *thick descending part of the loop* is a continuation of the proximal convoluted tubule lined with similar cells termed the straight part.

(iii) The *thin descending and thin ascending parts* are lined with low cuboidal to squamous cells. The cells have few organelles, indicating a passive, rather than active, role in ion movement.

(iv) The *thick ascending part* is lined with cuboidal epithelium representing the beginning of the straight part of the distal tubule.

C. The *distal convoluted tubule* is located in the cortex. It comprises thin and thick straight parts and a convoluted part. These are parts of the tubule returning to the proximity of the glomerular capsule from which it took origin.

(i) Cells of the distal tubule are like those of the proximal tubule but surface microvilli are few and short. Basal infoldings are very deep, almost reaching the apex of the cell.

(ii) At the junction of the straight and convoluted tubules, the distal tubule fits between the afferent and efferent arterioles of the glomerulus of the renal corpuscle from which the tube originated, forming the *macula densa*. The distal convoluted tubule begins at the macula densa.

(iii) *Macular cells* (15–40 in number) in the wall of the distal tubule are cuboidal in shape and have many lateral interdigitations and short apical microvilli. They are thought to act as osmoreceptors.

(iv) In the notch between arterioles are *mesangial (lacis) cells*. These are spindle or irregular shaped cells embedded in an amorphous basal lamina-like mesangial matrix or extraglomerular mesangium. The matrix continues into and between the loops of glomerular capillaries, forming an *intraglomerular mesangium*.

(v) *Juxtaglomerular cells* are modified smooth muscle cells in the tunica media of the afferent arteriole of glomeruli. They contain cytoplasmic PAS positive granules and receive adrenergic nerve fibers.

(vi) The *juxtaglomerular apparatus or complex* comprises:
   1. Juxtaglomerular cells.
   2. Mesangial cells.
   3. Cells of the macula densa.
   4. Extraglomerular mesangium.

(vii) A fall in blood pressure or decrease in extracellular fluid causes hypertrophy of juxtaglomerular cells. Cytoplasmic granules contain the enzyme *renin* which are liberated into the bloodstream.

(viii) Renin acts on a plasma globulin (*angiotensinogen*), converting it to a decapeptide angiotensin I, which is inactive.

(ix) *Angiotensin I* is acted on by endothelium associated enzyme in the lung and is changed to an octapeptide angiotensin II which causes arteriolar vasoconstriction and raises blood pressure.

(x) *Angiotensin II*:
   1. Has a direct effect on smooth muscle cells in the walls of arterioles, causing their contraction and a rise in blood pressure.
   2. Stimulates the suprarenal cortex to secrete aldosterone which acts on the DCT cells, causing them to reabsorb more sodium and water. This in turn increases fluid in the circulatory system.

(xi) Juxtaglomerular cells respond to:
   1. Degree of stretch in the wall of the afferent arteriole.
   2. Chloride concentration in filtrate, reaching the distal convoluted tubule. Chloride concentration is a function of glomerular filtration rate.
   3. Adrenalin from sympathetic nerve stimulation which causes

juxtaglomerular cells to release renin.

D. *Arched collecting tubules* connect the nephron with an excretory duct.

E. *Straight collecting tubules* begin in medullary rays and are joined by other arched collecting tubules to form larger *papillary ducts* (of *Bellini*). These open onto the top of papillae, giving it a sieve-like appearance (the *area cribrosa*).

    (i) *Collecting ducts* are lined with simple cuboidal epithelium comprising clear cells with few organelles and occasional surface microvilli and dark cells which have surface microridges, more mitochondria and dense cytoplasm.

    (ii) The essential function of collecting tubules and ducts is to reabsorb water.

5. Blood Supply

5.1. The *renal artery* divides into *interlobular arteries* which pass from the hilum radially between the pyramids.

5.2. Each interlobular artery becomes an *arcuate artery* which bends horizontally at the junction between the cortex and medulla.

5.3. Arcuate arteries give radial *interlobular arteries* into the cortex and these become *afferent arterioles* of the glomeruli.

5.4. *Efferent arterioles* which leave glomeruli have a smaller lumen than that of afferent arterioles. As *straight arterioles*, they pass into the medulla to supply it.

5.5. *Straight venules* drain the medulla directly into *arcuate veins*.

5.6. A number of *stellate veins* draining the superficial cortex drain into *interlobular veins*.

5.7. The descending and ascending medullary vessels prevent excessive loss of osmotically active solute from the extracellular space.

5.8. Both limbs of the vessels are permeable to solutes and water. Blood entering the loop becomes increasingly hyperosmotic toward the medulla, a process reversed toward the cortex.

5.9. Looping of the medullary vessels allows:

A. Blood to provide oxygen to tissue.

B. Removal of absorbed water and solutes while preserving an hypertonic environment of the medulla.

6. Further Functions of the Kidney

6.1. The kidneys can rid the body of water by producing copious volumes of dilute urine or conserve water by producing small amounts of concentrated urine. To achieve this, they contain a *countercurrent multiplier* (*the loop of Henle*) and two *countercurrent exchangers* (the descending and ascending limbs of looping medullary vessels (vasa recta) and large collecting ducts passing through medullary interstitium.

6.2. In the urinary space, the ultrafiltrate is isotonic with blood.

6.3. In the proximal tubule, sodium, glucose, protein, amino acids, sulphate, phosphate and bicarbonate are actively reabsorbed and urea and chloride ions follow passively. Water follows passively to maintain osmotic equilibrium. Although 70–80% of filtered sodium chloride is reabsorbed, the filtrate remains isotonic with blood plasma.

6.4. The ascending limb of the loop of Henle in the medulla, chloride ions move actively into the extracellular space. Sodium follows to establish electrical equilibrium. Water permeability is low in this segment and does not equilibrate.

6.5. The filtrate entering the distal tubule in the cortex is hypotonic relative to blood plasma. In the distal tubule, sodium is actively reabsorbed with chloride following passively.

6.6. *Aldosterone* from the zona glomerulosa of the suprarenal cortex promotes sodium reabsorption in the distal convoluted tubule.

6.7. *Atrial natriuretic factor* (*ANF*), a peptide released by atrial muscle cells in response to atrial distension, promotes renal sodium and potassium excretion.

6.8. Collecting ducts pass back through hypertonic medullary tissue so that urine is finally concentrated.

6.9. *Anti-diuretic hormone* (*ADH*) from the posterior lobe of the hypophysis increases the permeability of collecting ducts to water.

6.10. Urine is acidified by:

A. Reabsorption of bicarbonate with secretion of hydrogen ion into the distal nephron.

B. Conversion of ammonia to ammonium ions in the distal nephron.

KIDNEY

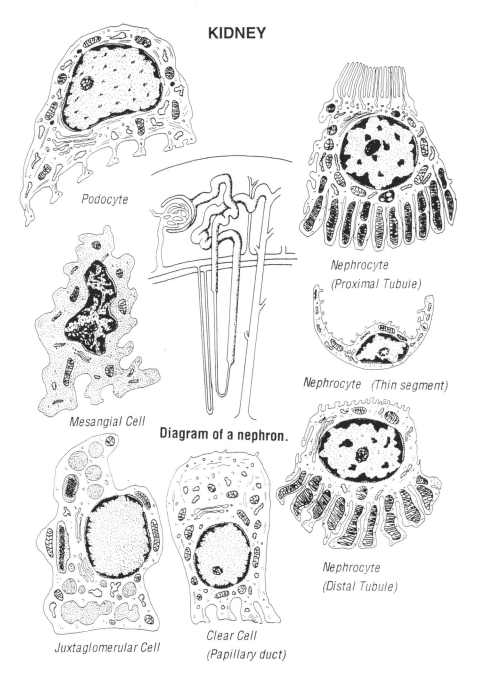

Podocyte

Nephrocyte
(Proximal Tubule)

Mesangial Cell

Diagram of a nephron.

Nephrocyte (Thin segment)

Nephrocyte
(Distal Tubule)

Juxtaglomerular Cell

Clear Cell
(Papillary duct)

Chapter 18

URINARY SYSTEM
2. RENAL PELVIS, CALYCES, URETER, BLADDER AND URETHRA

OBJECTIVES

After reading this chapter, you should be able to:

1. Give an account of the histologic structure of the ureter.
2. Describe the developmental origin of the ureter, its nerve supply and functions.
3. Describe the histologic structure of the bladder wall and how the epithelium (urothelium) adapts to changes in bladder distension.
4. Identify features observed in sections of the male and female urethra.
5. Give an account of the development of the urinary bladder.
6. Describe the sequential events in micturition.

CHAPTER OUTLINE

General structure of the renal pelvis, calyces and ureter. Ureters.

The bladder. General. Detailed structure of the bladder wall.

Male Urethra. Prostatic urethra. Membranous urethra. Cavernous (spongy) urethra.

Female Urethra.

Urination (Micturition).

Development of the bladder and urethra.

KEY WORDS, PHRASES, CONCEPTS

Renal pelvis
Transitional epithelium
(Urothelium)
Allantois
Muller's tubercle
Prostatic urethra
Urethral crest
Prostatic utricle
Spongy urethra
Corpus spongiosum penis
Micturition

Calyces
Plaques
Urogenital sinus
Cloacal septum
Trigone
Membranous urethra
Seminal colliculus
Prostatic sinus
Ureter
Corpora cavernosa penis
    Glans
    Tunica albuginea

RENAL PELVIS, CALYCES AND URETER

1. General Structure

The renal pelvis, calyces and ureter have the following basic structure:

1.1. The *adventitia* is a fibrous coat which blends with surrounding tissue. The fibrous coat of the renal pelvis is continuous with the renal capsule. The ureter lies beneath peritoneum where the adventitia is loose connective tissue containing adipocytes, blood and lymph vessels and nerves.

1.2. The *muscularis* of the pelvis, calyces and upper two thirds of the ureter comprises *inner longitudinal* and *outer circular layers* of smooth muscle.

   1.2.1. Circular muscle forms rings around the bases of renal papillae and their contraction causes a "milking" action.

   1.2.2. Peristaltic movements in the muscle layers of the ureter moves urine into the bladder at the rate of 15 drops per minute.

1.3. The *submucosa* is not clearly defined. Deeper layers of loose and elastic tissue permit formation of five characteristic major and minor longitudinal folds in the lamina propria. This produces a stellate-shaped lumen in cross sections.

1.4. The *mucosa* comprises:

   A. The *lamina propria*, which contains thin collagenous fibres. Papillae do not indent the epithelium.

B. The *basal lamina*, which is thin.

C. *Transitional epithelium* (urothelium), 2–3 cell layers thick in the calyx and 4–5 cell layers thick in the ureter.

    (i) The appearance of transitional epithelium in sections depends on degree of stretching. Relaxed epithelium is high with surface *facet cells* whose folded apical surfaces bulge into the lumen, a few layers of elongated *intermediate cells* and a single layer of *basal cells*.

    (ii) *Facet cells* have an apical cell membrane which contains alternate plaque and hinge-like interplaque regions. They contain discoid-shaped vesicles in their apical cytoplasm. When the bladder fills, these discoid vesicles fuse with the surface plasma membrane and hinge open, thereby allowing the surface to spread. The open halves of the discoid vesicles are known as plaques. Cytoplasmic filaments insert into the plaques which bear the strain of distension of the bladder.

    (iii) Fine processes of facet cells maintain contact with the basal lamina.

2. Ureters

2.1. *Ureters* follow an oblique course through the bladder wall and folds of bladder mucosa serve as covering flap valves. Stone impaction may occur at sites of ureteric constriction:

A. At its cranial end where the renal pelvis becomes the ureter.

B. Where the ureter crosses the brim of the lesser pelvis.

C. Where the ureter passes through the bladder wall.

2.2. The *muscularis* comprises inner longitudinal, middle circular and outer longitudinal layers of smooth muscle. The outer longitudinal muscle layer is most distinct in the lower third of the ureter where the inner longitudinal layer becomes less distinct.

2.3. The *blood supply* to the ureter is from several sources, the renal artery, aorta, testicular or ovarian artery, internal iliac artery, vesical and uterine arteries with much variation in the amounts supplied by each. There is a good longitudinal anastomosis in the adventitia.

2.4. The *nerve supply* is from contributions from the renal, aortic, superior and inferior hypogastric plexuses. A plexus of nerve fibres, small ganglia and isolated ganglion cells is found in the fibrous and muscular coats mostly in the lower parts of the ureter.

   A. Both sympathetic and parasympathetic systems are represented but their function is unclear. They can be stripped from the ureters without affecting muscle function.

   B. Excessive distension causes *renal colic* characterised by muscle spasm and spasmodic agonizing pain referred to cutaneous areas supplied by T11-L2.

3. The Bladder

3.1. The *urinary bladder* is a reservoir varying in size, shape, position and relationships with the amount of urine it contains.

3.2. The *mucous membrane* lining the interior of the bladder is only loosely attached to the subjacent muscular layer and develops folds when the bladder contracts.

3.3. The *trigone* is a smooth triangular area above and behind the internal orifice of the urethra and bounded by the points of entry of the ureters. The mucous membrane over the trigone is firmly bound to the subjacent muscle layer.

3.4. The *interureteric crest* connecting the ureteric openings is formed by a continuation of the muscle layers of the ureters into the bladder.

3.5. *Ureteric folds* laterally are caused by the ureters running obliquely through the bladder wall.

3.6. The *serous layer* (*serosa*) is a peritoneal cover limited to the superior surface only of the bladder.

3.7. The *muscular layer* consists of the detrusor muscle with external, internal longitudinal and middle oblique layers. There is much intermingling of fibres which are difficult to separate.

   A. The external longitudinal layer passes along the inferolateral border, over the apex on to the superior surface. Over the base, it blends with the capsule of the prostate or anterior wall of the vagina. On the front of the rectum, it forms the *rectovesical muscle*. Other fibres traverse the medial puboprostatic ligaments as the *pubovesical muscle*.

B. The middle circular layer is mostly oblique but circular near the neck of the bladder where it forms the *sphincter vesicae* or the *internal sphincter*. Continuous with prostatic muscle, fibres encircle the proximal urethra. The *sphincter urethrae* or the external sphincter is a circular band of striated muscle at the base of the prostate and part of the muscular urogenital diaphragm.

C. The inner longitudinal layer is thin. The *trigonal muscle* is a continuation of muscular coats of the ureter.

D. Two bands of oblique muscles fibres begin behind the ureters and converge to the median prostate. They maintain the oblique direction of the ureters, thereby preventing reflux of urine.

3.8. The *mucous membrane* of the bladder is pale pink in color and covered with urothelium 6–8 cell layers thick. There are no true glands in the mucous membrane but there are mucous follicles near the neck of the bladder.

3.9. The *lamina propria* is loose connective tissue and the mucosa is folded into *rugae* when the bladder is empty.

3.10. Autonomic and sensory nerves form a plexus, with ganglion cells, in the adventitia.

A. The vesical plexus comprises both sympathetic and parasympathetic motor nerves as well as sensory nerves.

B. Parasympathetic *nervi erigentes* (S2-4) are motor fibres to the fibres of the detrusor muscle. They inhibit the sphincter vesicae.

C. Striated muscle of the *sphincter urethrae* (external sphincter) is supplied by the internal pudendal nerve (S2-4).

D. Afferent nerves which respond to pain and bladder distension run with parasympathetic and sympathetic nerves. Section of nerves on only one side does not relieve pain originating from the bladder.

4. Male Urethra

4.1. The *prostatic urethra* is 3.5 cm long, fusiform in shape and crescentic in section. Epithelium is transitional with patches of stratified columnar epithelium.

A. On the posterior wall of the prostatic urethra is a prominent vertical ridge, the *urethral crest* with a gutter on each side, the *prostatic sinus*.

B. The *urethral crest* rises to a summit, the *seminal colliculus* onto which opens a diverticulum, the *prostatic utricle* formed from the entodermal vaginal plate.

C. On the lips of the utricle open the fine orifices of the *ejaculatory ducts*. These are formed by the union of the ductus deferens and duct of the seminal vesicle.

D. Many *prostatic ducts* open into the floor of the prostatic sinus.

4.2. The *membranous urethra* is 2 cm long, extending from the prostate to the penis. It pierces the striated muscles of the urogenital diaphragm and is lined with stratified columnar epithelium.

4.3. The *cavernous urethra* is 15 cm long, extending through the corpus spongiosum of the penis.

A. *Epithelium* lining the urethra is transitional near the bladder while the remainder is stratified or pseudostratified columnar containing scattered chromaffin cells. Near the meatus epithelium is stratified squamous.

B. *Glands* opening into the urethra are of three kinds:
   (i) Intraepithelial nests of mucous cells.
   (ii) *Urethral glands* (*of Littre*) branching mucous tubules extending into the lamina propria. They produce a secretion which contains glycosaminoglycans and protects the epithelium from acid urine.
   (iii) *Bulbourethral glands* are paired tubuloalveolar glands which open into the proximal cavernous urethra.

C. The *lamina propria* is loose connective tissue continuous with erectile tissue.

D. The *muscularis* in the prostatic and membranous urethra contains inner longitudinal and outer circular layers of smooth muscle. The cavernous urethra lacks a muscularis.

E. The *adventitia* is atypical. In the prostatic urethra, the layer is represented by the prostate. In the membranous urethra, it is the deep transverse perinei (skeletal) muscle and in the cavernous urethra, it is erectile tissue.

5. Female Urethra

5.1. The *female urethra* is 4 cm long and is homologous to the male prostatic and membranous urethrae.

5.2. *Epithelium* lining the lumen is transitional to stratified columnar then stratified squamous non-keratinized near the outlet. Nests of mucous cells and chromaffin cells are located in the epithelium and in diverticula (*urethral glands*).

5.3. The *lamina propria* is loose connective tissue containing venous plexuses. It is folded longitudinally, giving the lumen an irregular stellate shape.

5.4. The *muscular layer* comprises thick inner longitudinal and outer circular layers of smooth muscle. Near the neck of the bladder is a thickening of the circular layer (the involuntary sphincter) and below is circular skeletal muscle of the sphincter urethrae (the voluntary sphincter).

5.5. The *adventitia* is an indefinite layer of loose connective tissue which fuses with the fibrous coat of the vagina.

6. Urination (Micturition)

6.1. The abdominal wall and diaphragm first contract to increase intra-abdominal pressure.

6.2. Pubococcygeus muscle relaxes and the neck of the bladder then descends.

6.3. Downward movement of the bladder activates smooth muscle layers of the bladder wall (*detrusors*).

6.4. At the same time, longitudinal muscle fibres of the urethra (continuous with the detrusor) contract, shortening the urethra and widening its lumen.

6.5. Urine is expelled.

6.6. Pubococcygeus contracts, raising the neck of the bladder.

6.7. Detrusor and urethral muscles relax.

6.8. Finally the internal urethral orifice closes.

6.9. Clinically, if the pelvic floor is fixed so that the bladder cannot descend (e.g., with carcinoma), urination cannot be started or stopped voluntarily. Also:

A. With spinal cord transection, voluntary control of the bladder is lost.

B. With loss of autonomic motor nerves, no reflex function is possible and the detrusor acts independently and inefficiently.

C. With sensory nerve loss, sensation and reflex loss results in overdistension of the bladder.

7. Development of Bladder and Urethra

7.1. The common terminal part of the hindgut and allantois is the *cloaca*.

7.2. From 4–7 weeks, a wedge of mesenchyme, the *cloacal or urorectal septum* (formed in the angle between allantois and hindgut during cephalocaudal folding), pushes caudally and fuses with the cloacal membrane. This septum divides the cloacal membrane into a *urogenital membrane* anteriorly and an *anal membrane* posteriorly and the cloaca is divided into the *primitive urogenital* sinus anteriorly and the *rectum* dorsally.

7.3. Three parts of the urogenital sinus are distinguished:
   A. The *urinary bladder* connected to the allantois by a duct, the *urachus* (ouron (Gk) urine and cheo (Gk) I pour).
   B. The *vesicourethral canal* above the site of entry of the mesonephric ducts (pelvic part of the urogenital sinus).
   C. The *definitive urogenital sinus* below the entry of the mesonephric ducts (phallic part of the urogenital sinus).

7.4. The position of entry of the mesonephric ducts, changes through absorption of the ducts into the wall of the sinus. For a while, the absorbed wall is covered internally by mesoderm.
   A. The ureters, initially outbuddings of the mesonephric ducts, come to enter the bladder separately and with further absorption, their orifices move cranially and laterally.
   B. The mesonephric ducts then enter the upper part of the urethra.

7.5. In the adult, the bladder is connected to the umbilicus by the *median umbilical ligament* formed by obliteration of the *urachus* (the duct connecting the *allantois* and the *cloaca*).

7.6. The fate of the definitive urogenital sinus differs in the sexes:
   A. In the male, the small pelvic portion forms the lower part of the prostatic urethra and membranous urethra.
   B. In the female, the definitive urogenital sinus forms part of the urethra, lower one fifth of the vagina and vestibule.

7.7. At the end of the third month, epithelium of the cranial urethra proliferates and buds into surrounding mesoderm. In the male, this leads to formation of the prostate and in the female, to *urethral* and *paraurethral glands*.

URINARY BLADDER

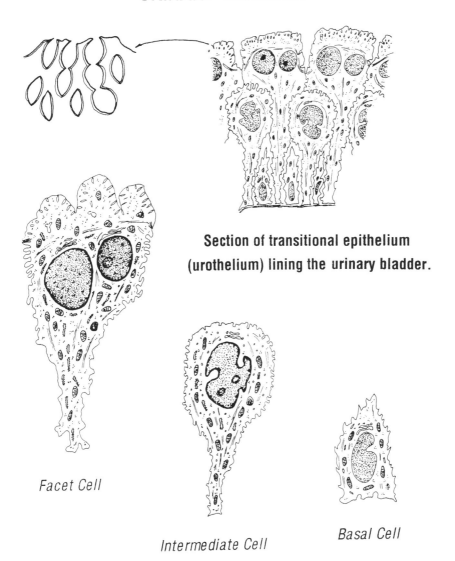

Section of transitional epithelium (urothelium) lining the urinary bladder.

Facet Cell

Intermediate Cell

Basal Cell

Chapter 19

MALE REPRODUCTIVE SYSTEM
1. THE TESTIS

OBJECTIVES

After reading this chapter, you should be able to:
1. Give a description of the histologic structure of the testis.
2. Give an account of the structure of a mature spermatozoon.
3. Describe the development of the testis.
4. Compare and contrast mitosis and meiosis.
5. Describe the stages of spermatogenesis.
6. Describe the process of spermiogenesis.
7. Discuss the concepts of a cycle of seminiferous epithelium and theduration of spermatogenesis.
8. Describe the histologic structure and function of Sertoli cells and the concept of the "blood-testis barrier"
9. Describe the histologic structure and function of Interstitial cells.
10. Outline the hormonal factors influencing testis function.

CHAPTER OUTLINE

General. Composition of the male reproductive system.

Internal genitalia.

The testes.

General.

Detailed structure. Seminiferous epithelium. Structure of mature spermatozoon. Terminology Spermatogenesis. Spermatocytogenesis. Spermiogenesis. Meiosis. Mitosis. Spermatogonia. Primary spermatocytes. Secondary spermatocytes. Spermatids.

Cycles of seminiferous epithelium. Sertoli cells. Functions of Sertoli cells. Interstitial cells (of Leydig). Functions of interstitial cells.

Boundary layers of Seminiferous Tubules.

Factors influencing testicular function.

Development of the testis.

KEY WORDS, PHRASES, CONCEPTS

Primordial germ cells
Primitive spermatogonia
(Prespermatogonia)
Spermatogonia (Pale type A,
 Dark type A, Type B)
Primary spermatocytes
Stem cells
Secondary spermatocytes
Spermatozoa
Spermatogenesis
Testis
Visceral layer of tunica
 vaginalis testis
Tunica albuginea
Mediastinum testis
Seminiferous tubules
Sertoli cells
Myoid cells
Testosterone
Meiosis
Spermiogenesis

Acrosome
 Acrosome vesicle
Head cap
Spermatozoon
 Head, Midpiece, Tail
Mitochondrial sheath
Principal sheath, End piece
 Axoneme, Coarse fibers
 Outer dense fibers,
 Dorsal and ventral columns
 Fibrous ribs
Interstitial cells (Leydig)
Hormonal basis of testis
 function
Androgen binding protein
Inhibin
Testicular fluid
Blood testis permeability
 barrier
Spermatids
Intercellular bridges

1. General

1.1. The male reproductive system comprises:
   A. Two *gonads* (gone (Gk) generation) the testes which produce germ cells and male sex hormone, located in the scrotum.
   B. A *tubular system* in which germ cells mature, are stored and delivered at ejaculation lead from each testis.
   C. *Accessory glands* which provide a vehicle for germ cells.
   D. A *copulatory organ*, the penis (penis (L) a tail).
1.2. The testis, ducts and accessory glands are the *internal genitalia* and the penis and scrotum are the *external genitalia.*
1.3. Internal genitalia comprise the testes, epididymes (epi (Gk) upon and didymos (Gk) double), ductus deferens, seminal vesicles, ejaculatory ducts, prostate gland and bulbourethral glands. The testes are both exocrine (cytogenic) and endocrine glands.
1.4. *Spermatozoa* (sperma (Gk) sperm and zoon (Gk) animal) produced in the testes pass to the epididymis for storage. At emission, they pass through the ductus deferens, ejaculatory duct and urethrae to the external urethral orifice.
1.5. The remaining glands, the seminal vesicles, prostate and bulbourethral glands add secretions to the composite seminal fluid.

2. Testes. General

2.1. Each *testis* (testis (L) a witness, an admissible witness in Roman law had to have testicles present) is an ovoid organ 4.5 cm long, 2.5 cm in breadth, and 3 cm in anteroposterior diameter weighing about 25 g.
2.2. The testis is suspended in a serous cavity, the *processus vaginalis*, a remnant of a peritoneal pouch which preceded the descent of the testis during development.
2.3. The serous membrane covering the front and sides of the testis and epididymis is the *visceral layer of the tunica vaginalis* which is reflected onto the inner lining of the scrotum as the *parietal layer of the tunica vaginalis.*
2.4. The *tunica albuginea* (albus (L) white) is a thick, dense white fibrous capsule surrounding the testis.

2.5. Ductules, vessels and nerves leave or enter the posterior margin of the testis through the *mediastinum testis*, a thickening of the tunica albuginea which is devoid of a visceral covering of tunica vaginalis.

2.6. The *tunica vasculosa* on the inner aspect of the tunica albuginea, is a loose connective tissue layer containing large blood vessels of the testis.

2.7. *Septulae testis* are fine strands of loose connective tissue radiating from the mediastinum to the tunica albuginea. They divide the testis into some 250 conical compartments (*lobules*).

2.8. *Lobules* of the testis each contain one to four sperm-producing convoluted *seminiferous tubules*. These are about 60 cm long, with a combined length of 250 meters.

2.9. Connective tissue spaces between seminiferous tubules contain blood vessels, nerves and extensive lymphatic sinusoids. There is also a population of macrophages, mast cells, fibroblasts and endocrine interstitial or Leydig cells.

3. Detailed Structure. Seminiferous Epithelium

3.1. *Seminiferous tubules* of the testis are lined with stratified *seminiferous (germinal) epithelium* comprising germinal cells which proliferate from the periphery of the tubule toward the lumen and a population of non-proliferating supporting (Sertoli) cells.

3.2. The *mature spermatozoon* comprises:

(i) The head of a spermatozoon in man is almond shaped, 4–5 μm long and 2.5–3.5 μm wide. It comprises a condensed nucleus and *acrosomal (head) cap* which contains glycoprotein and lysosomal enzymes.

(ii) The *neck region* is located behind the head and first gyre of the mitochondrial sheath of the middle piece. The neck contains some cytoplasm, the connecting piece, 9 *segmented columns* that fuse with 9 *outer coarse (dense) fibers* of the *middle piece* and a pair of *centrioles*. Two of the columns form *major columns*, one of which expands into a *capitulum* to fuse with an amorphous *basal plate* located in an *implantation fossa* at the caudal end of the head. *Minor columns* converge on major columns at the base of the head.

(iii) The *middle piece* is 5–7 μm long and 1 μm in diameter. It comprises:
- (a) Outer helicoidally arranged mitochondria in a *mitochondrial sheath*;
- (b) Nine *coarse outer fibers* (derived from the segmented columns of the connecting piece) of which fibers 1, 5 and 6 are largest; and
- (c) A *core* (*axoneme*) comprising a central pair of microtubules surrounded by nine peripheral pairs of microtubules.

The *annulus* is a dense ring to which the flagellar membrane is closely applied at the end of the middle piece.

(iv) The principal piece is 45 μm long and 0.5 μm in diameter but tapering. It has an outer fibrous sheath of branching circumferential fibers, nine longitudinal coarse outer fibers (reducing to seven as fibers 3 and 8 become apposed longitudinal columns) and a central axoneme. The fibers are accessory contractile elements.

(v) The *end piece* is 5 μm long, is the axoneme covered only by a cell membrane.

(vi) The fibrous sheath of the principal piece divides the tail into a minor compartment of 3 coarse fibers and a major compartment of 4 coarse fibers.

(vii) The principal plane of bending of the tail is perpendicular to the dorsoventral axis of the head. The longitudinal columns of the fibrous sheath are placed dorsally and ventrally and the tail has a more rapid power stroke toward the side of the four coarse fibers.

4. Spermatogenesis

4.1. Terminology:
- (a) *Spermatogenesis* is the development of the most immature germ cells from spermatogonia to spermatozoa.
- (b) *Spermatocytogenesis* refers to the cytological changes in the transformation of spermatogonia to spermatids.
- (c) *Spermiogenesis* refers to the cytological transformation (metamorphosis) of spermatids to spermatozoa.
- (d) *Meiosis* is the particular nuclear division reserved for germ cells. It consists of a reductional division in which the number of

chromosomes is halved (haploid or n) with 2n DNA content followed by an equatorial division. The resulting cells are called *gametes (ova or sperm)*.

(e) *Mitosis* is the method of cell division of all somatic cells (except germ cells) consisting of indirect nuclear division followed by division of the cell body. It results in the formation of two daughter cells with an identical (diploid) number of chromosomes (2n) and same content of DNA as the original cell.

4.2. *Spermatogonia* (sperma (Gk) sperm and gone (Gk) generation) are immature stem cells bordering the outer basal lamina of the seminiferous tubule.

(a) *Dark type A (Ad) spermatogonia* have dark nuclei with fine chromatin and irregular nucleoli. The cytoplasm has no RER and the Golgi complex is inconspicuous or absent. These cells are thought to be reserve stem cells or long cycling cells.

(b) *Pale type A (Ap)* spermatogonia have pale nuclei and divide mitotically to become type B cells.

(c) *Type B spermatogonia* are pear-shaped cells contacting the basal lamina by a narrow base. They have spherical nuclei with chromatin adjacent to the nuclear membrane and a central nucleolus. They divide mitotically into primary spermatocytes.

(d) *Cytokinesis* in type A and B spermatogonia is incomplete, leaving protoplasmic intercellular bridges 2–3 μm wide between four primary spermatocytes, eight secondary spermatocytes and sixteen spermatids. Divisions within a syncytium of partly separated cells are synchronous but a few of the component cells do not divide at all.

(e) Proliferation of spermatogonia is regulated by a metabolic inhibitor *chalone* which is produced by dividing spermatogonia and which inhibits mitosis of remaining stem cells.

4.3. *Primary spermatocytes* (sperma (Gk) sperm and kytos (Gk) cell) are larger cells than spermatogonia. They have a nucleus with conspicuous heterochromatin strands and a diploid chromosome content. The cytoplasm contains centrioles, peripheral mitochondria, RER and Golgi complex and is interconnected to adjacent spermatocytes by intercellular bridges. Primary spermatocytes pass through the leptotene, zygotene, pachytene and diplotene stages of the first meiotic division to become secondary spermatocytes.

4.4. *Secondary spermatocytes* are much smaller than primary spermatocytes. Their nucleus is spherical with pale granular chromatin and contains a haploid (23) number of chromosomes. Interphase of secondary spermatocytes is very brief (circa 8 hrs) so they are infrequently seen in sections. They enter the second maturation division to become spermatids.

4.5. *Spermatids* mature into spermatozoa through a series of nuclear and cytoplasmic modifications or metamorphosis known as spermiogenesis. These sequentially are:

(a) The *Golgi Phase* in which secretion granules rich in glycoprotein (proacrosomal granules) appear in the Golgi complex. The granules coalesce to form a large single granule (the acrosomal granule). The Golgi complex forms an acrosomal vesicle around the granule. The acrosome thus formed contains lysosomal enzymes hyaluronidase and a trypsin-like enzyme used when the spermatozoon penetrates between cells of the corona radiata and through the amorphous zona pellucida to reach the ovum. Opposite the acrosome, a basophilic fibrogranular chromatoid body transforms into the annulus. Two centrioles move to a position near the nucleus opposite the developing acrosome. The proximal centriole attaches to the caudal pole of the nucleus in the implantation fossa. The distal centriole induces production of the flagellum.

(b) In the *Cap Phase*, the acrosomal vesicle flattens to form the head cap of the spermatozoon and spreads thinly over the anterior half of the nucleus. The Golgi complex disengages from the acrosomal vesicle and the distal centriole gives rise to rudiments of the axial filament (9 + 2 microtubule pairs). The nucleus elongates and chromatin condenses.

(c) The *Acrosome Phase* is characterized by orientation of the anterior pole of the spermatid toward the base of the seminiferous tubule. Contents of the acrosomal vesicle condense over the nucleus, forming the acrosome. Microtubules form a cylindrical sheath attached to the caudal pole of the nucleus and form the manchette (manchette (Fr) a cuff). The annulus migrates down the tail. Coarse outer fibers form in the neck region. Mitochondria wrap around the coarse outer fibers. Nuclear chromatin condensation increases.

(d) The *Maturation Phase* is characterized by pinching off and phagocytosis of residual spermatid cytoplasm by Sertoli cells. Sertoli cells permit release of late spermatids into the lumen of seminiferous tubules and finally, intercellular bridges are broken.

5. Cycles of Seminiferous Epithelium

5.1. A repeating sequence of characteristic groupings of germ cells around a Sertoli cell seen in sections is a stage in a cyclic process of spermatogenesis.

5.2. Six such consecutive sequential groupings (stages) are identified in man and upon the reappearance of the first stage, the seminiferous epithelium has undergone a cycle.

5.3. In man, different stages occupy small patch-like areas along the length of the tubule.

5.4. The duration of a cycle in man is about 16 days.

5.5. Spermatogenesis requires four cycles or about 64 days.

6. **Sertoli cells** (*Sustentacular or Supporting cells, Sustentocytes*) are non dividing, tall, pyramidal cells attached to the basal lamina of seminiferous tubules.

6.1. The nucleus is ovoid and infolded with characteristic tripartite nucleolus.

6.2. The cytoplasm contains long slender mitochondria, lipid droplets, glycogen granules, filaments and microtubules surrounding the nucleus, RER and SER, lysosomes, inclusion bodies (of Charcot-Bottcher) and a very large Golgi complex.

6.3. Tight junctions between adjacent Sertoli cells subdivide the seminiferous epithelium into a *basal compartment* (containing spermatogonia, preleptotene and leptotene spermatocytes) and an *adluminal compartment* (containing more advanced spermatocytes and spermatids).

6.4. Spermatogenic cells lie in deep, membrane-lined recesses of Sertoli cells. Around spermatids, the cytoplasm of Sertoli cells contains filaments and flattened cisternae of endoplasmic reticulum.

6.5. Functions of Sertoli cells:

(a) They provide *mechanical support* and *structural cohesion* between elements of seminiferous epithelium.

(b) *Provide nutrients* to germ cells (but there is no direct evidence for this function).

(c) *Phagocytose degenerating cells* and cytoplasmic remnants of developing spermatozoa.

(d) *Move germ cells* from the basal lamina toward the lumen and release spermatids. They contain actin and possibly are contractile.

(e) *Secrete androgen binding protein (ABP)* under the control of FSH and testosterone. ABP concentrates testosterone in seminiferous epithelium.

(f) Produce *calmodulin* which modulates calcium dependent functions in eukaryotic cells.

(g) *Produce plasminogen activator* which temporarily breaks Sertoli cell tight junctions and allows spermatocytes to migrate adluminally.

(h) *Produce anti-Müllerian hormone* which causes regression of the Müllerian (paramesonephric) duct system, which give rise to most of the female internal genitalia.

(i) Sertoli cells *resist heat, radiation and some toxic agents* that destroy spermatogenic cells.

7. **Interstitial cells (of Leydig)** are irregular polyhedral acidophilic cells 14–21 μm in diameter found singly or in clusters between seminiferous tubules and adjacent capillaries.

7.1. The nucleus is eccentric, poor in heterochromatin and contains one or two nucleoli.

7.2. Cells have abundant cytoplasm, contain relatively few free ribosomes and RER cisternae, have a distinct Golgi complex, numerous lysosomes, lipid droplets, lipofuscin granules, lipochrome, crystalloids (of Reinke) and an extensively developed SER.

7.3. Functions of Interstitial cells:

They produce *testosterone* from the precursor cholesterol which has the effects of:

(a) *Stimulating spermatogenesis*.

(b) Stimulating *development and maintenance of male secondary sex characteristics*.

(c) Acting on the brain to *maintain male sexual behavior*.

(d) By negative feedback, *inhibiting secretion of hypothalamic*

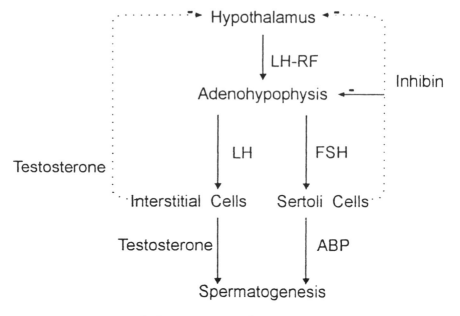

Control of testosterone and spermatogenesis.

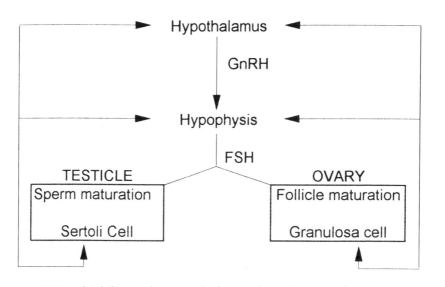

FSH and Inhibin in the control of testicular and ovarian functions.

gonadotrophin releasing factor and hypophyseal gonadotrophin.
(e) *Stimulating protein synthesis* (the anabolic effect).
(f) Characteristic structure and endocrine functions of interstitial cells are controlled by the hypophyseal gonadotrophic hormone luteinizing hormone (LH), also known as *interstitial cell stimulating hormone (ICSH)*.
(g) Negative feedback of testosterone *inhibits gonadotrophin releasing factor* from the hypothalamus and LH secretion.
(h) High concentrations of testosterone near seminiferous tubules are necessary to maintain spermatogenesis. Lower concentrations in the peripheral circulation are sufficient to maintain libido and secondary sex characteristics.

8. *Boundary layers of seminiferous tubules* comprise:
   (i) *Basal lamina* adjacent to seminiferous epithelium.
   (ii) *Clear zone* containing collagen fibrils.
   (iii) A *layer of flattened, actin-containing myoid cells* which may contract and contribute to the propulsion of sperm and testicular fluid to the rete testis.

9. Factors Influencing Testicular Function

9.1. *Noxious factors* such as infections, alcohol, dietary deficiencies (vitamins A and E).

9.2. *Local factors*: Testicular temperature is normally maintained at about 2 degrees centigrade cooler than that of the abdominal cavity by counter current cooling of the testicular arterial blood by the surrounding draining pampiniform venous plexus. Cryptorchidism or undescended testis leads to irreversible changes if not corrected by 5 years of age.

9.3. *Age*: Some degenerating tubules occur in men older than 35 years of age. Spermatogenesis decreases after 55 years but continues into the senile period. With increasing age, the numbers of abnormal, non-viable sperm increase in the ejaculate.

9.4. *Vasectomy* may result in antibodies entering the lumen of the rete testis and epididymis, thereby affecting the fertilizing capacity of spermatozoa. Epididymal macrophages are involved in sperm resorption.

10. Development of the Testis

10.1. At 5–6 weeks, the sex of the individual cannot be determined macroscopically or microscopically. Both male and female have a double set of ducts and the gonads (testis and ovary) are indistinguishable. This is known as the *indifferent stage*.

10.2. Peritoneum (coelomic epithelium) thickens into longitudinal *gonadal (or genital) ridges* situated medial to the mesonephric ridges and lateral to the dorsal mesentery.

10.3. Gonadal ridges comprise a superficial "germinal" epithelium and central mesenchymal blastema.

10.4. Surface epithelium proliferates, penetrating the mesenchyme to form *sex cords*.

10.5. *Primordial germ cells* are first identifiable in the wall of the yolk sac near the allantois. They migrate via the entoderm through the dorsal mesentery to the genital ridge until some 1400 cells are present in the testis at the 4 mm stage.

10.6. Primordial germ cells associate with sex cords which branch and anastomose in the blastema as *testis cords*.

10.7. Surface epithelium becomes separated from the cords by a thickening of the mesenchyme which condenses into the *tunica albuginea*.

10.8. Testis cords become horseshoe-shaped. The proximal part remains as straight *tubuli recti* and the distal part arches and convolutes, becoming *tubuli contorti*. They converge on the *rete testis* in the *mediastinum* of the testis.

10.9. Sex cords remain solid until puberty when they acquire a lumen and become *seminiferous tubules*.

10.10. *Interstitial cells* differentiate from the mesenchyme.

TESTIS – SPERMATOGENESIS

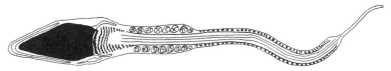

Spermatozoon

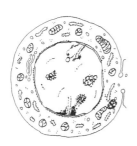

Primary spermatocyte

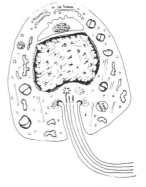

Spermatid

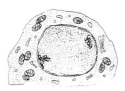

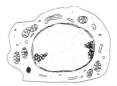

Spermatogonium A

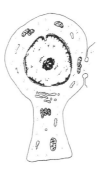

Spermatogonium B

MALE REPRODUCTIVE SYSTEM

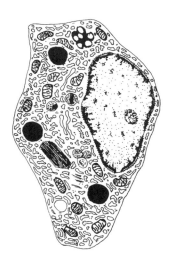

Interstitial Cell

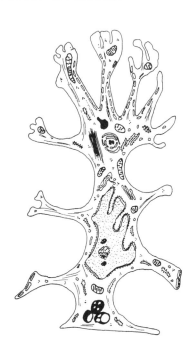

Sustentacular Cell
(Sertoli Cell)

MALE REPRODUCTIVE SYSTEM

EFFERENT DUCTULES

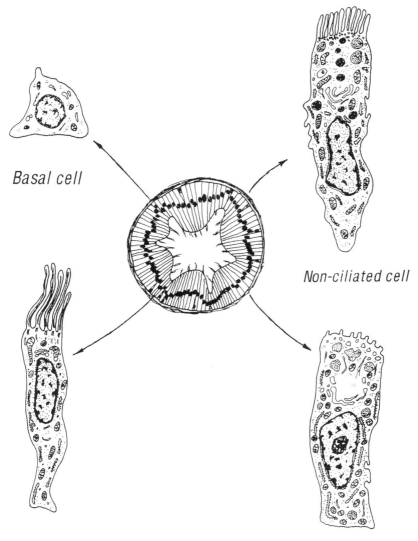

Basal cell

Non-ciliated cell

Ciliated cell

Non-ciliated cell

Chapter 20

MALE REPRODUCTIVE SYSTEM
2. GENITAL DUCT SYSTEM, ACCESSORY GLANDS AND EXTERNAL GENITALIA

OBJECTIVES

After reading this chapter, you should be able to:

1. Describe the development of the male genital duct system and give an account of the remnants of the mesonephric and paramesonephric ducts in the adult.
2. Identify the histologic features of all segments of the male genital duct; tubuli recti, rete testis, ductuli efferentes, ductus deferens, ejaculatory duct and urethra.
3. Describe the histologic structure and functions of the accessory glands; the prostate, seminal vesicles and bulbo-urethral glands.
4. Describe the composition of seminal fluid and glandular and muscular events in ejaculation.
5. Describe the histologic structure of the penis and its blood supply in detumescence and erection.
6. Discuss the development of the urogenital sinus and penis as well as the descent of the testis.

CHAPTER OUTLINE

Detailed structure. Rete testis. Straight tubules. Efferent ductules.

Duct of the Epididymis.

Ductus Deferens. Functions of the ductus deferens. Composition of the spermatic cord.

Development of the duct system.

Accessory Glands. Seminal Vesicles. Prostate. Bulbourethral glands. Seminal fluid.

External genitalia. Scrotum.

Development of genital ligaments.

Cryptorchidism.

Penis. Blood supply of the cavernous bodies. Erection and ejaculation.

Development of the external genitalia.

KEY WORDS, PHRASES, CONCEPTS

Rete testis
Efferent ductules
Appendix testis
Superior aberrant ductules
Paradidymis
Appendix epididymis
Ductus epididymis
Ductus deferens
Spermatic cord
Seminal vesicle
Ejaculatory ducts
Prostatic urethra
Urethral crest
Prostatic sinus
Seminal colliculus
Prostatic utricle
Prostate

Penis
Corpus cavernosum urethrae
(corpus spongiosum)
Corpora cavernosa penis
Erectile tissue
Helicine arteries
Nutrient arteries
Arteriovenous anastomoses
Cloacal eminence
Cloacal fold
Genital swelling
Urethral fold
Scrotal folds
Prepuce
Ligamentum testis
Gubernaculum testis
Vaginal process

Principal cells

Basal cells

Bulbourethral glands

Seminal fluid

Tunica vaginalis

Suspensory ligament of the testis

Cryptorchidism

Ejaculation

1. Detailed Structure

1.1. *Convoluted seminiferous tubules* drain into *straight tubules* (*tubuli recti*) approaching the *mediastinum testis*. Straight tubules are lined with simple columnar or cuboidal epithelium comprising only Sertoli cells without seminiferous epithelium.

1.2. The *rete testis* (rete (L) a net) is an anastomosing network of tubules located in the mediastinum testis. They are lined with simple cuboidal to columnar cells, some of which bear a single flagellum.

1.3. *Efferent ductules* are 15–20 tubules which pass laterally into the *head of the epididymis* after perforating the tunica albuginea. At first, straight in the mediastinum, efferent ductules become convoluted, forming conical masses or *lobules of the epididymis* which together form the *head of the epididymis*.

    1.3.1. The lining of efferent ductules comprises alternating groups of simple and pseudostratified epithelium. Columnar ciliated cells alternate with shorter non-ciliated cells with surface microvilli which are absorptive cells and secretory. Cilia on the ciliated cells beat towards the epididymis and are the only cilia in the entire male duct system.

    1.3.2. Externally, the tubule contour is smooth and surrounded by a basal lamina, a thin layer of smooth muscle and elastic fibers.

1.4. The *epididymis* is a comma-shaped body on the lateral and posterior surface of the testis comprising:

    A. An enlarged *head* which contains the efferent ductules in lobules of the epididymis.

    B. A *body* containing the highly convoluted duct of the epididymis.

    C. A *tail* containing the duct of the epididymis which continues into the ductus deferens.

    1.4.1. The *duct of the epididymis* is a single, slender, coiled duct about 4 meters long which develops from the mesonephric duct.

1.4.2. Epithelium lining the duct is pseudostratified columnar comprising:

    A. *Basal cells* believed to differentiate into principal cells.

    B. *Principal cells* characterized by an infolded basal nucleus, basal RER, supranuclear SER, lipofuscin granules, a large Golgi complex, lysosomes and micropinocytotic vesicles. The apical plasmalemma bears a tuft of stereocilia which are 40–80 μm long non-motile microvilli.

1.4.3. The duct is surrounded by a circular layer of smooth muscle.

1.4.4. *Functions* of the epididymis include:

    A. It acts as a *storage site for spermatozoa*. Passage through this tube segment takes about 6 weeks.

    B. *Principal cells secrete enzymes* necessary for metabolism and maturation of spermatozoa.

    C. *Principal cells resorb fluid* leaving the testis.

1.5. The *ductus deferens* (defere (L) to carry down) is a thick walled muscular tube extending from the tail of the epididymis ascending from the scrotum in the spermatic cord to enter the pelvis at the deep inguinal ring.

1.5.1. In the pelvis, its lumen enlarges behind the bladder into an ampulla. It narrows and joins the excretory duct of the seminal vesicle to form the *ejaculatory duct*.

1.5.2. *Ejaculatory ducts* pierce the base of the prostate to open on the summit of the *urethral crest* on the posterior wall of the *prostatic urethra* on each side of the *prostatic utricle*, a remnant of the Müllerian duct.

1.5.3. Epithelium lining the ductus deferens is pseudostratified. Columnar cells bear surface *stereocilia* while basal cells are considered to replace the columnar cells.

1.5.4. The *lamina propria* is a thin layer of dense connective tissue. The mucosa forms 4–6 longitudinal folds which gives a stellate shape to the lumen of the duct in cross sections.

1.5.5. The outer *muscularis* consists of thick layers of smooth muscle (1–5 mm) arranged in thin inner longitudinal, thick middle circular and thick outer longitudinal layers.

1.5.6. *Functions* of the ductus deferens.

    A. Contraction of the longitudinal fibers in the muscle wall shortens and widens the ductus immediately before ejaculation, sucking epididymal contents into the ductus. The ejaculatory duct remains closed.

   B. At ejaculation, contraction of the entire wall forces contents into the ejaculatory duct and prostatic urethra.

   C. The ductus depends for its normal morphology and function on hormonal support.

1.6. The *spermatic cord* is a composite structure extending from the posterior border of the testis to the deep inguinal ring. Its *contents* are:

A. Ductus deferens posteriorly.

B. Artery of the ductus deferens, a branch of the umbilical artery.

C. Testicular artery, a branch of the abdominal aorta.

D. Cremasteric artery, a branch of the inferior epigastric artery.

E. Testicular veins which form the pampiniform plexus which surrounds the testicular artery and cools arterial blood before it reaches the testis.

F. Nerves including branches of the genital branch of the genitofemoral nerve and the testicular and deferential autonomic plexuses.

G. Lymphatics draining to lumbar nodes on the aorta.

H. Remnants of the vaginal process, a peritoneal sac which evaginated into the scrotum in advance of the descent of the testis.

Coverings of the cord are:

Internal spermatic fascia from fascia transversalis.

Cremasteric fascia from the internal oblique muscle.

External spermatic fascia from external oblique muscle.

2. Development of the Duct System

2.1. At 6 weeks in the indifferent stage when both male and female gonads and ducts are indistinguishable, there are two parallel, longitudinal ducts in the gonadal ridges which reach the cloaca caudally.

2.2. The *paramesonephric duct* arises as a longitudinal invagination of the coelomic epithelium. It remains open cranially. Caudally, it crosses in front of the mesonephric duct, fuses with its opposite in the midline and contacts the posterior wall of the *urogenital sinus* between the mesonephric ducts at the Müllerian tubercle. The paramesonephric duct largely degenerates in the male but leaves a small vesicular appendage, the *appendix testis* attached to the upper end of the testis.

2.3. Of the mesonephric duct:

A. Excretory tubules disappear except opposite the testis where they become the *efferent ductules*. The cranial 5–12 excretory tubules may remain as vestigal *cranial aberrant ductules,* a narrow tube in the head of the epididymis attached to the rete testis. The caudal tubules leave the *paradidymis,* a few blind tubules above the head of the epididymis in the spermatic cord.

B. The mesonephric duct leaves a pedunculated appendage on the head of the epididymis, the *appendix epididymis*. It also gives rise to the convoluted, elongated epididymis, ductus deferens and ejaculatory duct.

3. Seminal Vesicles

3.1. *Seminal vesicles* develop as diverticula from the wall of the ductus deferens near its entry into the prostate.

3.2. Each is a convoluted glandular sac 5–10 cm long situated behind the prostate and lateral to the ampulla.

3.3. The central lumen is irregular and highly recessed with saclike evaginations but no real alveoli.

3.4. The *mucosa* is thrown into complex deep branched infoldings which appear like diverticulae in sections. The mucosa comprises:

A. *Pseudostratified non-ciliated epithelium. Columnar (Principal) cells* contain secretory granules, lipofuscin granules and lipid droplets. *Basal cells* rest on the basal lamina. The epithelium depends on testosterone support while its secretion is yellowish, gelatinous, sticky, mucoid and weakly alkaline containing prostaglandins and fructose.

B. The *lamina propria* is thin in branching folds of loose connective tissue which contains elastic fibers.

3.5. The *muscularis* is arranged in inner circular and outer longitudinal layers of smooth muscle.

3.6. The adventitia is loose connective tissue containing elastic fibers forming a capsule.

4. Prostate

4.1. The *prostate* (from pro (Gk) before and istanai (Gk) to stand, i.e., the organ that stands before the bladder) is a chestnut-shaped gland contacting the base of the bladder and surrounding the first or prostatic part of the urethra.

4.2. It comprises three lobes divided into *mucosal glands*, short invaginations of urethral epithelium, *submucosal glands*, tubuloalveolar glands beneath the urethral epithelium and *main prostatic glands*, an aggregate of 30–50 tubuloalveolar glands.

4.3. The glands open into the prostatic urethra through 15–30 ducts into the prostatic sinus on either side of the seminal colliculus.

4.4. A thin fibroelastic *capsule* contains smooth muscle fibers which penetrate between lobules. A loose outermost sheath is derived from visceral pelvic fascia and contains the prostatic venous plexus.

4.5. Secretory alveoli and tubules vary greatly in size, degree of branching and in shape.

4.6. Glandular epithelium is simple columnar or pseudostratified:

A. *Principal cells* are columnar, secretory cells which contain supranuclear secretory granules and have a high content of acid phosphatase.

B. *Basal cells* are thought to be precursors of principal cells.

4.7. Secretion of the prostate is thin, colorless and slightly acid (pH 6.5). It contains proteolytic enzymes (notably fibrinolysin which liquifies semen, zinc, citric acid and acid phosphatase, the latter two being the basis of sensitive tests of prostate function).

4.8. *Prostatic concretions* (*corpora amylacea*) are small, concentric lamellated bodies 2–20 μm in diameter. They are thought to be secretory condensations around cell fragments. They may calcify and are more common with increasing age.

4.9. Prostatic epithelium requires testosterone support.

5. Bulbourethral Glands

5.1. Bulbourethral glands are pea-sized, compound tubuloalveolar glands situated on each side of the bulb of the urethra. They connect by long ducts with the penile urethra.

5.2. They have a dense connective tissue capsule within skeletal muscle of the urogenital diaphragm.

5.3. The stroma is dense connective tissue dividing the parenchyma into small lobules.

5.4. Parenchyma is simple cuboidal or columnar mucus secreting cells.

5.5. Secretion is clear and viscous, contains galactose, galactosamine, galacturonic acid, sialic acid and methylpentose and acts as a lubricant of the urethra.

6. Seminal Fluid

6.1. *Seminal fluid* is a yellowish, slightly opalescent viscous fluid mixture of secretions of the testis, epididymis, seminal vesicles, prostate, bulbourethral glands and urethral glands.

6.2. Spermatozoa make up 10% of the 3.5 ml ejaculate (60 000 per ml). In addition, seminal fluid normally contains occasional epithelial cells, Sertoli cells, spermatogonia, lymphocytes, prostatic concretions, pigment granules, lipid droplets, amino acids, cholesterol, lactic acid, fructose, hyaluronidase and prostaglandins.

7. External Genitalia

7.1. The *scrotum* (scortum (L) a skin or hide) contains the testes, epididymes and spermatic cords and a division of the original coelom, the tunica vaginalis testis.

7.1.2. The wall comprises layers represented in the anterior abdominal wall:

A. *Skin*

B. *Dartos muscle* and fascia (equivalent to abdominal fatty and membranous layers of superficial fascia).

C. *External spermatic fascia* (equivalent to external oblique aponeurosis).

D. *Cremaster muscle* (equivalent to the fleshy fibers of internal oblique and transversalis muscles).

E. *Internal spermatic fascia* (equivalent to fascia transversalis).

F. *Areolar tissue and fat* (equivalent to extraperitoneal fatty tissue).

G. *Processus vaginalis* (equivalent to peritoneum).

8. Development of Genital Ligaments

8.1. The mesentery of the testis is the *mesorchium*. In the adult, it is a fold between the testis and epididymis.
8.2. The cranial part of the genital ridge degenerates, leaving the *suspensory ligament of the testis*.
8.3. The caudal part of the genital ridge degenerates, leaving the *ligamentum testis*. This extends from the caudal testis to the transverse bend in the urogenital ridge.
8.4. A ligament develops in a fold (the *inguinal fold*) that bridges from the bend in the genital ridge to the anterior body wall. The ligament continues into the scrotal swelling.
8.5. The *gubernaculum* of the testis is a combination of:
   A. Ligamentum testis.
   B. A connecting cord in the urogenital ridge in the region of regression of the mesonephros.
   C. A ligament extending from this ridge into the scrotal swellings. The gubernacular cord is a mesenchymatous column and keeps the pathway for descent open; however, the exact role of the gubernaculum in descent of the testis is not clear.

9. Cryptorchidism (Undescended Testis)

9.1. About 10% of newborn males have testes not fully descended into the scrotum but most proceed to descend spontaneously.
9.2. Progressive degeneration of germ cells is irreversible if the testes are not moved to the scrotum before 5 years of age.
9.3. Beyond 30 years of age, fibrosis impairs interstitial cell function.
9.4. Causes of *cryptorchidism* (from kryptos (Gk) hidden and orchis (Gk) testicle) suggested include low levels of androgen (not shown) or failure of traction of the gubernaculum. Although the gubernaculum shortens, it does not exert traction.

10. Penis

10.1. The *penis* comprises three cylinders of erectile tissue:
   A. The unpaired *corpus cavernosum urethrae* (*corpus spongiosum*)

encloses the *cavernous urethra* and enlarges terminally as the *glans*.

    B. The *corpora cavernosa penis* are paired dorsal bodies which extend from crura proximally to abut the glans distally.

10.2. *Tunica albuginea* forms a dense fibroelastic connective tissue layer and binds the three bodies together. This layer is thinner around the corpus spongiosum. The *pectiniform septum*, formed by fusion of the tunica albuginea, surrounds the corpora cavernosa medially. It is incomplete distally.

10.3. *Erectile tissue* which forms the core of the erectile bodies is a network of venous spaces separated by trabeculae of connective tissue and smooth muscle and lined with vascular endothelium.

10.4. *Skin* covering the penis is thin with small sweat glands and sparse lanugo hairs. It is reduplicated terminally over the glans as the *prepuce (foreskin)*.

10.5. *Subcutaneous tissue* has no fat but contains smooth muscle.

10.6. *Smegma* is odoriferous epithelial debris retained by the prepuce.

10.7. *Blood supply of the cavernous bodies.*

    10.7.1. In the flaccid state, blood flows toward the corpora cavernosa through the *deep artery of the penis*. This vessel contains *intimal cushions* which can regulate blood flow.

    10.7.2. Almost all blood flows to *AVAs*, which connect to efferent veins.

    10.7.3. Inside the corpora, the deep artery divides into:
        (i) *Helicine arteries* which empty into blood spaces; and
        (ii) *Nutritive arteries* of the trabeculae which reform to a small vein emptying into cavernous space.

    10.7.4. Cavernous spaces are drained by veins with intimal cushions.

    10.7.5. Veins pierce the tunica albuginea.

    10.7.6. During *erection*, blood flow in the deep artery of the penis increases.
        (i) AVA opening is reduced by active vasoconstriction.
        (ii) Helicine arteries dilate the cavernous spaces while nutritive arteries and the venous junction with cavernous spaces is compressed. The blood flow leaving cavernous bodies is not reduced during erection.

10.7.7. Relaxation of autonomic activity reduces flow to cavernous spaces, leading to flaccidity or detumescence. Most blood is shunted to peripheral venous vessels.

10.8. *Ejaculation* refers to sequential events occurring during orgasm:

10.8.1. Bulbourethral glands discharge during erection and their mucus lubricates the urethra.

10.8.2. The prostate discharges. Its alkaline secretion reduces acidity of urine bathed urethra, it dilutes thicker constituents and augments sperm motility. Note that sperms are highly susceptible to acid.

10.8.3. Sperms are forced down the ducts by contractions of the ductus epididymis.

10.8.4. Finally, the seminal vesicle adds its thick secretion and sperm are pushed by it, clearing the urethra and adding fructose, the main nutrient for sperm.

10.8.5. Contraction of bulbocavernosus compresses the bulb of the penis, forcing semen out of the urethra.

11. Development of the External Genitalia

11.1. In the third week, the *cloacal membrane* is surrounded by *cloacal folds* meeting rostrally in the genital tubercle. Descent of the *urorectal septum* and its fusion with the cloacal membrane divides the membrane into a *urogenital membrane* anteriorly and *anal membrane* posteriorly. The *cloacal fold* is divided into *urethral folds* anteriorly and *anal folds* posteriorly.

11.2. Lateral to the genital swellings are paired elevations, the *scrotal swellings*. These move caudally and make up halves of the scrotum (in the female, they are known as labial swellings and remain separated and form the labia majora).

11.3. The *genital tubercle* elongates, forming the *phallus*.

11.4. *Genital or urethral folds* form the lateral walls of the *urogenital or urethral groove* which extends along the caudal aspect of the phallus.

11.5. Entoderm at the bottom of the groove proliferates, forming the *urethral plate*.

11.6. By the third month, the urethral folds close over the urethral plate, forming the *urethral canal*.

11.7. In the fourth month, ectodermal cells from the tip of the glans form a solid epithelial cord and penetrate inward. The cord canalizes, forming the *glandular portion of the penile urethra*.

11.8. *Genital swellings* fuse caudally to become the scrotum which remains fused but internally separated from its opposite number by a *scrotal septum*.

DUCTUS EPIDIDYMIS

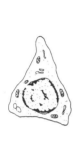

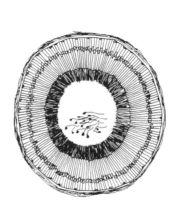

Basal cell

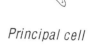

Principal cell

MALE REPRODUCTIVE SYSTEM

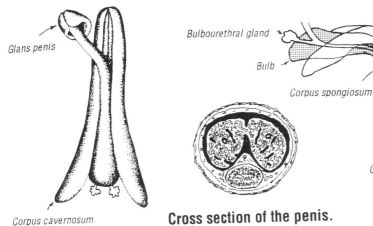

Glans penis

Bulbourethral gland

Bulb

Corpus spongiosum

Glans penis

Corpus cavernosum

Cross section of the penis.

Schematic representation of the penis.

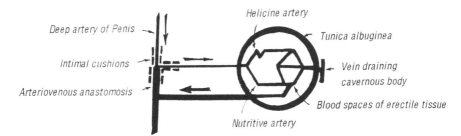

Deep artery of Penis

Helicine artery

Tunica albuginea

Intimal cushions

Vein draining cavernous body

Arteriovenous anastomosis

Blood spaces of erectile tissue

Nutritive artery

Blood flow in the flaccid penis.

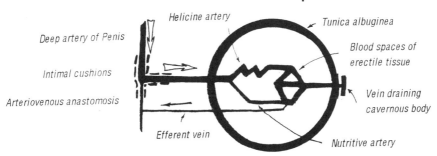

Helicine artery

Tunica albuginea

Deep artery of Penis

Blood spaces of erectile tissue

Intimal cushions

Arteriovenous anastomosis

Vein draining cavernous body

Efferent vein

Nutritive artery

Blood flow in the erect penis.

MALE REPRODUCTIVE SYSTEM

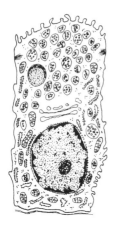

Principal cell
(Prostate)

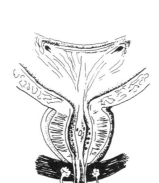

Basal cell
(Prostate)

Trigone of the bladder and prostatic urethra.

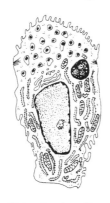

Principal cell
(Seminal Vesicle)

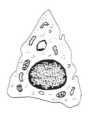

Basal cell
(Seminal Vesicle)

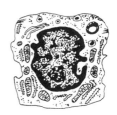

Duct cell
(Seminal Vesicle)

Chapter 21

FEMALE REPRODUCTIVE SYSTEM 1. OVARY

OBJECTIVES

After reading this chapter, you should be able to:
1. Give an account of the general structure of the ovary and identify the histologic features observable in sections.
2. Describe the process of oogenesis correlating stages in development of ova with mitotic and meiotic divisions and development of follicles.
3. Describe the process of development of ovarian follicles.
4. Give an account of the histology of thecae surrounding follicles and of their origin, function and fate.
5. Describe the histological features of ovulation and hormonal factors which control it.
6. Give an account of the functional and histologic changes that occur in cells contributing to the corpus luteum.
7. Describe regressive or degenerative changes in ovarian follicles.
8. Describe and indicate the significance of the hormonal background to the ovarian cycle.

CHAPTER OUTLINE

General. Description of female external and internal genitalia.

General structure of the ovary.

Oogenesis. Multiplication phase, Growth phase, Maturation phase. Oogonia. Primary oocytes. Primary (primordial or unilaminar) follicles. Secondary solid follicles. Secondary vesicular (antral) follicles. Interstitial cells. Hilum cells.

Ovulation.

Corpus Luteum (Luteal gland). Corpus luteum of ovulation. Corpus luteum of pregnancy. Corpus albicans. Atresia.

Blood supply of the ovary.

Nerve supply.

Lymphatics.

Hormonal background of the ovarian cycle.

Development of the ovary.

KEY WORDS, PHRASES, CONCEPTS

Cortex
Germinal epithelium
Stroma
Medulla
Tunica albuginea
Oogonia
Oogenesis
Multiplication phase
Growth phase
Maturation phase
Corpus luteum of pregnancy
Polar bodies
Primary follicles
Zona pellucida
Basal lamina (Glassy membrane)
Follicular (Granulosa) cells
Follicular fluid
Antrum
Folliculostatin

Cumulus ovaricus (oophorus)
Theca externa
Theca interna
Corona radiata
Ovulation
Corpus luteum
Granulosa lutein cells
Theca lutein cells
Corpus luteum of ovulation
Primary oocyte
Secondary oocyte
Corpus albicans
Atresia
Interstitial cells
Gonadotrophins
Estrogen
Progesterone
Negative feedback

1. General

1.1. The female reproductive system comprises *external genitalia* collectively known as the *vulva* (from volva (L) a cover or wrapper) and *internal genitalia*.
1.2. The *mammary glands* (mamma (L) a breast) are specialized integumentary compound tubuloalveolar glands for feeding the infant.
1.3. In addition, the transitory *placenta* has important hormone-secreting functions.
1.4. Of the external genitalia:
   A. *Labia majora* (labium (L) a lip) are elongated folds which enclose the pudendal cleft and are homologous to the halves of the scrotum. They are covered by pigmented skin containing sebaceous glands and covered with coarse hairs after puberty.
   B. *Labia minora* are two folds of skin which bound the vestibule of the vagina.
   C. The *clitoris* (kleio (Gk) to close or kleitorizein (Gk) to tickle) is an erectile body homologous to the corpora cavernosa of the penis.
   D. *Bulb of the vestibule* (vestibulum (L) a forecourt or entrance) comprise paired, elongated erectile bodies covered by a thin layer of skeletal muscle (Bulbospongiosus m.). They are located on each side of the vaginal opening and are homologous to the corresponding halves of the bulb of the penis.
   E. The *mons pubis* (mons (L) a mountain) is the median swelling over the pubes. It is covered with skin bearing coarse hairs after puberty and contains subcutaneous fibro-fatty tissue.
1.5. Of the internal genitalia:
   A. *Ovaries* (ovum (L) an egg) are cytogenic and hormone secreting glands.
   B. A *tubular system* comprises the *uterine tubes*, *uterus* (uterus (L) a womb) and *vagina* (vagina (L) a scabbard or sheath). The system is concerned with reception, transport and union of ova and sperm, accommodation of the fertilized ovum and fetus and with expelling the fetus at term.
   C. The *placenta* (placenta (L) a cake) is a transient hormone-secreting organ responsible for physiological exchange between the mother and embryo/fetus.

2. General Structure of the Ovary

2.1. The *ovary* is attached to the broad ligament of the uterus by a mesentery, the *mesovarium*. Blood vessels enter and leave the *hilum* of the ovary through the mesovarium.

2.2. The ovary is covered by a dull, grey surface layer of cuboidal cells, the *germinal epithelium*, a layer of reflected peritoneum which, contrary to its name, does not produce primordial germ cells or oogonia.

2.3. The *tunica albuginea* (albus (L) white) is a layer of dense connective tissue situated beneath the germinal epithelium.

2.4. The stroma of the cortex is loose connective tissue containing reticular fibers and a few smooth muscle cells which, by their contraction, may have a role in ovulation. *Stromal cells* contribute to the growth of sheaths (thecae) around growing and mature ovarian follicles. They may also secrete *androgens*. Stromal cells also contribute to the formation of the thecal cone, a wedge of cells which attaches the developing ovarian follicle to the surface of the ovary and acts like a gubernaculum.

3. Oogenesis

3.1. *Primordial germ cells* first appear in the wall of the yolk sac at the end of the third week and migrate into the developing ovary by the fifth week. In the cortex of the ovary, they differentiate into *oogonia*, primary germ cells which are some 20 μm in diameter. They undergo a series of mitotic divisions but most die before birth.

3.2. *Oogenesis* is the process of development of *oogonia* (oon (Gk) an egg and gonos (Gk) offspring), to a mature *ovum or secondary oocyte*. It is divided into phases:

A. The *multiplication phase* is the series of mitotic divisions of oogonia up to birth. This phase results in formation of primary oocytes surrounded by follicular cells which together form primordial ovarian follicles. As fetal life ends, primary oocytes enter the long dictyotene stage of the first (reductional) meiotic division. Primary oocytes have a large vesicular nucleus with a prominent nucleolus containing a diploid number of chromosomes in the dictyotene (resting) stage of the first meiotic division. Their cytoplasm (ooplasm) contains a few granules of yolk, a moderate number of small mitochondria, annulate lamellae and a single Golgi complex.

B. The *growth phase* is the period of increase in size of one primary oocyte up to ovulation. Meiotic division of the primary oocyte at the end of the growth phase results in equal division of chromatin (haploid number of chromosomes) but unequal division of cytoplasm. One daughter cell, the first polar body, remains very small. The other daughter cell, the secondary oocyte, receives almost all of the cytoplasm.

C. The *maturation phase* extends from the end of the *first meiotic division* (just before ovulation) to fertilization. After expulsion of the *first polar body* at the end of the growth phase, the nucleus of the *secondary oocyte* commences the second (equatorial) meiotic division but progresses only to metaphase unless it is fertilized. The secondary oocyte is a large spherical cell with a cytoplasm which contains many Golgi profiles, small mitochondria, short RER cisternae and granules concentrated beneath the cell membrane. The surface of the cell is covered with microvilli which contact microvilli of surrounding granulosa cells.

The result of the *second meiotic division* (which occurs in the uterine tube) is the formation of a *second polar body* and an ovum. The result of oogenesis is the formation of one *secondary oocyte* and three *polar bodies*. The first polar body also divides into two second polar bodies.

3.3. *Follicles* (*folliculus* (L) a little bag) undergo regular development and/or destruction in the ovary until there are none left at about 50 years of age. Only 420–480 mature completely and ovulate, the remainder will undergo degeneration at any stage in their development toward mature (vesicular) follicles.

3.3.1. *Primary* (*primordial or unilaminar*) *follicles* contain a primary oocyte surrounded by a single layer of cuboidal *follicular* (*granulosa*) *cells*. The greatest number of primary follicles (300–400 000) is seen in late fetal life.

3.3.2. *Growing solid follicles* (*secondary solid follicles or multilaminar primary follicles*) contain a primary oocyte surrounded by a solid mass of stratified follicular (granulosa) cells.

A. The *zona pellucida* (*mucoid oolemma*), is a transparent, refractile, extracellular amorphous glycoprotein membrane which surrounds the oocyte. It is thought to be a secretory product of follicular cells and/or of the oocyte. Microvillous processes of the oocyte and of follicular cells cross the zona pellucida.

B. A *basal lamina* (*glassy membrane*) separates follicular cells from stromal cells which begin to organize into thecae (theca (L) an enclosure or sheath).

3.3.3. *Vesicular follicles* (*secondary vesicular or antral follicles*) arise when follicle cells begin to secrete *follicular fluid* (*liquor folliculi*). Fluid from individual cells coalesce into a single extracellular space, the *follicular antrum* within the follicle cell layer.

A. *Call Exner bodies* are small 3–10 μm cavities which appear among follicle cells and are filled with PAS positive material. Electron micrographs show that they contain basal lamina material and they appear to be channels for the circulation of liquor folliculi.

B. Fluid accumulates, crowding the primary oocyte (ovum) and neighboring follicle cells to one side of the follicle. The eccentric cellular mound formed containing the ovum and surrounding follicular cells is the *cumulus ovaricus* (*or cumulus oophorus*).

C. The peripheral shell of cuboidal *follicular* (*granulosa*) *cells* surrounding the antrum forms the *stratum granulosum*.

D. The zona pellucida around the primary oocyte is surrounded by a continuous layer of follicular (granulosa) cells (the *corona radiata*).

E. The surrounding stroma forms a double layered capsule:

   (i) *Theca interna* consists of ovoid or spindle-shaped cells, some with extensive RER and others, especially before ovulation, with branched SER and lipid droplets. They are situated close to the basal lamina (glassy membrane).

   (ii) *Theca externa* comprises fibroblast-like cells (myofibroblasts) which contain myofilaments and by their contraction, contributes to postovulatory collapse of the follicle.

4. **Interstitial cells (Interstitiocytes)** are clusters or cords of large, epithelioid cells in the ovarian stroma present before birth but which disappear after menopause. Together, they represent an interstitial gland. Their cytoplasm contains lipid droplets and they resemble luteal cells cytologically. They produce estrogen which controls prepuberal development of secondary sex characteristics. They are thought to arise from hypertrophied cells of the theca interna of atretic secondary follicles.

5. **Hilum cells** (hilum (L) a little thing) are epithelioid cells found in the region of the hilum. They increase in number during pregnancy and at the onset of menopause. The cytoplasm contains lipid droplets, lipochrome pigment and Reincke crystals. They are associated with vascular spaces and unmyelinated nerves and are believed to secrete androgens since tumors of these cells occur with a masculinizing effect.

6. Ovulation

6.1. *Ovulation* is the process of rupture of a vesicular ovarian follicle with expulsion of the secondary oocyte.

6.2. The vesicular follicle attains a diameter of 10–20 mm and bulges from the surface of the ovary.

6.3. The oocyte, surrounded by corona radiata (granulosa cells) is loosened from the cumulus oophorus. At this time, it completes the first meiotic division.

6.4. Stratum granulosum, thecae and tunica albuginea adjacent to the follicle become weaker and thinner toward the surface of the ovary (the *stigma*) and the blood supply is restricted in this area.

6.5. The stigma ruptures and the secondary oocyte and adherent corona radiata flows into the infundibulum of the uterine tube. Rupture is followed by weak hemorrhage into the follicle.

6.6. The secondary oocyte enters the uterine tube and begins the second maturation division advancing to metaphase but completing the division only if fertilized.

6.7. Ovulation occurs approximately every 28 days at about mid (13th–15th day) menstrual cycle.

7. Corpus Luteum (Luteal Gland)

7.1. The *corpus luteum*, is a highly vascular temporary gland which arises from the collapsed follicle wall. Upon rupture, the follicle becomes prominently folded and contains some transuded serum and blood.

7.2. Stratum granulosum cells enlarge (but rarely divide) and arrange in cords separated by capillaries. Their cytoplasm increases in content of SER and acquires lipid droplets. They become *progesterone* secreting *granulosa lutein* (*luteal*) cells.

7.3. Theca interna cells become smaller, darker staining *theca lutein cells* which begin to secrete *androgen*.

7.4. Capillaries and spindle cells invade the main cell mass. Fibroblasts form a reticulum throughout and line the central cavity of the collapsed follicle.

7.5. The *corpus luteum of ovulation* (*of menstruation, cyclicum or corpus luteum spurium*) forms when fertilization and implantation do not occur. It reaches its maximum development after 9 days and involutes by 14 days.

7.6. The *corpus luteum of pregnancy* (*Corpus luteum verum, gravidatus*) is the corpus luteum that persists in the event of pregnancy. Under the influence of *human chorionic gonadotrophin* (*HCG*) from the cytotrophoblast of the placenta, it becomes larger (up to 2.5 cm in diameter) and persists to the 5th–6th month of pregnancy before beginning to involute.

7.7. The *corpus albicans* is a well delineated oval, white scar deep in the ovarian stroma. It results from gradual involution of a corpus luteum and is seen only after the onset of puberty. Epithelium of the corpus luteum is replaced by dense connective tissue proliferated from the theca externa and leaves a white hyaline scar.

7.8. *Atresia* (a (Gk) without and tresis (Gk) a hole) refers to interruption of the growth of follicles and their subsequent degeneration.

   A. Atresia is prominent from the fetal period to puberty and slows thereafter.

   B. It can occur at any stage of development of the follicle.

   C. Factors causing atresia are unknown. It may be related to the need for many follicles to begin to develop so as to raise the blood estrogen levels to provide feedback for the hypothalamus.

D. In an active sex life span of 30–35 years, some 400 follicles reach maturity. Unsuccessful follicles become atretic and disappear.

E. Atresia of primary follicles firstly involves degeneration of the ovum, then of follicular cells, and stromal tissue replaces the follicle.

F. Atresia of vesicular follicles involves firstly degeneration of the ovum, then the zona pellucida swells, follicular cells show fatty degeneration, theca interna cells become epithelioid and finally the center of the follicle becomes fibrotic.

8. Blood Supply of the Ovary

8.1. *Helicine arteries* from the ovarian arteries penetrate the hilum and form a plexus at the periphery of the medulla.

8.2. *Radial vessels* form a network in the follicular thecae.

8.3. The density of vascularization follows changes in the ovarian cycle.

9. Nerve Supply

9.1. Non-myelinated nerves follow blood vessels and form a plexus around follicles.

9.2. Some of the nerves are sensory.

10. Lymphatics

10.1. Large lymphatic vessels surround follicles.

10.2. Vessels have open intercellular junctions so that material from interstitial spaces can readily penetrate.

11. Hormonal Background of the Ovarian Cycle

11.1. Primordial follicles have not yet responded to *follicle stimulating hormone* (FSH).

11.2. Cyclic FSH secretion by gonadotrophs begins at puberty, stimulating groups of follicles:

A. To undergo further development.

B. To produce enough estrogen to support reproductive function.

11.3. Every 28 days, approximately 20–50 primordial follicles respond to

FSH. Follicle cells acquire more FSH receptors and show hyperplasia and hypertrophy.

11.4. Estrogen production at this stage is from two main sources, theca interna cells and interstitial cells:

A. *Theca interna cells* produce *estrogen* which passes into vessels of the theca interna.

B. *Theca interna cells also produce nutritive follicular fluid and secrete androgen substrates.* These pass through the follicular fluid to non-vascularized granulosa cells, which convert them to estrogen.

C. *Interstitial cells produce androgen substrate* which is used by granulosa cells for conversion to estrogen. In addition, interstitial cells produce estrogen directly.

11.5. Follicle maturation is largely controlled by the *luteinizing hormone* (*LH*) which causes final maturation of the follicle and triggers ovulation (ovulation follows the LH surge). Granulosa and thecal cells have surface *LH receptors* induced by FSH acting with estrogen.

11.6. In the first half of the ovarian cycle:

A. Gonadotrophin releasing factor producing cells in the hypothalamus cause gonadotrophs in the anterior lobe of the hypophysis to produce and accumulate gonadotrophins (FSH and LH).

B. FSH brings on follicle development and hence estrogen production.

C. Blood borne estrogen promotes LH and FSH accumulation in gonadotrophs.

D. A day before midcycle, estrogen exerts a positive feedback effect at the hypophysis and gonadotrophs release accumulated gonadotrophins which causes the LH surge responsible for ovulation.

11.7. In the second half of the ovarian cycle:

A. Intrafollicular estrogen acts on granulosa cells, inducing *LH receptor formation* in their cell membranes.

B. Shortly before ovulation, LH directs granulosa cells to begin producing progesterone.

C. LH reduces availability of FSH and *estradiol receptor sites* on granulosa cells. Granulosa cells reduce estrogen production and shift to progesterone production.

D. Granulosa cells also produce *folliculostatin*, which acts as a feedback inhibitor of FSH secretion from gonadotrophs.

12. Development of the Ovary

12.1. The ovaries develop from paired *gonadal (genital) ridges*. In its earliest stages (the *indifferent stage*), male and female ridges are indistinguishable. Differentiation in the ovary occurs later (week 7) than in the testis.

12.2. In the eighth week, the ovary consists of a dense *primary cortex* beneath the germinal epithelium, a *primary medulla* and a *rete ovarii* comprising a compact cellular mass that bulges into the mesovarium. The blastema shows clusters of small indifferent cells and one or more primordial germ cells.

12.3. By 3–4 months, the ovary enlarges because of deposition of a new *definitive cortex*. This arises by proliferation of the surface germinal epithelium but true cortical cords do not form.

12.4. Most cells of the original internal cell mass become young *oogonia.*

12.5. The tunica albuginea of loose connective tissue becomes distinguishable by 6 months at the end of deposition of new cortex.

12.6. Oogonia of the primary medulla and cortex decline and are replaced by the vascular, fibrous stroma of the permanent medulla.

12.7. *Primary follicles* comprise *germ cells (oogonia)* surrounded by cells derived from surface epithelium *(follicular cells). Vesicular follicles* do not appear until sexual maturity.

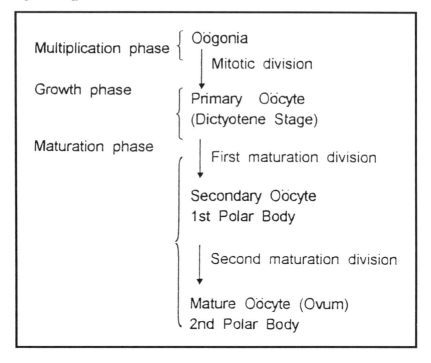

Stages in oögenesis.

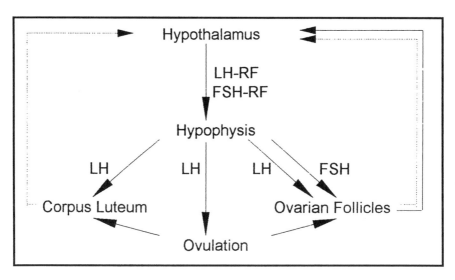

Control of ovarian function.

OVARY

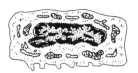

*Follicular cell of
Primordial Follicle*

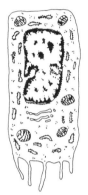

*Follicular cell of
Primary Follicle*

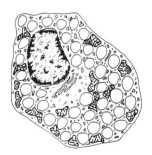

Interstitial cell of Ovary

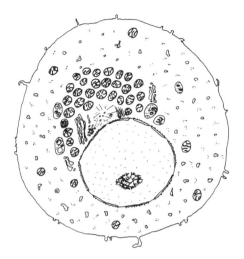

Oocyte

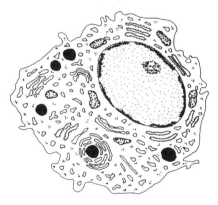

Lutein cell of Corpus Luteum

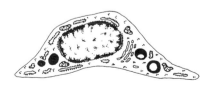

Theca interna cell

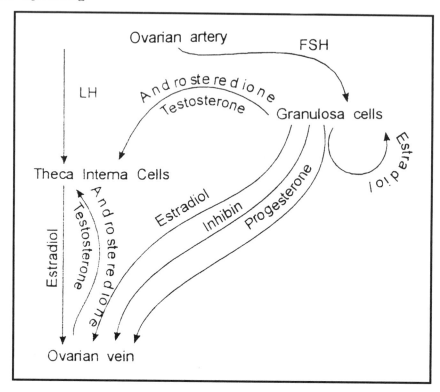

Gonadotrophnin interaction in the ovary regulating follicle maturation and steroidogenesis.

Chapter 22

FEMALE REPRODUCTIVE SYSTEM
2. UTERINE TUBES, UTERUS AND VAGINA

OBJECTIVES

After reading this chapter, you should be able to:
1. Describe the histologic features of the uterine tubes and give an account of its histophysiology.
2. Describe the structure of the endometrium of the uterus and its changes in the menstrual cycle.
3. Give an account of the hormonal basis of the menstrual cycle.
4. Describe the blood supply of the endometrium and its significance.
5. Compare the structure of the cervix with that of the body of the uterus.

CHAPTER OUTLINE

Uterine tubes

General. Parts of the tubes.

Detailed structure.

Functions of the tubes.

The Uterus

General. Parts of the uterus.

Peritoneal relationships. Perimetrium, Parametrium, Paracervix.

Detailed structure. Myometrium. Histophysiology. Mucosa (Endometrium). Uterine glands. Endometrial zones. The menstrual cycle. Blood supply of the endometrium. Phases of the menstrual cycle. Proliferative phase, Secretory phase, Menstrual phase.

The Cervix.

Functions of the uterus.

Vagina.

Development of the uterine tubes, uterus and vagina.

KEY WORDS, PHRASES, CONCEPTS

Uterine tubes	Infundibulum
Ampulla	Mesosalpinx
Isthmus (of the tube)	Fimbriae
Interstitial (uterine) part	Uterus
Body (corpus)	Cervix
Isthmus (of the uterus)	Fundus
Perimetrium (serosa)	Parametrium
Myometrium (muscularis)	Relaxin
Stratum submucosum	Stratum vasculosum
Stratum supravasculosum	Supravaginal cervix
Vaginal cervix	Subserosa
Oxytocin	Endometrium (mucosa)
Uterine glands	Arcuate arteries
Straight (basal) arteries	Coiled arteries
Lamina functionalis	Lamina basalis
Cervix	Endocervix
Ectocervix	Cervical glands
Palmate folds	Prostaglandins
Paracervix	Vagina
Vaginal rugae	Vaginal cycle
Müllerian tubercle	Vaginal plate

UTERINE TUBES

1. General

1.1. The *uterine tubes* are located in the upper edge of the broad ligament, the segment between the ovary and the tube being known as the *mesosalpinx* (salpinx Gk. a trumpet or tube).

1.2. They are 10–12 cm long and divided into four parts:

    A. *Infundibulum* (infundibulum (L) a funnel) is the funnel-shaped end of the tube bounded by 20–30 tentacle like fimbriae (fimbria (L) a fringe or thread). The ovarian fimbria is one of the longest processes close to the tubal end of the ovary. The abdominal ostium or pelvic opening of the uterine tube is located at the base of the funnel.

    B. *Ampulla* (ampla (L) full and bulla (L) a vase) is the longest and widest distal part of the tube.

    C. *Isthmus* (isthmos (Gk) a narrow passage) is the narrower and thicker walled segment adjoining the uterus.

    D. *Interstitial part* (intramural or uterine part) lies in the wall of the uterus, ending in the cavity of the uterus as the uterine ostium.

2. Detailed Structure

2.1. *Tunica mucosa (endosalpinx)* comprises:

    2.1.1. Epithelium is simple columnar epithelium comprising equal numbers of ciliated and non-ciliated secretory cells.

        A. *Ciliated cells* have numerous tall cilia which beat toward the uterus on their apical border. They are more frequent in the distal tube and may transport ova through the ampulla to the site of fertilization at the ampullo-isthmic junction. Some consider that the prime role of cilia is to orient spermatozoa and that movements of the tubes are mainly responsible for movement of ova. The presence of cilia depends on the presence of estrogen and there are few ciliated cells remaining after menopause (they reappear with estrogen therapy).

        B. *Secretory cells* are non-ciliated and vary in height and number with the uterine cycle. Estrogen promotes secretory activity and synthesis while progesterone inhibits it.

2.1.2. *Lamina propria* is cellular and contains a thin collagenous network. It is thrown into longitudinal folds which subdivide the lumen into narrow clefts. The folds decrease in height, number and complexity towards the uterus.

2.2. *Tunica muscularis* comprises inner circular and outer longitudinal layers of smooth muscle which increases in thickness toward the uterus. Progress of the zygote towards the uterus is delayed, apparently insuring that it is at a sufficient developmental stage to implant. No intramural sphincter that could account for this delay has been shown. It is thought that stretch of the tube delays progress of the zygote.

2.3. *Tunica subserosa* is loose connective tissue containing blood vessels, nerves and lymphatics.

2.4. *Tunica serosa* is a simple squamous mesothelium of the peritoneum.

3. Functions of the Uterine Tubes

3.1. *Fimbriae* are engorgable with blood (cf. erectile tissue) and can be moved by their subperitoneal smooth muscle. This adapts their position relative to the preovulatory ovarian follicle.

3.2. Secretion provides nutrition for the fertilized ovum.

3.3. Segmental movements biased toward the uterus result from nervous and hormonal modulation and move the ovum toward the uterus.

3.4. *Sperm transport* in the tube is divided into:

A. *A rapid phase* induced by oxytocin and prostaglandins in semen, which results in muscular contractions in the tract, allowing some sperms to reach the distal tube within 5 min of coitus.

B. A *sustained phase* in which sperm colonized in reservoir areas (cervical mucus) are sequentially distributed.

3.5. *Capacitation*, the process by which spermatozoa acquire the ability to fertilize an oocyte, occurs in the tube and requires 1–6 h.

3.6. *Fertilization* occurs mostly at the junction of the ampulla and isthmus.

THE UTERUS

1. General

1.1. The *uterus* (uterus (L) a womb) is a piriform, hollow, muscular organ comprising a part protruding above the entrance of the uterine tubes, the fundus, a corpus or body, the main or upper two thirds extending downwards to a constriction, the isthmus and a lower third extending down to the opening within the vagina, the cervix.

1.2. The main portion of the cervix is the *supravaginal part* while that penetrating the vagina is the *vaginal part*.

2. Peritoneal Relationships

2.1. The uterus gives the impression that it has invaginated the peritoneal cavity from below so that the body has acquired a serous coat on most of its anterior and all of its posterior surface. The two layers become continuous to enclose the uterine tube and spread laterally as the broad ligaments.

2.2. *Perimetrium* is the outer coat (tunica serosa) corresponding to peritoneum.

2.3. *Parametrium* and *paracervix* are loose connective tissue (tunica adventitia) on the lateral sides of the uterus and cervix continuous with similar tissue into the broad ligaments. It contains the uterine arteries, lymph vessels and nerves lateral to the cervix.

3. Myometrium

3.1. *Tunica muscularis or myometrium* consists of crossed and helicoidally arranged bundles of smooth muscle capable of great hypertrophy and hyperplasia during pregnancy.

3.2. It is arranged in three poorly defined layers, a thick *middle circular layer* and *thinner inner and outer longitudinal or oblique layers*. Because of their common origin from the fused Müllerian ducts, the muscle layers are confluent with those of the uterine tubes.

3.3. There are three *vascular layers* in the myometrium:

A. An *innermost layer* (*stratum submucosum*) contains small calibre vessels forming a network immediately below the endometrium.

B. A *middle layer* (*stratum vasculosum*) contains thick-walled muscular arcuate arteries and veins.

C. An *outermost layer* (*stratum supravasculosum*) of small vessels occupies the external zone.

3.4. *Histophysiology*

3.4.1. Estrogen controls the differentiation of smooth muscle cells of the myometrium and maintenance of cell size.

3.4.2. During pregnancy, cells increase in size from 25 μm to 5 mm in length. New muscle cells arise from undifferentiated cells.

3.4.3. The myometrium has some inherent rhythmicity of its own; however, contractions during pregnancy are inhibited by a hormone, relaxin,, produced by granulosa lutein cells and the basal plate of the placenta.

3.4.4. *Oxytocin* from the posterior lobe of the hypophysis and prostaglandins initiate and maintain contractions at the end of pregnancy.

3.4.5. At menopause, smooth muscle cells of myometrium atrophy because of the lack of estrogens.

3.4.6. Contractions of the myometrium are related to ovarian activity. There is a peak at ovulation and another at menstruation (low progesterone and endometrium prostaglandin release). These can orient the ovary relative to the infundibulum. Contractions are increased with coitus from oxytocin release and prostaglandins in seminal fluid.

4. Mucosa (Endometrium or Tunica Mucosa)

4.1. Epithelium is simple columnar comprising both non-ciliated secretory and ciliated cells (cilia beat toward the vagina).

A. *Uterine glands* are simple, slightly branched tubular, mucus secreting glands whose cells are identical with surface cells. They extend through the mucosa, almost reaching the myometrium, and undergo a monthly cycle of activity (see below).

4.2. The lamina propria is cellular connective tissue with spindle-shaped fibroblasts, reticular fibers and abundant ground substance, lymph vessels and occasional nerves.

4.3. *Endometrial zones*:
- A. *Compact layer* is nearest the surface, contains the straight necks of uterine glands and enlarged stromal cells (cf. decidual cells of pregnancy).
- B. *Spongy layer* contains dilated portions of glands.
  The compact and spongy layers comprise the functional layer of the endometrium which participates in the menstrual cycle.
- C. *Basal layer* contains the blind ends of glands. This layer (and the distal end of glands) does not participate in the menstrual cycle.

5. The Menstrual Cycle

5.1. In sexually mature women, the endometrium undergoes cyclic changes (the *menstrual cycle*). This involves building up followed by destruction and repair of the bulk of the endometrium if the secondary oocyte is not fertilized and the blastocyst implanted.

5.2. The cycle recurs every 21–35 days (average 28 days) with days of the cycle numbered from the appearance of menstrual flow (the first day is day 1).

5.3. The cycle is driven hormonally by the ovary. *Estrogens* (*estradiol*) causes proliferation of the endometrium and *progesterone* causes increase in cell secretion and glycogen accumulation in uterine glands. As a result, the endometrium dilates with fluid and glands coil and sacculate.

5.4. *Blood supply* of the endometrium:
  5.4.1. The *uterine artery* in the broad ligament gives off 6–10 arcuate arteries to the uterus.
  5.4.2. Radial branches pass through the inner muscular layer of myometrium and basal endometrium (lamina basalis or basal layer) where they divide into:
    - A. *Basal* (*straight*) *arteries* supplying the lamina basalis of the endometrium.
    - B. *Coiled* (*spiral*) *arteries* which run parallel to uterine glands supplying the outer endometrium (lamina functionalis or functional layer) and ending in a subepithelial capillary network. These branches supply the stroma, invest the glands and form arteriovenous anastomoses. Coiled arteries show marked changes in response to hormonal stimulation.

5.5. Lymphatics form plexuses but are absent from the superficial mucosa.

5.6. *Phases in the menstrual cycle*:

   A. *Proliferative phase*, days 5–14 (also known as the *follicular phase, Reparative phase or estrogenic phase*).

     (i) This is a period of growth induced by estrogen and coincides with growth of the ovarian follicle.

     (ii) The mucosa increases from less than 1 mm to more than 2 mm in thickness.

     (iii) Glands proliferate increasing in length, waviness and accumulate glycogen. Gland cells produce a thin, mucoid secretion.

     (iv) Connective tissues increase mostly by the production of new reticular fibers.

     (v) Coiled arteries grow slowly.

   B. *Secretory phase*, days 15–28 (also known as the progravid phase, progestational phase or luteal phase).

     (i) This phase coincides with production of progesterone by the corpus luteum.

     (ii) The uterus reaches a stage where it can accept a fertilized ovum.

     (iii) Glands swell and secrete profusely.

     (iv) Coiled arteries lengthen, spiral tightly and reach almost to the surface of the endometrium.

     (v) Fibroblasts of the stroma become decidual cells, large polygonal cells containing RER, lysosomes, glycogen and aggregated lipid droplets. Their surface bears microvilli and cells connect through nexuses with adjacent cells. They may synthesize proteins and provide nutritive substances to the blastocyst during implantation.

     (vi) The endometrium reaches 4–6 mm thick from oedema of the stroma and accumulation of secretion in glands.

     (vii) The time from the start of the secretory phase to the onset of bleeding is 14 days and is uniform regardless of the length of the cycle.

   C. Menstrual phase, days 1–4.

     (i) Menstruation occurs in the absence of fertilization (i.e., in the absence of HCG).

     (ii) The functional layer shrinks and coiled arteries are compressed.

Shrinkage appears to result from resorption of interstitial fluid with withdrawal of estrogen and progesterone as a result of degeneration of the corpus luteum.

(iii) Coiled arteries constrict intermittently 1 day before bleeding starts. Vasoconstriction is compounded by buckling of coiled arteries and the effects of tissue metabolites from ischemia. The result is necrosis of the superficial (functional) layer of endometrium which sloughs off.

(iv) Coiled arteries relax locally and blood escapes. Pools of uncoagulated blood appear in the lamina propria.

(v) Tissue separation exposes torn glands, arteries and veins. The discharge (menses) is about 35 ml in volume consisting of blood, disintegrated epithelium and stroma and glandular secretion.

(vi) Straight arteries to the basal endometrium do not constrict during the menstrual cycle so that the blood supply to this zone is never compromised.

6. Cervix

6.1. The *cervix* is the tube-like lower part of the uterus. It has a central canal (the cervical canal) extending from the internal os at the beginning of the cervix near the isthmus to the external os at the lower end of the cervix protruding into the vagina.

6.2. The cervix differs from the corpus uteri in the following respects:

A. Epithelium of the cervical canal (endocervix) is simple columnar with some cells ciliated but most are mucus-secreting cells. Epithelium abruptly becomes stratified non-keratinizing squamous lining the vaginal portion of the cervix (ectocervix). The area medial to the junction (the transformation zone) may undergo squamous metaplasia. When this zone is visible by colposcopy, it is incorrectly known as an "erosion".

B. Epithelium of the endocervix forms branched tubular mucous cervical glands which may contain retention cysts (Nabothian cysts). The amount of mucous secretion varies with the menstrual cycle and the glands enlarge and proliferate in pregnancy. Glands produce a highly viscous mucus in the proliferative phase of the cycle which becomes watery at midcycle, facilitating spermatozoan migration.

C. The myometrium in the cervix contains spiral bundles of smooth muscle and many elastic fibers.

D. Mucosa is thrown into complicated palmate folds.

E. The endocervix does not participate in the menstrual cycle.

7. Functions of the Uterus

7.1. The uterus is *specialized to receive and rear the fertilized ovum* in the mucosa. Here, it is nourished and protected before it is finally expelled.

7.2. The *menstrual cycle anticipates possible pregnancy*.

7.3. In pregnancy, the secretory phase continues under the influence of progesterone from the corpus luteum and later, the placenta. The hormonally supported mucosa is the decidua of pregnancy and its stromal cells, the decidual cells of pregnancy. Part of the endometrium (decidua basalis) becomes the maternal part of the placenta.

7.4. An *anovulatory cycle* is one in which there is an ovarian cycle of normal duration without ovulation so that a corpus luteum is lacking. Endometrial epithelium remains in the proliferative phase until menstrual bleeding occurs. It is believed that a normal healthy woman has 3–4 anovulatory cycles.

8. Vagina

8.1. General

    8.1.1. The *vagina* (vagina (L) a scabbard or sheath) is a tubular fibromuscular sheath extending from the cervix of the uterus to the vestibule of the vagina. The lumen is H-shaped in transverse section with a transverse folds of mucosa (vaginal rugae).

    8.1.2. In most virgins, the opening of the vagina into the vestibule is partly closed by an annular fold of mucosa, the *hymen* (hymen (Gk) a membrane).

8.2. Detailed Structure

    8.2.1. Of the mucosa:

        A. *Epithelium* is thick, non-keratinized, stratified squamous epithelium with numerous indenting epithelial (dermal) ridges.

Layers of the epithelium are:

(i) *Basal and parabasal cells* from the deep zone.

(ii) *Transitional or intermediate cells* and *precornified cells* from the middle zone.

(iii) *Spinal or prickle cells* from the superficial zone.

The transition from cervical to vaginal epithelium is abrupt. Glands are absent; lubrication of the epithelium depends on mucus from the cervical glands.

B. *Lamina propria* is dense connective tissue containing elastic fibers and a plexus of small veins. Lymphocytes and macrophages are present during the menstrual cycle and some invade the epithelium. Mucosal folds form transverse *rugae* (ruga (L) a wrinkle).

8.2.2. *Tunica muscularis* comprises inner circular and outer longitudinal layers of smooth muscle. Some skeletal muscle (bulbocavernosus m.) surrounds the bulb of the vestibule and the external entrance, forming an external sphincter.

8.2.3. *Tunica adventitia* is loose connective tissue; however, the posterior fornix of the vagina is covered with peritoneum.

8.3. Functions of the vagina

8.3.1. The vagina acts as:

A. A copulatory organ; and

B. A birth canal.

8.3.2. The *vaginal cycle* is a sequence of changes occurring in vaginal epithelium throughout the 28 day menstrual cycle. Changes are, however, minimal in the human.

A. From menstruation (the early proliferative phase), cells in vaginal smears are polygonal, precornified and not folded at the edges. Nuclei are vesicular and the cytoplasm, basophilic. There are also some polymorphs and bacilli in the smear.

B. A few days before ovulation (under the influence of estrogens), vaginal epithelium is thickest (250 μm). At ovulation (the late proliferative phase), superficial and spiny cells accumulate glycogen and begin to desquamate. Liberated glycogen is fermented by lactobacilli to lactic acid (pH 4) which protects the vagina from other bacteria. Smears show all cells to be acidophilic and very swollen with pyknotic nuclei.

    C. During the secretory phase (under the influence of progesterone), desquamation continues and the epithelium is thinner (150 μm). The amount of glycogen (and acidity) decreases. Smears show clumped cells with folded borders.

9. Development of the Uterine Tubes, Uterus and Vagina

9.1. The *paramesonephric duct* arises on the lateral side of the mesonephros as an invagination of the coelomic epithelium. Rostrally, it opens into the coelomic cavity but caudally, it crosses ventrally to the mesonephric duct to join the paramesonephric duct from the other side. The two ducts then run longitudinally to end blindly on the dorsal wall of the urogenital sinus between the mesonephric ducts at an elevation, the Müllerian tubercle.

9.2. In the absence of stimuli from the fetal testis, the paramesonephric ducts form most of the female genital ducts.

9.3. The cranial longitudinal part of the paramesonephric ducts forms the uterine tubes.

9.4. The intermediate unfused parts of the ducts expand and are incorporated into the fundus and body of the uterus.

9.5. The caudal fused parts of the ducts form the cervix while the caudal blind end of the fused ducts is initially at the Müllerian tubercle (site of the future hymen).

9.6. Proliferation of the epithelium on the posterior wall of the urogenital sinus at the Müllerian tubercle forms the *vaginal plate*, which separates the Müllerian tubercle from the urogenital sinus.

9.7. Central cells of the plate break down, forming the vaginal lumen from the hymen to the vaginal fornices.

9.8. The mesonephric duct in the female remains as vestiges located in the broad ligament:

    A. The cranial end forms the *vesicular appendages*.

    B. The intermediate part together with excretory ducts connect with the rete ovarii to form the duct and tubules of the *epoophoron* (epi (Gk) upon, oon (Gk) egg and phoros (Gk) bearing).

    C. Caudal tubules end blindly, forming the *paroophoron*, a small collection of blind sacs in the broad ligament.

D. The caudal mesonephric duct forms *Gartner's duct* which may persist as cyst like structures in the walls of the uterus and/or vagina.

UTERINE TUBE

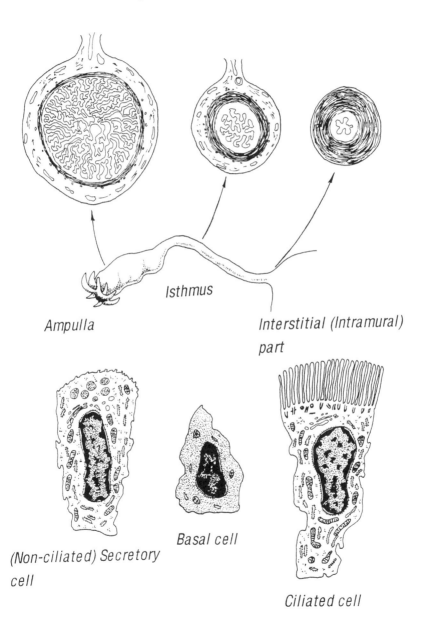

Ampulla

Isthmus

Interstitial (Intramural) part

(Non-ciliated) Secretory cell

Basal cell

Ciliated cell

UTERUS

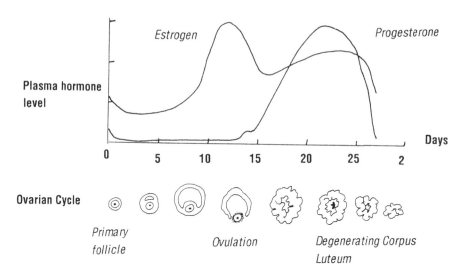

Plasma hormone level

Estrogen *Progesterone*

Days

0 5 10 15 20 25 2

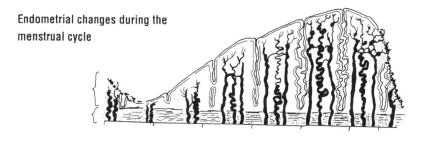

Ovarian Cycle

Primary follicle *Ovulation* *Degenerating Corpus Luteum*

Endometrial changes during the menstrual cycle

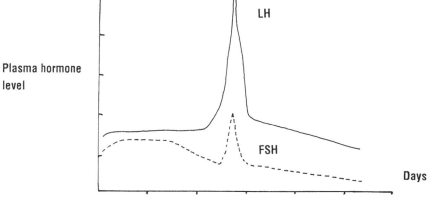

Plasma hormone level

LH

FSH

Days

Chapter 23

FEMALE REPRODUCTIVE SYSTEM
3. EXTERNAL GENITALIA AND
MAMMARY GLANDS

OBJECTIVES

After reading this chapter, you should be able to:

1. Describe the composition and histologic features of the female external genitalia.
2. Discuss the embryologic development of the external genitalia.
3. Give an account of the histologic structure of the non-lactating breast.
4. Describe the histologic changes that occur in the breast during pregnancy and after parturition.
5. Describe the hormonal and nervous control of lactation.
6. Give an account of the development of the breast from initiation to puberty.

CHAPTER OUTLINE

External genitalia

General. Mons pubis. Labia majora. Clitoris. Labia minora. Major vestibular glands. Minor vestibular glands. Bulbs of the vestibule. Development of the external genitalia.

Mammary glands

General.

Detailed structure. Nipple. Areola. Duct system. Epithelium of ducts and of alveoli.

Colostrum, Milk.

Endocrine and neural control of the mammary gland.

Development of the mammary gland.

KEY WORDS, PHRASES, CONCEPTS

Vulva

Mons pubis

Labia minora

Vestibule of the vagina

Minor vestibular glands

Mammary glands

Lactiferous ducts

Galactophores

Areola

Secretory (alveolar) cells

Prolactin

Milk

Pudendum

Labia majora

   Clitoris

   Crus, Glans,

   Corpora cavernosa

Major vestibular glands

Bulbs of the vestibule

Nipple

Lactiferous sinus

Involution

Areolar glands

Myoepitheliocytes

Oxytocin

Colostrum

1. General

The external genitalia in the female are:

1.1. The *mons pubis*, a mass of adipose tissue covering the symphysis pubis. After puberty it is covered with hair.

1.2. The *labia majora*, two elongated folds running down and backward from the mons pubis to enclose the pudendal cleft. The outer aspect tends to be pigmented and the epithelium contains hair follicles, sweat glands and sebaceous glands. The core of the labia contains adipose tissue and some smooth muscle. They are homologues of the halves of the scrotum.

1.3. The *clitoris* (kleio (Gk) I close or kleitorizein (Gk) to tickle), homologous to the penis in the male. It comprises two small corpora cavernosa affixed to the os pubis as crura clitorides. The crura unite, ending in a short *corpus (body) clitoridis*. A rudimentary *glans clitoridis* is a rounded elevation on the end (beneath) of the body related to the *bulbs of the vestibule*. Unlike the penis, the clitoris is not traversed by the urethra and it lacks a corpus spongiosum. It is covered with thin stratified, squamous non-keratinized epithelium with high papillae over a vascular stroma. The wall of the clitoris is a dense tunica albuginea. The core contains erectile tissue. The glans is very rich in Meissner's, Ruffini's, Kraus' and Pacinian corpuscles as well as intraepithelial nerve endings.

1.4. *Labia minora* are homologous with the undersurface of the penis but unlike that region of the penis, remain ununited. They are two elongated folds of skin running downward and backward from the mons pubis and enclose the pudendal cleft. They divide at the clitoris into:
Medial part, passing below the clitoris to form the frenulum of the clitoris; and
Lateral part, which forms the hoodlike prepuce of the clitoris over the glans.
Labia minora bears no hairs but do contain sebaceous glands and sweat glands. Skin on the inner surface is thin and pink like a mucous membrane.

1.5. The *major vestibular glands* (of Bartholin also known as *vulvovaginal glands*) are small, paired tubuloalveolar mucus-secreting glands found on either side of the vestibule. Fibromuscular septa divide the parenchyma into small lobules. Tubuloalveoli are lined with large, clear, columnar cells. The duct opens into the groove between the hymen and labium minus. Major vestibular glands are homologous to the bulbourethral glands in the male. After 30 years of age, they undergo involution.

1.6. *Minor vestibular glands* are clusters of mucus secreting cells in the epithelium surrounding the clitoris and urethra. Gland cells are tall columnar one or two cells deep. They lubricate the epithelium of the vagina.

1.7. The *bulbs of the vestibule* are elongated masses of erectile tissue at the sides of the pudendal cleft beneath the bulbospongiosus muscle. They are homologues of the bulb of the penis and adjacent parts of the corpus spongiosum.

2. Development of the External Genitalia

2.1. Female external genitalia go through an indifferent stage in which they are indistinguishable from those of the male.

2.2. At this stage (4 weeks), a cranial *genital tubercle* leads to *cloacal folds*, which surround the *cloacal membrane*. On either side of the cloacal folds are another pair of elevations, the *genital swellings*.

2.3. When the urorectal septum reaches the cloacal membrane at 6 weeks, it establishes the perineal body. It also divides the cloacal membrane into a cranial *urogenital membrane* and caudal *anal membrane* and the cloacal folds into cranial *urethral folds* and caudal *anal folds*.

2.4. The genital tubercle elongates only slightly to form the *clitoris*.

2.5. The urethral folds do not close (fuse) as in the male but develop into the *labia minora*. The urogenital groove remains open to the surface, forming the *vestibule*.

2.6. The genital swellings enlarge greatly to form the *labia majora*.

MAMMARY GLANDS

1. General

1.1. The *mammary glands* (mamma (L) a breast) contain a parenchyma of compound tubulo alveolar gland tissue, subcutaneous fibrous tissue stroma connecting its lobes, adipose tissue between, and a nipple where the gland's ducts open onto the skin surface.

1.2. They are of cutaneous origin, developing in pairs along embryonic milk lines which extend from the axilla to the groin.

1.3. Glands consist of 15–20 lobes that radiate from the *nipple* to occupy the central portion of the breast. Each lobe has a single *lactiferous duct* (*galactophore*). Fat and fibrous tissue subdivide lobes into lobules which consist of a series of rounded alveoli whose ducts open to the smallest branches of lactiferous ducts.

1.4. Ducts converge toward the *areola* beneath which each is dilated to form a secretory reservoir, the *lactiferous sinus*. Ducts then narrow and directly traverse the nipple to its summit where they open in constricted individual orifices.

2. Detailed Structure

2.1. The *nipple* is a columnar elevation traversed by 15–20 *lactiferous ducts* (*galactophores*) which open independently onto its crest.

    2.1.1. It is covered by pigmented epidermis with deep epidermal ridges and dermal papillae. There are numerous sebaceous glands in the epidermis and many free nerve endings and Meissner's corpuscles.

    2.1.2. The core contains helical bundles of smooth muscle around lactiferous ducts. Contraction of the muscle in response to cold, touch or suckling elevates the nipple.

2.2. The *areola* (dim of area (L) an open space) is a circular area of hairless skin surrounding the nipple. Its stratified squamous keratinized epithelium has long, branched dermal papillae, is pigmented from puberty, and particularly during and after pregnancy. Smooth muscle bundles in the dermis contract and wrinkle the skin.

    2.2.1. *Areolar glands* (*of Montgomery*) are tubuloalveolar cutaneous glands in the areola that moisten the nipple.

    2.2.2. The areola also contains sebaceous glands and Meissner's corpuscles.

2.3. *Fascia* covering the breast loosely envelopes the entire gland and extends into its substance to enclose the parenchymal units. It gives fibrous processes that fuse with the superficial layer of subcutaneous tissue. These are well-developed in the upper part of the breast as the *suspensory ligaments*. Areolar tissue in the stroma predominates in the periphery of the breast, filling the intervals between lobes.

2.4. The structure of the breast varies with age and whether or not pregnancy has occurred.

    2.4.1. Before puberty, mammary glands contain only a few lobules of short, sparsely branched and poorly canalized ducts, but no alveoli. The stroma is relatively abundant comprising groups of adipocytes (lipocytes). Slight breast enlargement is the result of deposition of fat and stroma.

2.4.2. At puberty, under the influence of estrogen, ducts proliferate and branch. Granular, polyhedral cells at the ends of branches may show some development into blunt tubular or spherical outgrowths under the influence of progesterone, but decline with collapse of the corpus luteum.

2.4.3. With pregnancy, multiplication and branching of tubuloalveoli begins but they remain collapsed. Lobules increase in volume in parallel with a diminution in stroma. Intralobular connective tissue becomes infiltrated with lymphocytes, eosinophils and plasma cells. There is also an increase in adipose tissue and in circulating blood.

2.4.4. At menopause, the parenchyma reduces (especially at the periphery of the gland) and tubuloalveoli almost totally disappear (senile involution). Connective tissue becomes less cellular and there may be an increase in adipose and elastic tissues.

2.5. *Secretory or alveolar cells* are cuboidal cells with surface microvilli rich in mitochondria and RER. During lactation, vacuoles containing casein separate from the Golgi complex and lipid droplets bulge from the surface of the cells. Droplets separate, still surrounded by a rim of cytoplasm.

2.6. *Myoepitheliocytes* contain actin microfilaments and their contraction in response to oxytocin causes extrusion of milk toward the duct system (the milk ejection reflex).

2.7. Secretion increases in the later half of pregnancy. Cells become cuboidal and produce colostrum a few days after parturition.

2.7.1. *Colostrum* (witch's milk) is similar to blood plasma. It contains cells thought to be macrophages filled with fat globules, colostral corpuscles and cell fragments and is rich in lactoproteins and antibodies, but poor in lipids. Its secretion continues for 1–3 days.

2.7.2. True milk appears a few days after parturition. Alveolar cells at this stage are low cuboidal to columnar and show increased numbers of organelles. Alveoli are distended and the stroma reduced to narrow strands containing lymphocytes, plasma cells and eosinophilic granulocytes. Lactation decreases 5–6 months after birth.

2.7.3. *Milk* is an emulsion comprising water (88%), lactose (7%), fat and mostly long chain fatty acids (4%) synthesized by alveolar cells, protein (1%), vitamins, ions (calcium, phosphate, sodium, potassium and chloride) and immunoglobulins. IgA assists in maintaining the sterility of milk during secretion and IgG gives passive immunity to the young.

2.8. *Involution* follows cessation of nursing. Milk particles are phagocytosed by macrophages and epithelial cells autophagocytose casein granules and lipid droplets. Epithelial cells degenerate and are phagocytosed but the duct system remains.

3. Endocrine and Neural Control of the Mammary Gland

3.1. Mammary gland growth from birth to puberty follows body growth.

3.2. Sometime before puberty, growth of all tissues in the mammary gland accelerates. Estrogen is responsible for ductal growth and with the onset of the ovarian cycle, progesterone stimulates development of tubuloalveoli. Small amounts of other hormones (STH, LTH, ACTH, prolactin, insulin, corticoids and parathormone) are also required for normal breast growth.

3.3. The above hormones are needed to establish and maintain lactation but lactation begins after a decrease of estrogen and progesterone from the placenta causes the mammary gland to become more sensitive to LTH.

3.4. *Maintenance of lactation* results from the influence of LTH, thyroxin and STH. The suckling reflex stimulates production of prolactin releasing factor, LTH, ACTH and oxytocin, the latter of which causes contraction of myoepithelial cells.

4. Development

4.1. The mammary gland first appears at 13 mm as a localized thickening of surface epithelium, the *mammary ridge* which extends from the base of the forelimb toward the base of the hindlimb.

4.2. Much of this ridge disappears except in the pectoral region where some 15–20 solid epithelial cords grow into the underlying mesenchyme.

4.3. The cords canalize, forming *lactiferous ducts* which at first open
into a pit in the epithelium. Near birth, the mesenchyme around the
pit proliferates, elevating the pit to the crest of the nipple.

MAMMARY GLAND

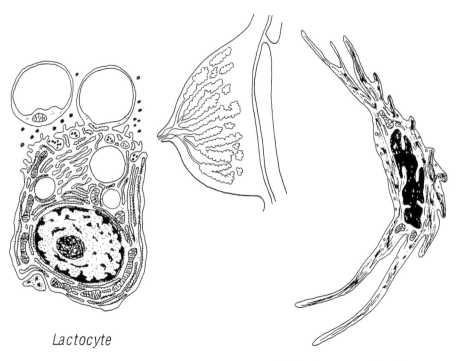

Lactocyte

Stellate myoepitheliocyte

Chapter 24

FEMALE REPRODUCTIVE SYSTEM 4. PLACENTA

OBJECTIVES

After reading this chapter, you should be able to:

1. Give an account of some of the processes preliminary to fertilization such as transport and viability of sperm and ova, fate of sperm and ova, and factors governing fertility.
2. Identify the location of fertilization, describe the process of entry of sperm into the oocyte and the results of fertilization.
3. Describe the implantation period.
4. Describe the lacunar stage in the development of the trophoblast.
5. Describe the formation of chorionic villi.
6. Give an account of the regional differences in the decidua and chorion up to and including the formation of decidual septa and cotyledons.
7. Identify the macroscopic and microscopic features of the full term placenta.
8. Discuss the nature of the placental barrier and placental circulation.
9. Discuss the histophysiology of the placenta including its hormones and factors involved in the initiation of parturition.

CHAPTER OUTLINE

General.

Processes preliminary to fertilization.

Fertilization (Zygote formation).

Cleavage. Morula formation. Blastocyst formation.

The implantation period.

The lacunar stage of placental development.

The trabecular stage of placental development.

Development of villi. Primary villi. Stem villi. Secondary villi. Boundary zone. Tertiary villi. Cytotrophoblastic shell. Chorion frondosum. Chorion laevae.

Decidua.

Structure of the placenta. Decidual septae. Cotyledons.

Blood supply of the placenta.

Structure of the full term placenta.

Functions of the placenta.

The umbilical cord. General. Detailed structure.

KEY WORDS, PHRASES, CONCEPTS

Ovulation
Seminal fluid (Semen)
Capacitation
Zygote
Blastomeres
Morula
Trophoblast
Inner cell mass (embryoblast)
Embryotrophe
Syncytiotrophoblast
Cytotrophoblast

Boundary zone
Chorion frondosum
Chorion laevae
Decidua basalis
Decidual plate
Decidua capsularis
Decidua parietalis
Placenta
Decidual septa
Cotyledons
Placental circulation

Lacunae
Decidual cells
Trabeculae
Primary villi
Blastocyst
Tertiary villi
Stem villi

Placental barrier
Human chorionic
gonadotrophin (HCG)
Human placental lactogens (HPL)
Secondary villi
Cytotrophoblastic shell

THE PLACENTA

1. General

1.1. The *placenta* (placenta (L) a flat cake) is a transient organ comprising a *fetal portion* derived from an extraembryonic membrane, the chorion, and a *maternal portion* derived from the decidua basalis, a portion of the endometrium. It serves as a source of hormones during pregnancy and is the site of exchange between maternal and fetal bloodstreams.

2. Processes Prior to Fertilization

2.1. There are two phases of *spermatozoon transport*:
   A. *Rapid phase* in which some spermatozoa reach the distal uterine tube within five minutes of insemination. This phase results from uterine and tubular contractions enhanced by coitally induced release of oxytocin and prostaglandins (present in semen).
   B. *Sustained phase* in which spermatozoa, colonized in the cervical mucus reservoir, are slowly released from cervical crypts over 15 to 45 minutes following insemination.

2.2. *Capacitation* is a molecular change to spermatozoa during which they acquire the ability to fertilize an ovum. The process occurs in the female genital tract and requires 1 to 6 hours. It is reversible and probably entails removal of components attached to the surface of spermatozoa or activation of enzymes.

2.3. The *acrosome reaction* refers to a series of changes in the capacitated spermatozoon head when near the secondary oocyte. The anterior part of the acrosome cap swells, vesiculates and enzymes (hyaluronidase

PLACENTA

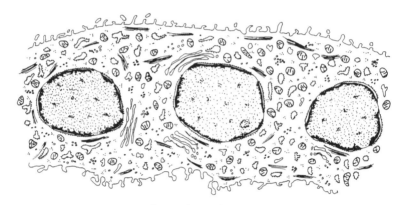

Syncytiotrophoblast

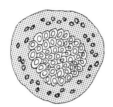 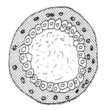 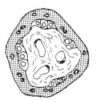

Primary stem villus   *Secondary stem villus*   *Tertiary villus*

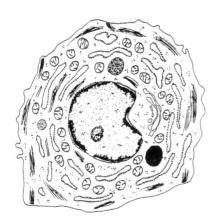

Cytotrophoblast cell

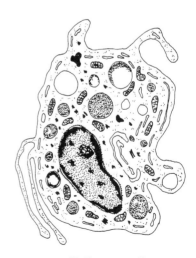

Hofbauer cell

and esterases) are released, which assist penetration between corona radiata cells and through zona pellucida.

2.4. While motile spermatozoa have been recovered from the female genital tract up to 6 days after coitus, their ability to fertilize probably lasts not more than 48 hours. The ovum can be fertilized for a period of 24 hours.

2.5. Transport of ova through the uterine tube results from ciliary action and tubal contractions. The tube shows segmental contractions with preferential directionality of muscle activity imposed by neuronal and hormonal modulation. Cilia beat at a constant speed toward the uterus.

3. Fertilization

3.1. *Fertilization* occurs most commonly at the junction of the ampulla with the isthmus of the uterine tube.

3.2. Spermatozoa attach to the zona pellucida then penetrate it by enzyme action (released from the acrosome) and their own motility to reach the perivitelline space.

3.3. The proacrosomal cell membrane fuses with microvilli of the oocyte and bulges induced from the oocyte surface envelop the spermatozoon head.

3.4. The secondary oocyte reacts by:

A. Depolarization of the cell membrane following sperm entry which causes the release of cortical granules containing a trypsin-like enzyme. This modifies the membrane and digestibility of the zona pellucida, thereby blocking the entry of other sperms.

B. Completing the second meiotic division with expulsion of the second polar body. The nucleus of the oocyte is called the female pronucleus.

3.5. The sperm looses its tail and the head enlarges, forming the male pronucleus.

3.6. Male and female pronuclei approach in the center of the ovum, lose their nuclear membranes, and their chromosomes intermingle.

3.7. The *results of fertilization* are:

A. *Restoration of a diploid number of chromosomes.*

B. *Determination of the sex* of the embryo which depends on whether the oocyte is fertilized by a sperm carrying an X or Y chromosome.

C. *Initiation of cleavage* — a series of rapid cell divisions by the fertilized ovum (zygote).

4. Cleavage

4.1. *Cleavage* involves a series of mitotic divisions of the zygote into smaller cells (blastomeres).

4.2. The zygote normally enters the uterus at the 8–12 cell stage some 80 hours after ovulation. Sphincter-like closure of circular muscle of the isthmus together with thick glycoprotein secretion persisting for several days after ovulation functionally occludes the isthmic lumen and temporarily prevents entrance of the zygote into the uterus.

4.3. By 72–96 hours, the fertilized ovum has divided into 16 cells, the *morula* (from morula (L) a mulberry) inside the zona pellucida. The innermost cells of the morula are the *inner cell mass* (*embryoblast*) which forms the embryo and outermost cells, the *outer cell mass* (*trophoblast*) which contributes to the placenta.

4.4. In the uterine cavity:

4.4.1. The zona pellucida disappears. The zona pellucida had kept *blastomeres* together and prevented their adherence to the wall of the uterine tube.

4.4.2. Fluid passes into the morula from the uterine cavity, forming a central *blastocoel* (*blastocyst cavity*). The cell mass and its fluid-filled core is called a blastocyst.

4.4.3. Cells of the *blastocyst* are separable into:

A. *Trophoblast* (*outer cell mass*) — flat cells forming the wall of the blastocyst.

B. *Embryoblast* (*inner cell mass*) located at one pole of the blastocyst.

4.4.4. Uterine glands produce "uterine milk" (*embryotrophe*), a secretion rich in glycogen and carbohydrates which nourishes the blastocyst.

5. The Implantation Period

5.1. The blastocyst attaches to the endometrium at the embryonic pole between (sometimes in) the mouths of uterine glands.

5.2. Implantation occurs mostly in the upper posterior (55.5%) or upper anterior (44.5%) median uterine wall.

5.3. Abnormal implantation sites include:

    A. Near the internal os where the placenta develops bridging the os (*placenta praevia*).

    B. Below the internal os (*cervical pregnancy*).

    C. In the uterine tube (*tubal pregnancy*).

    D. In the ovary (*primary ovarian pregnancy*).

    E. In the abdominal cavity, commonly in the rectouterine pouch (*primary abdominal pregnancy*).

5.4. Trophoblast cells over the embryoblast penetrate between epithelial cells of the uterine mucosa. This is probably a result of activity of proteolytic enzymes produced by the trophoblast by the 10th–11th postovulatory day.

5.5. The endometrium is at the progestational (secretory) stage (day 22). Stroma is edematous, uterine glands are secreting and capillaries prominent. Fibroblast-like cells of endometrial stroma transform into large, round or polygonal protein-secreting decidual cells and the transformation process is known as decidualization. There is no maternal tissue necrosis.

5.6. Implantation is *interstitial,* i.e., in the stratum compactum beneath surface epithelium by days 10–12.

5.7. Trophoblast cells at the embryonic pole form a solid disc separable into:

    A. *Syncytiotrophoblast* (*syncytium*), an outermost dark multinucleated zone.

    B. *Cytotrophoblast*, an innermost layer of pale discrete mononucleated cells. Mitotic figures in these cells (but not in the syncytiotrophoblast) suggest that cytotrophoblast gives rise to syncytiotrophoblast.

6. The Lacunar Stage of Placental Development

6.1. At this stage, intercommunicating clefts (*lacunae*) appear in the syncytiotrophoblast between the 10th and 13th postovulatory days. These spaces become partially confluent to form the precursors of the intervillous spaces.

7. The Trabecular Stage of Placental Development

7.1. Between days 14–21, *trabeculae* (trabs (L) a wooden beam) or columns of syncytiotrophoblast incompletely separate lacunae.

7.2. Trabeculae become radially oriented and come to possess a cellular core which arises from proliferation of cytotrophoblast cells from the chorionic plate.

7.3. These *trabecular columns* (*primary stem villi*) are not true villi but the framework from which the villous tree later develops. *Stem villi* are trabeculae that extend from the chorionic plate to the cytotrophoblastic shell (see below).

7.4. Trabeculae are thickest because of their better nutrition at the embryonic pole away from the uterine lumen. At the abembryonic pole, the trophoblast comprises mostly cytotrophoblast with few lacunar spaces.

7.5. Maternal blood (*hemotrophe*) enters lacunae, thereby coming into direct contact with syncytiotrophoblast.

8. Development of Villi

8.1. *Cytotrophoblast cores* extend to the region of attachment of syncytiotrophoblast to endometrium and spread laterally to form a continuous cytotrophoblast shell.

8.2. *Syncytiotrophoblast* is split into:

A. *Definitive syncytium* on the fetal side which persists as the limiting layer of the intervillous space; and

B. *Peripheral syncytium* between cytotrophoblastic shell and decidua. This portion degenerates and is replaced by fibrinoid material (*Nitabuch's membrane*).

8.3. Villi develop a loose mesenchymal core formed by a distal extension of extraembryonic mesenchyme and are then known as secondary stem villi.

8.4. The villous core contains fibroblasts and macrophages (*Hofbauer cells*) which play a number of roles but importantly trap maternal antibodies crossing the placenta.

8.5. Trophoblast and the primary mesenchyme is now referred to as the *chorion*.

8.6. Cytotrophoblast cells migrate into the endometrium. Some invade and partially replace endothelial cells which line maternal spiral arteries, causing distension of the vessels.

8.7. Distal cytotrophoblast spreads to join the cytotrophoblast of other villi. It penetrates the syncytium and comes into contact with maternal tissue.

8.8. Villi next develop a capillary system in their core and are now referred to as tertiary stem villi.

8.9. Cytotrophoblast cells of the shell never develop a mesenchymal core so that fetal blood vessels do not penetrate the shell.

8.10. Cytotrophoblast cells on villi decreases in amount in the second trimester (except at the zone of attachment) to a single broken layer of cells between syncytium and mesenchyme. Some have contributed to syncytium and some to connective tissue cores of villi.

8.11. Syncytium is also reduced in the third trimester. Nuclei are irregularly dispersed and often aggregated to form *syncytial "knots"*. Fetal capillaries appear to dilate.

8.12. The *boundary between maternal and fetal blood supplies* comprises:
   A. Attenuated syncytiotrophoblast cytoplasm.
   B. Basal lamina.
   C. Attenuated fetal endothelial cytoplasm.

8.13. Villi on the side of the chorion toward the decidua basalis (embryonic pole) proliferate and arborize, forming the *chorion frondosum* (frondosum (L) shaggy) which develops into the definitive placenta.

8.14. Villi oriented toward the uterine cavity (abembryonic pole) degenerate and, by the 3rd month, this part of the chorion is smooth and non-vascular, the *chorion laevae* (laevae (L) smooth).

9. Decidua (Endometrium)

9.1. Beneath the chorion frondosum, the *decidua basalis* (*decidual plate*) is the compact and spongy layers of endometrium. It contains spiral arteries and dilated uterine glands.

9.2. *Decidua capsularis* is the thin layer of endometrium over the abembryonic pole which borders the uterine lumen.

9.3. *Decidua parietalis* is the endometrium lining the remainder (opposite side) of the uterine cavity.

9.4. Chorion laevae and decidua capsularis project into the uterine cavity.
9.5. By 3.5 months, the decidua capsularis atrophies and chorion laevae contacts and fuses with decidua parietalis, thereby obliterating the uterine lumen.
9.6. By 4.5 months, decidua capsularis disappears except at the margins of the placenta.

10. Structure of the Placenta

10.1. The only functional part of the chorion is the chorion frondosum.
10.2. The placenta has two parts:
     A. Chorion frondosum — the fetal portion.
     B. Decidua basalis — the maternal portion.
10.3. *Placental (decidual) septa* appear during the 3rd month. They protrude into the intervillous space from the basal plate and divide the maternal surface of the placenta into 15–20 lobes.
10.4. *Septae* are folds of basal plate formed partly by pulling up of basal plate into the intervillous space by anchoring trabeculae and partly by regional variability of placental growth.
10.5. Septae comprise basal plate tissue (decidual tissue covered by trophoblast-remnants of cytotrophoblast embedded in fibrinoid). They do not reach the chorionic plate.
10.6. *Cotyledons* (kotyledon (Gk) a cup-like hollow) are 15–20 compartments of the placenta formed by one stem villus and its branches. Each cotyledon is incompletely surrounded by decidual septa and provided with a separate blood supply.

11. Blood Supply of the Placenta

11.1. The maternal blood supply to the placenta is through spiral arteries enlarged by invading cytotrophoblast. These open into intervillous spaces most probably into the central villus-free space of the fetal lobule.
11.2. Blood flows in a funnel-shaped stream, is baffled by villi, and is laterally dispersed returning into basally placed wide inlets of an endometrial venous network.

12. Structure of the Full Term Placenta

12.1. The mature placenta is shaped like a flattened cake approximately 15–20 cm in diameter, 3 cm in thickness and weighing 500 g.

12.2. It is described as:

 A. *Chorioallantoic* — it is vascularized on the fetal side by umbilical vessels analogous to allantoic vessels in some animals.

 B. *Hemochorial* — describing the direct relationship of maternal blood supply to the villi.

 C. *Villous* — referring to the particular presence of villi in the human placenta.

 D. *Deciduate* — since some maternal decidua is shed at birth with the placenta; and

 E. *Discoidal* — referring to its circular shape.

13. Functions of the Placenta

13.1. *Exchange of substances* across the placenta including:

 A. Oxygen and carbon dioxide which cross by simple diffusion from differences in partial pressures. These are intervillous space 90 mm Hg, uterine vein 50 mm Hg, fetal blood 15–30 mm Hg.

 B. Glucose crosses by facilitated diffusion.

 C. Amino acids are actively transported through the syncytium.

13.2. *Excretion*: Urine voided by the fetus into amniotic fluid is swallowed, enters the fetal circulation, and thereby reaches the maternal circulation. Urea passes the placental barrier.

13.3. *Placental hormone production*:

 A. Syncytiotrophoblast synthesizes *progesterone* and (with enzymes produced by the fetal suprarenal cortex), *estrogen*. Progesterone inhibits myometrial contractions and with estrogen, stimulates fetal genital and breast development, and growth of decidual vasculature. Estrogen stimulates growth of the uterus.

 B. Cytotrophoblast produces *human chorionic gonadotrophin* (HCG) as early as the 8th day after ovulation, i.e., 1 day after implantation. HCG maintains the corpus luteum until the 4–5th month of pregnancy.

 C. Syncytiotrophoblast produces *human chorionic somatotrophin*

(HCS, or *human placental lactogen*, HPL) the "growth hormone of pregnancy".

D. *Human chorionic thyrotrophin* (HCT) increases the secretion of thyroid hormone.

E. *Placental luteinizing hormone releasing factor* (LH-RF) produced by cytotrophoblast regulates HCG secretion by adjacent syncytiotrophoblast.

13.4. As an *immunologic barrier*: Separation of maternal and fetal circulations and lymphatic systems protects the immunocompetent fetus from sensitizing the mother.

A. Trophoblast lacks major histocompatability antigens and fibrinoid secretion by trophoblast cells masks surface antigens.

B. Antigen-antibody complexes bind receptors on trophoblast.

C. Trophoblast hormones suppress the immune response.

D. Maternal antibodies (IgG) cross the syncytiotrophoblast by pinocytosis, giving the fetus passive immunity against some diseases.

THE UMBILICAL CORD

1. General

1.1. The *umbilical cord* forms at the ventral aspect of the embryo as a result of cephalocaudal folding at the junction of the amnion and ectoderm.

1.2. It comprises gelatinous connective tissue covered by amnion and transmits, depending on age,

1.2.1. At 5 weeks:

A. Connecting stalk containing allantois and umbilical vessels.

B. Yolk sac stalk with vitelline vessels.

C. A canal joining intra and extraembryonic coeloms.

1.2.2. At 10 weeks (in which time the cord has elongated):

A. Yolk sac stalk.

B. Umbilical vessels (two arteries and a vein).

C. Remnant of the allantois.

D. Some loops of intestine.

1.2.3. By the end of the 3rd month:

A. Umbilical vessels.

B. Intestinal loops withdraw into the abdominal cavity and the fetal coelomic cavity in the cord is obliterated.

1.3. At birth, the cord is 2 cm in diameter, 50–60 cm long and tortuous forming "*false knots*".

2. Detailed Structure

2.1. In sections, the cord has:
   A. An outermost layer of amnionic epithelium ,simple cuboidal to stratified squamous, continuous with the abdominal epidermis.
   B. A core of gelatinous("mucous") connective tissue comprising primitive stellate fibroblasts in a proteoglycan ground substance with collagen fibers (Wharton's jelly).
   C. Two umbilical arteries with relatively thick muscular walls and diffuse elastic fibers but no internal or external elastic laminae.
   D. One umbilical vein (the left) with a relatively thick muscular wall.
   E. A remnant of the allantois.

Chapter 25

THE EYE

OBJECTIVES

After reading this chapter, you should be able to:

1. Describe the relationship between the three layers (coats) of the wall of the eye, their modifications in different parts of the eyeball and their developmental origin.
2. Describe and contrast the structures of the cornea and sclera.
3. Give an account of the formation and drainage of aqueous humor.
4. Give an account of the histologic structure of the choroid and ciliary body.
5. Describe the formation, growth and structure of the lens.
6. Discuss the mechanism of, and structures involved, in accommodation.
7. Give an account of the histologic structure of the retina with particular reference to the structure of component cells, layering of the retina, blood-retina barrier and turnover of photoreceptor disk membrane proteins.
8. Give a histologic account of structures seen with an ophthalmoscope in the living retina (macula lutea and optic disk).

CHAPTER OUTLINE

Development of the optic cup and lens vesicle.

Development of the retina, iris and ciliary body.

Detailed structure of the eye.

Cornea.

Sclera.

Limbus (Sclerocorneal junction).

Anterior chamber.

Posterior chamber.

Uvea. Iris. Choroid and Ciliary Body.

Lens.

Ciliary Zonule.

Vitreous Body.

Retina. Blood-retina barrier. Layers of the retina. Cells of the retina. Photoreceptor disk membrane protein turnover, disk shedding.

Macula lutea and Fovea centralis.

Optic papilla (disc).

Retinal vessels.

Optic nerve.

KEY WORDS, PHRASES, CONCEPTS

Cornea
Bowman's layer
Substantia propria
Endothelium
Sclera
Choroid
Suprachoroidal space
Choriocapillaris
Ciliary body
Ciliary muscle
Lens vesicle
Lens fibers
Primary lens fibers
Crystallins

Anterior corneal epithelium

Descemet's membrane
Corneal grafting
Lamina cribrosa
Suprachoroid
Vessel layer of choroid
Bruch's membrane
Scleral spur
Lens
Lens epithelial cells
Germinal zone of lens
Secondary lens fibers
Lens capsule

Zonule (suspensory ligament)
Iris
Pupillary margin
Stromal cells
Dilator pupillae
Limbus
Internal scleral sulcus
Trabecular sheets
Trabecular spaces (Fontana)
Vitreous body
Retina, Macula lutea
Outer and inner segments
   of photoreceptors
Outer plexiform layer
Inner plexiform layer
Retinal (optic) nerve fiber layer
Rods
Cones
Bipolar cells
Ganglion cells
Fovea centralis

Accommodation
Pupil
Pigmented epithelial cells
Sphincter pupillae
Iridocorneal angle
Scleral spur
Sinus venosus sclerae
(Canal of Schlemm)
Aqueous humor
Hyaloid canal
Retinal pigment epithelium
External limiting membrane
Outer nuclear layer
Inner nuclear layer (bipolars)
Ganglion cell layer
Internal limiting membrane

Horizontal cells
Amacrine cells
Disk shedding
Papilla (optic disk)

THE EYE

1. Development of the Optic Cup and Lens Vesicle

1.1. At 22 days, the eyes develop from shallow grooves on each side of the invaginating forebrain.

1.2. With closure of the neural tube, the grooves form outpocketings of the forebrain, the *optic vesicles*.

1.3. The vesicles contact surface ectoderm, then invaginate, forming a double-walled *optic cup*.

1.4. An *intraretinal space* separates inner and outer layers of the cup.

1.5. Invagination also involves the inferior surface of the optic cup, forming the *choroidal fissure* which allows the *hyaloid artery* (a branch of the ophthalmic artery) to reach the inner chamber of the eye.

1.6. At 7 weeks, the lips of the choroidal fissure fuse and the mouth of the optic cup forms the *pupil*.

1.7. Surface ectoderm cells, upon contact with the optic vesicle, elongate, becoming the *lens placode*.

1.8. The placode invaginates and looses contact with the surface epithelium, becoming the *lens vesicle* which is located at the mouth of the optic cup.

2. Development of the Retina, Iris and Ciliary Body

2.1. Cells of the outer layer of the optic cup accumulate small pigment granules and become the *pigment layer of the retina*.

2.2. The inner layer of the optic cup is separable into:
   A. A posterior four fifths, the *pars optica retinae*.
      (i) Cells bordering the intraretinal space give rise to the photoreceptor rods and cones.
      (ii) Adjacent cells give rise to the mantle layer in turn, differentiating into neurons of the inner nuclear and ganglion cell layers.
   B. An anterior fifth, the *pars caeca retinae*, which remains one cell thick and later is divisible into:
      (i) *Pars iridica* retinae forms the inner layer of the iris.
      (ii) *Pars ciliaris retinae* which participates in formation of the ciliary body.

2.3. The region between the optic cup and overlying surface epithelium is filled with mesenchyme.

2.4. The *sphincter and dilator pupillae muscles* develop from underlying ectoderm of the optic cup.

2.5. The *iris* is formed by:
   A. The pigment containing outermost layer of the optic cup.
   B. The unpigmented internal layer of the optic cup.
   C. A layer of richly vascularized connective tissue containing pupillary muscles.

2.6. The *pars ciliaris* becomes markedly folded.
   A. Externally, it is covered by mesenchyme, forming the *ciliary muscles*.
   B. Internally, it is connected to the lens by a network of elastic fibers, the *ciliary zonule or suspensory ligament of the lens*.

3. The Cornea

3.1. The *cornea* (cornu (L) a horn and corneus (L) horny) is the avascular anterior part of the eye wall. It is about 0.5 mm thick in the center, 1.0 mm thick at the periphery and 11 mm in diameter. Although corneal stroma appears like that of the white sclera, it is optically homogeneous because it contains more mucopolysaccharide and interstitial fluid. The fluid is continuously pumped across semipermeable membranes which keeps the cornea turgescent.

3.2. Anterior *corneal epithelium* is stratified squamous non-keratinized about 5 cells thick. Superficial cells have surface microplicae which may serve to keep the layer moist. The surface of the cornea is highly innervated and stimulation leads to blinking and flowing of tears.

3.3. *Bowman's membrane* is an acellular layer beneath the surface epithelium, which contains randomly arranged collagen bundles.

3.4. The *stroma* (*substantia propria*) comprises laminae of collagen fibers which are parallel to the surface. Fibrils of one lamina run at right angles to those of the next lamina. There are also some elastic fibers in the stroma. Flattened fibroblasts (keratocytes or stromal cells) lie between laminae as well as some macrophages and leucocytes.

3.5. *Descmet's membrane* beneath the inner endothelial layer is an acellular basal lamina which contains collagen. It takes up the slack during reversible swelling of the cornea.

3.6. *Endothelium* (*posterior corneal epithelium*) is a simple squamous, metabolically active epithelium with complex interdigitations that protects the cornea from swelling.

4. Sclera

4.1. The *sclera* (skleros (Gk) hard) is the dense outer connective tissue tunic of the eyeball extending from the limbus of the cornea. It comprises an outer layer of dense bundles of collagen with scattered elastic fibrils, interspersed flattened fibroblasts and a thin, less dense inner layer containing melanocytes. Mucopolysaccharide is almost absent so the sclera does not imbibe water like the cornea.

4.2. Near the cornea, there is a rich plexus of blood vessels that anastomoses with Schlemm's canal and the anterior ciliary vessels.

4.3. At the site of exit of the optic nerve, the sclera is reduced to a thin fenestrated membrane, the *lamina cribrosa*.

4.4. The sclera becomes continuous posteriorly with the dural sheath of the optic nerve.

4.5. A narrow *suprachoroid space* separates the sclera from the choroid and an *episcleral space* from the ocular fascia (capsule of Tenon).

5. Limbus (Sclerocorneal Junction)

5.1. The *limbus* is the boundary zone of abrupt optical change between sclera and cornea.

5.2. On the outer side is the boundary between conjunctival and corneal epithelial epithelium (*external scleral sulcus*).

5.3. On the inner side is the internal scleral sulcus which contains a trabecular meshwork continuous with Descemet's membrane and the posterior corneal epithelium.

5.4. A trabecular strand of the meshwork contains a central core of collagenous and elastic fibers covered by basal lamina and endothelium.

5.5. The *trabecular meshwork* is the site of drainage of *aqueous humor* (humor (L) a liquid) from the anterior chamber of the eye. Spaces of Fontana within the meshwork communicate with an endothelial lined circumferential venous channel at the anterior edge of the sclera (*Schlemm's canal*) which in turn drains through fine channels into episcleral veins. Obstruction of this system causes a rise in intraocular pressure (*glaucoma*) which leads to impaired vascular perfusion of neural tissues and blindness.

6. The Anterior Chamber

6.1. The boundaries of the *anterior chamber* are the cornea anteriorly, and iris and lens posteriorly.

6.2. The anterior chamber contains *aqueous humor* and communicates with the posterior chamber through a fine channel between the iris and lens.

7. The Posterior Chamber

7.1. The boundaries of the *posterior chamber* are anteriorly, the posterior surface of the iris and posteriorly, the anterior surface of the lens, ciliary zonules and the ciliary body laterally.

7.2. The *posterior chamber* contains aqueous humor and communicates with the anterior chamber through a fine channel between the iris and lens.

7.3. The pupillary margin of the iris rests on the lens and acts as a ball valve so that aqueous humor passes from the posterior to anterior chamber and not in the reverse direction.

7.4. *Aqueous humor* is secreted by ciliary epithelium. It contains most soluble constituents of blood but far less protein (0.02% compared with 7%) urea and glucose. It penetrates the vitreous body and is responsible for metabolic supply of the lens and maintenance of intraocular pressure.

8. The Uvea

8.1. The *uvea* (uva (L) a grape)is a pigmented, predominantly vascular coat of the eye comprising the iris, ciliary body and choroid.

8.2. The *iris* (iris (Gk) a rainbow or halo) is an annular diaphragm extending from the angle of the anterior chamber to the pupillary margin.

  A. The anterior surface lacks an endothelial cover so that the spongy connective tissue core is exposed to the anterior chamber.

  B. The posterior surface is lined with a double layer of pigmented epithelium resting on the lens at the pupil margin. The anterior layer of this epithelium forms the dilator muscle. Both layers are pigmented regardless of the color of the skin of the individual. They extend further toward the border of the pupil than the stroma, which accounts for the collarette of pigment at the edge.

  C. The *stroma* is pigmented, vascular loose connective tissue containing fibroblasts, melanophores (absent from blue eyes) and phagocytes (clump cells) which are rounded and heavily pigmented.

  D. Bundles of the *sphincter pupillae* muscle near the pupil margin are of epithelial origin and innervated by the parasympathetic nervous system.

  E. Fibers of the *dilator pupillae* muscle just anterior to the epithelium of the iris are innervated by the sympathetic nervous system.

8.3. The *choroid* is a heavily vascularized, variably pigmented layer which extends posteriorly from the ora serrata between the pigmented layer and the sclera.

From within it comprises:

A. *Bruch's membrane*, the basal lamina of the pigment layer which limits the access of macromolecules from capillaries of the choriocapillaris to the outer retinal layer.

B. *Choriocapillaris,* a dense fenestrated capillary network responsible for nourishing the photoreceptors. The stroma is a pigment-containing connective tissue containing fibroblasts, macrophages, melanophores and some mast cells. It also contains unmyelinated nerve fibers.

C. The vessel layer containing large muscular arteries from the ciliary arteries and draining into vortex veins.

D. The *suprachoroid*, which contains layers of fibroblasts, macrophages and melanophores in a collagenous and elastic fiber meshwork.

8.4. The *ciliary body* is a fibromuscular body located between the ora serrata and the base of the iris (scleral spur). It comprises:

An anterior part (*pars plicata*) comprising 70–80 ciliary processes which give attachment to fibers of the ciliary zonule.

A posterior part (*pars plana*) which has a smooth surface.

The *ora serrata* is the irregular dentate line between the optic and ciliary parts of the retina.

A. The ciliary body is covered by a double layer of epithelium comprising an *inner layer of cuboidal pigmented* cells and *outer layer of non-pigmented cells* which are phagocytic and responsible for the formation of zonule fibers.

B. The *stroma* consists of a vascular loose connective tissue which contains smooth muscle fibers.

C. A *circular muscle bundle* supplied by the parasympathetic nervous system, is located along the inner edge of the ciliary body close to its base.

D. A *meridional muscle bundle* innervated by the sympathetic nervous system attaches to the scleral spur.

E. Contraction of ciliary muscles is responsible for *accommodation* of the lens. Contraction of ciliary muscles relaxes tension on ciliary zonule fibers and the lens assumes a more relaxed (convex) shape.

F. Ciliary epithelium produces aqueous humor.

9. The Lens

9.1. Cells of the posterior wall of the lens vesicle elongate in an anterior direction, eventually filling the lumen of the vesicle, and are known as *primary lens fibers*.

9.2. Growth of the lens continues by addition of cells (*secondary lens fibers*) to the central core from a germinal zone at the rim (*equatorial region*) of the lens.

9.3. The *capsule* of the lens, the basal lamina of the lens fibers, is thicker on the anterior surface (10 μm) than on the posterior surface (< 0 5 μm).

9.4. Anterior lens cells (*lens epithelium*) is a single layer of cuboidal cells complexly interdigitated and joined by junctional complexes.

9.5. The lens substance contains *lens fibers* (*cells*) and is divisible into a *cortex* and *nucleus*. Individual fibers are 7–10 mm long, 5–12 μm wide and 2–4 μm thick. They are arranged in concentric layers meeting end to end at Y-shaped sutures on the anterior and posterior surfaces of the lens. Individual cells are held together by ball and socket interdigitations of the cell membrane.

10. The Ciliary Zonule or Suspensory Ligament of the Lens

10.1. The *ciliary zonule* is a system of radial fibers suspending the lens and consisting of:

A. Long fibers arising near the ora serrata which insert into the anterior surface of the lens; and

B. Short fibers arising from the ciliary body which insert into the posterior surface of the lens.

10.2. Fibers are dense aggregates of fibrils made of the same glycoprotein as elastic fibers.

11. Vitreous Body (Humor)

11.1. The *vitreous body* is a colorless, amorphous, transparent and gelatinous material filling the space between the lens and the retina. It is a connective tissue containing minute amounts of fibrils in hydrophilic polysaccharides.

11.2. The inner limiting membrane is condensed vitreous at the boundary with the retina.

11.3. The *hyaloid membrane* is a dense packing of fibrils in the anterior border of the vitreous body.

11.4. The *hyaloid canal* between the optic papilla and lens is a remnant of the hyaloid vessels which disappear when differentiation of the eye is complete.

11.5. Cells in the vitreous body are:
  A. *Vitreous cells* (*hyalocytes*).
  B. *Macrophages* (occasionally).

11.6. Fibrils are collagenous microfibrils.

12. Retina

12.1. The *retina* is a photosensitive part of the central nervous system 0.5 mm thick attached within the eyeball to the optic head posteriorly and ciliary epithelium anteriorly. The remainder has no cytological attachment to underlying tissue.

12.2. It is divided into a functional posterior portion (*pars optica retinae*) and a non-functional anterior portion (*pars caeca retinae*) covering the ciliary body.

12.3. *Pigment epithelium* forms a single layer of cuboidal cells of neuroepithelial origin absent from the head of the optic nerve posteriorly and transforming into the pigment layer of the ciliary epithelium anteriorly.
  A. The apical cytoplasm contains a heavy concentration of melanin granules during periods of darkness. In periods of light, granules stream into short microvilli which extend between and surround outer segments of photoreceptors. This has the effect of decreasing sensitivity of the retina but of increasing its resolving power.
  B. The cytoplasm also contains primary and secondary lysosomes as the cells phagocytose used membranous discs of photoreceptors.
  C. Cells are joined to one another by junctional complexes but there is no specialized attachment to photoreceptors.
  The *subretinal space* separates the pigment and photoreceptor layers.

12.4. *Muller's cells* are tall, slender glial cells attached to the basal lamina (inner limiting membrane) whose cytoplasm extends throughout the complete thickness of the retina (to the outer limiting membrane).

EYE – RETINA

Rod cell

Cone cell

Bipolar cell

Pigment epithelial cell

Muller cell
(Radial glyocyte)

A. Muller's cells are broad at their base, tapering apically to microvilli which penetrate between photoreceptors. They are attached near their apex to adjacent photoreceptors and to one another near their base, by junctional complexes.

B. Their cytoplasm contains microfilaments, glycogen particles and RER consistent with a role in structural and metabolic support.

12.5. *Photoreceptors* are highly differentiated neuroepithelial cells sensitive to light. Two types are:

A. *Rods* (120 million). Slender cells at the periphery of the retina which, because of their higher content of photoabsorptive pigment (rhodopsin or visual purple) and cumulative neural connections, are most sensitive to low levels of light.

B. Cones (5 million) are more flask-shaped, situated at the central part of the retina and because of their less summating neural connections, are capable of greater resolution. They contain the visual pigment iodopsin and are functionally but not morphologically divisible into red, blue and green sensitive cells.

Parts of photoreceptor cells are:

(i) Outer segments are the finger-like portions of both rods and cones containing closely packed membranous discs (lamellar plates) or flattened sacs of lipid and visual pigment. Discs are produced at the ciliary connection zone by photoreceptor cells. In rods, they move peripherally to be phagocytosed by pigment cells in the course of 10–13 days. Cones do not have such turnover.

(ii) Ciliary connection absorbs light and triggers visual stimulus.

(iii) Inner segments are divided into an outer ellipsoid containing many mitochondria and inner myoid containing RER and Golgi complex.

(iv) The outer and inner fibers are parts of photoreceptor cytoplasm outside and inside of the nucleus respectively.

(v) Both photoreceptors end in bulb-shaped synaptic enlargements (rod spherules and cone pedicles) which contain synaptic ribbons and synaptic vesicles.

12.6. The *outer nuclear layer* of the retina contains rod and cone nuclei.

12.7. The *outer plexiform layer* contains photoreceptor terminals, dendrites of bipolar cells and dendrites of horizontal cells.

12.8. The bipolar layer (inner nuclear layer) contains bipolar neurons (intrinsic neurons) which relay impulses from photoreceptors to the next layer containing ganglion cells or principal neurons of the retina. The layer also contains nuclei of Muller cells, horizontal (intrinsic neuron) cells and amacrine (intrinsic neuron) cells.

12.9. Bipolar neurons extend from the outer plexiform layer where they make synaptic connections with photoreceptors to the *inner plexiform layer* where they contact ganglion cell and amacrine cell dendrites. Three types are:

A. Rod bipolar cells which connect with several rod cells.

B. Midget bipolar cells which connect with one cone cell.

C. Flat or diffuse bipolar cells which connect with several cone cells.

12.10. *Horizontal cells* are intrinsic neurons whose axons run horizontally and outwardly to contact spherules and pedicles of rods and cones and dendrites of bipolar cells. Two types are described:

A. Luminosity horizontal cells which respond to illumination with hyperpolarization.

B. Chromaticity horizontal cells which hyperpolarize or depolarize depending on the wavelength of light.

12.11. *Amacrine cells* (a (Gk) not and makros (Gk) long) are intrinsic neurons without axons which send all of their processes inwardly to the inner plexiform layer where they synapse with axons of bipolar cells and dendrites of ganglion cells. There are two types:

A. Wide field diffuse amacrine cells whose dendrites spread throughout the thickness of the inner plexiform layer.

B. Narrow field diffuse (stratified) amacrine cells whose dendrites ramify in one or two horizontal layers of the inner plexiform layer.

12.12. The *inner plexiform layer* contains the connections between bipolar axons and amacrine cells with the dendrites of ganglion cells.

12.13. The *ganglion cell layer* contains the nuclei of ganglion cells which are the principal cell of the retina.

A. There are approximately 1 million *ganglion cells* whose axons form the innermost layer of the retina (the nerve fiber layer). They converge as unmyelinated fibers on the optic papilla (nerve head) where they combine to form the optic nerve and extend to

EYE

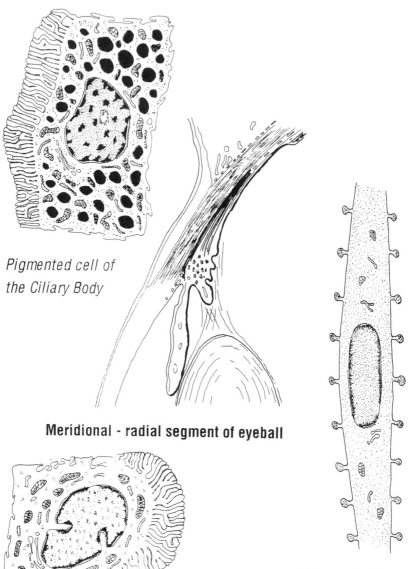

Pigmented cell of
the Ciliary Body

Meridional - radial segment of eyeball

Non-pigmented cell
of the Ciliary Body

Segment of Lens Cell
(fibre)

the lateral geniculate body in the thalamus.

B. Ganglion cell dendrites synapse with axons of bipolar cells and extensions of amacrine cells in the inner plexiform layer.

C. Three types are described:

   (i) *Midget ganglion* cells located near the fovea have a single dendrite contacting a single bipolar cell.

   (ii) *Diffuse giant ganglion cells* whose dendrites spread throughout the inner plexiform layer.

   (iii) *Stratified giant ganglion cells* whose dendrites branch in strata of the inner plexiform layer.

13. Macula Lutea and Fovea Centralis

13.1. The *fovea centralis* (fovea (L) a pit) is the deepest part of the *macula lutea* (macula (L) a spot and luteus (L) yellow), a depression in the retina about 1.5 mm in diameter in the optic axis of the eyeball. It is the site of greatest visual acuity.

13.2. At the macula, all retinal layers, except for elongated macular cones, are displaced laterally so that there is a decreased amount of tissue overlying the photoreceptors.

14. Optic Papilla (Optic Disc or Nerve Head)

14.1. The *optic papilla* is the site of exit of the as yet unmyelinated optic nerve fibers and of exit and entry of retinal vessels. It is 1 mm in diameter situated 3 mm nasal to the macula lutea.

14.2. The retina is absent at the papilla (the "blind spot").

14.3. Optic nerve fibers converge to form an annular ridge at the edges of the papilla (physiological cup) which is flattened with increased intraocular pressure.

15. Retinal Vessels

15.1. Blood supply to the retina is from two sources:

A. *Choriocapillaris* supplies the pigmented epithelium, photoreceptors and outer half of the outer plexiform layer.

B. The *central artery of the retina* supplies the remainder of the retina. Two major branches in the layer of nerve fibers supply a capillary network in the inner nuclear layer and these are end arteries.

15.2. *Mural cells* (*intramural pericytes*) control blood flow through capillaries.

15.3. The "*blood-retinal barrier*" prevents unrestricted flow of substances through vessel walls. It comprises:

A. Endothelial cells of the choroid and their basal lamina.

B. Pigmented epithelium joined by zonulae occludentes.

C. Endothelial cells of retinal capillaries and their basal laminae.

D. Perivascular feet of retinal glial cells.

16. Optic Nerve

16.1. The *optic nerve* is a collection of the axons of ganglion cells of the retina which combine after passing through the sieve-like lamina cribrosa of the sclera where they acquire a myelin sheath.

16.2. The nerve (in reality, a tract of the brain) comprises 0.4–1 million myelinated fibers of irregular size. They are separated by septa which extend from the pia mater and bear blood vessels. Between the fibers are bundles of astrocytes and oligodendroglia.

16.3. The optic nerve is surrounded by dura mater (continuous with the sclera), arachnoid and pia mater. There is an enlarged subarachnoid space (the vaginal space).

Chapter 26

THE EAR

OBJECTIVES

After reading this chapter, you should be able to:

1. Define the composition, histology and development of the auricle.
2. Describe the anatomy and histology of the external acoustic meatus.
3. Describe the histologic structure and development of the tympanic membrane.
4. Give an account of the anatomy and histology of the auditory tube.
5. Give an account of the structure and relationship of the bony and membranous labyrinths.
6. Describe the anatomical composition and development of the middle ear.
7. Give an account of the fate of the otocyst.
8. Describe the detailed histology and function of the maculae.
9. Describe the detailed histology and function of the cristae ampullares.
10. Identify histologic features of the cochlear duct exclusive of the spiral organ.
11. Give an account of the histologic structure of the spiral organ.
12. Describe the nerve and blood supply of the spiral organ.

CHAPTER OUTLINE

General.

The external ear. Development of the auricle. Structure of the auricle (pinna). Development of the external acoustic meatus. Structure of the external acoustic meatus.

The middle ear. Development. The tympanic membrane. The tympanic cavity. Auditory tubes.

The internal ear. General. Detailed structure.

The membranous labyrinth. Utricle. Saccule. Ductus reuniens. Endolymphatic duct (sac).

Development of the membranous labyrinth. Otic placode. Otocyst.

Endolymph.

Perilymph.

Detailed structure of the saccule and utricle. Maculae. Neuroepithelium.

Detailed structure of the semicircular ducts. Cristae. Neuroepithelium.

Detailed structure of the cochlear duct. Vestibular membrane. Spiral (basilar) membrane. Stria vascularis. Spiral ligament. Spiral limbus.

Detailed structure of the spiral organ (of Corti). Supporting cells. Sensory cells. Tectorial membrane. Interdental cells.

Nerves of the labyrinth.

Blood supply of the labyrinth.

KEY WORDS, PHRASES, CONCEPTS

External acoustic meatus
Ceruminous glands
Cerumen
Auricle
Tympanic membrane
  Pars tensa
  Pars flaccida
Auditory tube

Basilar membrane
(Spiral membrane)
Auditory strings
Spiral organ (of Corti)
Inner pillar cells
Outer pillar cells
Inner phalangeal cells
Border (internal limiting) cells

Tympanic cavity (tympanum)
Vestibule
Bony labyrinth
Cochlea
Semicircular canals
Perilymphatic duct
Scala vestibuli
Scala tympani
Modiolus
Spiral lamina
Cochlear duct (scala media)
Endolymphatic duct
Endolymphatic sac
Saccule
Utricle
Ductus reuniens
Membranous labyrinth
Macula
Otolithic membrane
Otoconia
Type I Vestibular cells (Hair cells, Cells with calyciform synapses)
Type II Vestibular cells (Hair cells, Cells with disseminated synapses)

Claudius (sustentacular) cells
Hensen (external Limiting) cells
Bottcher (sustentacular) cells
Inner hair cells
Outer hair cells
Tectorial membrane
Interdental cells
Spiral limbus
Stria vascularis
Marginal cells
Basal cells
Intermediate cells
Auditory placode
Auditory pits
Otocyst
First pharyngeal pouch
Auricular hillocks
Malleus
Incus
Stapes
Cristae
Cupula of crista ampullaris
Endolymph
Perilymph

THE EAR

1. General

1.1. The human *ear or vestibulocochlear organ* is concerned with hearing and equilibration. It comprises a sound conducting apparatus and a sense organ.

1.2. Reception and transmission of sound waves is the function of the external (auricle and external auditory meatus) and middle ear (tympanic membrane, tympanic cavity, auditory ossicles and auditory tube).

1.3. The internal ear is a complex fluid-filled, interconnected duct system (the membranous labyrinth) situated within a bony labyrinth in the temporal bone receptive to stimulation by sound waves (auditory sense), to the effects of gravity (static sense) and movements of the head (kinetic sense).

2. The External Ear

2.1. The *external ear* is a composite of the auricle and the external auditory meatus.

2.2. Development of the auricle or pinna

    2.2.1. The *auricle* (auris (L) an ear) or pinna (penna (L) a feather) develops around the first branchial groove with contributions from the first (mandibular) arch and second (hyoid) arches.

    2.2.2. At 6 weeks, six hillocks numbered 1, 2 and 3 on the cranial (mandibular arch) side and 4, 5 and 6 on the caudal (hyoid arch) side form the boundaries of the external acoustic meatus.

    2.2.3. Hillock 1 gives rise to the *tragus* (tragos (Gk) a goat cf. hair growing from behind like a goat's beard) while hillocks 2 and 3 combine to form the *helix* (helix (Gk) a coil or snail).

    2.2.4. Hillocks 4 and 5 give rise to the ***anti-helix*** while hillock 6 gives rise to the ***anti-tragus***.

    2.2.5. There may be considerable variation on this pattern.

2.3. Structure of the auricle

    2.3.1. The auricle is covered by thin skin with a hypodermis only on the posterior surface. Large sebaceous glands are associated with small hairs in the covering skin.

    2.3.2. The core of the auricle is an irregular plate of elastic cartilage which does not extend into the lobule.

    2.3.3. The hypodermis of the lobule is rich in adipose tissue and blood vessels.

    2.3.4. Six intrinsic (vestigial) muscles extend between parts of the cartilage. Three extrinsic muscles (auricularis anterior, superior and posterior) pass from the epicranial aponeurosis and mastoid process to the auricular cartilage.

2.4. Development of the external acoustic meatus

    2.4.1. The *external acoustic meatus* develops from the dorsal part of the ectodermal first pharyngeal cleft which is, for a time, in contact with the entoderm of the first pharyngeal pouch. The definitive tympanic membrane does not form at this region of contact but at one end added secondarily after loss of initial contact through expansion of the meatus by epithelial proliferation (below).

2.4.2. By the end of the second month, the groove deepens and an ectodermal cellular plate grows deeper to reach the wall of the tympanic cavity.

2.4.3. In the seventh month, the epithelial plate divides, forming the innermost part of the external meatus. A plug of desquamated epithelial cells may persist in the meatus at birth.

2.4.4. Mesodermal tissue between the end of the external acoustic meatus and the tympanic cavity thins so that the tympanic membrane is established.

2.4.5. At birth, the tympanic membrane is close to its final size but set at a more oblique angle than in the adult. It gradually becomes more erect as the external acoustic meatus lengthens.

2.5. Structure of the external acoustic meatus

2.5.1. The outer half of the external acoustic meatus (or cartilaginous part) is lined with elastic cartilage while the remainder (the deep or osseous part) is a bony tunnel in the temporal bone.

    A. The *cartilaginous part* of the external acoustic meatus is lined with thin skin containing fine hairs, large sebaceous glands and branched, tubuloalveolar ceruminous glands.

       (i) *Ceruminous glands* (from cera (L) wax) are branched tubuloalveolar glands lined with cuboidal cells which contain lipid and brown pigment granules. The cell surfaces are studded with cytoplasmic processes which separate during the apocrine secretion. Alveoli are surrounded by myoepitheliocytes.

      (ii) *Cerumen* is a mixture of thin secretion of ceruminous gland cells, of sebaceous cells and desquamated epithelial cells.

    B. The *bony part* of the external acoustic meatus is lined with very thin skin.

3. The Middle Ear

3.1. Development of the middle ear

    3.1.1. The auditory tube and tympanic cavity develop from the first pharyngeal pouch (the tubotympanic recess).

    3.1.2. At the end of the second month, the proximal stalk of the pouch constricts, forming the auditory tube.

    3.1.3. The blind outer end of the pouch enlarges, forming the primitive tympanic cavity and mastoid antrum.

    3.1.4. Auditory ossicles develop in surrounding mesenchyme of the first and second pharyngeal arches chondrifying from single centers.

    3.1.5. The *malleus* (malleus (L) a hammer) and *incus* (incus (L) an anvil) differentiate in serial order from the dorsal end of the first pharyngeal arch. Tensor tympani muscle attached to the medial border of the handle of the malleus is supplied by the nerve of the first pharyngeal arch (the mandibular division of the trigeminal nerve).

    3.1.6. The *stapes* (stare (L) to stand and pes (L) a foot) is derived from the second pharyngeal arch, its shape being related to early perforation by the stapedial artery (the artery of the first pharyngeal arch). The stapedius muscle, attached to the neck of the stapes, is innervated by the nerve of the second arch (the facial nerve).

    3.1.7. Spongy tissue surrounding the ossicles degenerates and epithelium lining the tympanic cavity wraps around the ossicles like a mesentery. Supporting ligaments of the ossicles develop in the mesenchyme of the mesenteries and are covered by entoderm.

    3.1.8. Epithelium of the posterior wall of the tympanic cavity begins to invaginate the mastoid process of the temporal bone to form the mastoid air cells at the close of fetal life.

3.2. *The tympanic membrane*

    3.2.1. The *tympanic membrane* is a thin (0.1 mm) membrane separating the external acoustic meatus from the tympanic cavity.

    3.2.2. It is thickened peripherally into a fibro cartilaginous ring and inserted into a groove in the osseous portion of the external meatus.

    3.2.3. The membrane is placed obliquely across the meatus, facing at an angle of 55 degrees to the anterior wall and floor. Being attached to the handle of the malleus, it bulges into the middle ear.

3.2.4. The major tightly stretched part (*pars tensa*) comprises:
  A. An outer (cutaneous) layer of thin skin.
  B. A fibrous layer disposed in outer radial and inner circular layers of collagen fibers.
  C. Low cuboidal epithelial layer (the mucous layer) lining the tympanic cavity.

3.2.5. The minor flaccid part (*pars flaccida*) occupies an upper triangular region above the attachment of the malleus. In this region, the fibrous layer is absent.

3.2.6. Sensory nerves enter the membrane peripherally, a bundle following the handle of the malleus.
  A. The auriculotemporal branch of the trigeminal nerve and auricular branch of the vagus supply the outer surface of the membrane.
  B. The glossopharyngeal nerve (through the tympanic plexus) supplies the inner surface (as well as the remainder of the tympanic cavity, mastoid air cells and the auditory tube).

3.3. The tympanic cavity

3.3.1. The tympanic cavity is an irregular air-filled space belonging to the middle ear located in the temporal bone.
  A. Its upper part, the epitympanic recess, communicates posteriorly with the tympanic antrum by the aditus and so with the mastoid air cells.
  B. Anteriorly, the tympanic cavity communicates with the auditory tube.
  C. It is bounded laterally by the meatus and tympanic membrane and medially by the lateral wall of the internal ear.
  D. The *vestibular* (*oval*) *window* (*fenestra vestibuli*) on the medial wall leading to the vestibule is closed by the foot plate of the stapes and a ligament anchoring the foot plate within the window.
  E. The *cochlear* (*round*) window (*fenestra cochleae*) in the medial wall is closed by the secondary tympanic membrane which covers the aperture in the bone, leading to the scala tympani of the cochlea.

F. The cavity of the middle ear contains the tendons of tensor tympani and stapedius muscles, auditory ossicles and the chorda tympani nerve.

3.3.2. Simple squamous to cuboidal epithelium lines the tympanic cavity with some patches of pseudo-stratified epithelium around the opening of the auditory tube. The epithelium comprises ciliated cells, secretory cells, non-ciliated and basal cells.

3.3.3. The *lamina propria* is richly vascularized and innervated loose connective tissue containing lymphocytes and some mucous glands, particularly in the anterior part of the cavity.

3.4. The auditory tubes

3.4.1. The auditory tubes are paired canals, partly bony and partly cartilaginous, joining the tympanic cavity with the pharynx.

3.4.2. The *bony part* along the angle of union of the squamous and petrous parts of the temporal bones is lined with columnar ciliated epithelium on a thin lamina propria.

3.4.3. The *cartilaginous part* is elastic near the junction with the bony part and hyaline near the pharynx. It is lined with a thicker mucous membrane than in the bony part and contains compound tubuloalveolar seromucous glands. Lymphocytes aggregate near the pharyngeal opening (the *tubal tonsil*).

3.4.4. Cartilage forms part of the tube wall and a fibrous membrane completes the wall.

3.4.5. Epithelial lining is pseudo-stratified ciliated with goblet cells near the pharynx and columnar ciliated near the tympanic cavity.

4. The Internal Ear

4.1. General

4.1.1. The *internal ear or labyrinth* is divided into bony and membranous parts, the former enclosing the latter.

4.1.2. Within the membranous labyrinth is a fluid, the *endolymph*, and outside, between the membranous and bony labyrinths (in the peri lymphatic space), is another fluid, the *perilymph*.

4.1.3. *Endolymph* is a watery fluid filling the membranous labyrinth produced by the stria vascularis in the cochlear duct and eliminated by cells of the endolymphatic sac into the subarachnoid space. It is poor in protein and sodium but rich in potassium.

4.1.4. *Perilymph* is the liquid circulating in the perilymphatic space. It is richer in sodium chloride and proteins than endolymph but contains less potassium.

4.2. The bony labyrinth is a compact bony capsule in which the membranous labyrinth is suspended. It comprises the vestibule, semicircular canals and the cochlea.

A. The *vestibule* is the central part of the labyrinth whose lateral wall corresponds to the medial wall of the middle ear.

(i) The *vestibular* (*oval*) window is closed by the foot plate of the stapes.

(ii) On the medial wall is a depression, the spherical recess perforated by holes for branches of the *vestibulocochlear nerve*.

(iii) Posteriorly and medially is the opening of the *aqueduct of the vestibule* for transmission of the endolymphatic duct.

(iv) At the posterior part are five openings of the *semicircular canals* and at the anterior part is an opening which leads to the scala vestibuli.

B. The *semicircular canals* are three arched osseous canals placed above and behind the vestibule, opening into it by five rounded apertures (two adjacent canals having one common opening).

(i) Each canal forms about two thirds of a circle and presents a dilation at one end, the *ampulla* (ampla (L) full and bulla (L) a vase).

(ii) The *anterior* (*superior*) *canal* is vertical (transverse to the long axis of the petrous temporal bone). Its medial extremity joins the opening of the posterior canal.

(iii) The *posterior canal* is vertical in a plane at right angles to the anterior canal, its upper end being joined to the lower opening of the superior canal.

(iv) The *lateral canal* slopes upward from horizontal just above the oval window.

C. The *cochlea* is cone-shaped with the base turned to the internal meatus and the apex opposite the canal for tensor tympani.

(i) It comprises a tapering spiral canal of two and a half turns around a bony axis, the *modiolus* (modiolus (L) a cylindrical borer, also a hub).

(ii) The canal is divided into two *scalae* (*scala* (L) a flight of stairs) by a partition of bone and membrane, the spiral lamina.

(iii) The enclosed arched extremity of the cochlea is called the *cupola* (cupola (Gk) a hole or hollow).

(iv) At the apex of the cochlea, the scalae vestibuli and tympani communicate with one another through the *helicotrema* (helix (Gk) a snail and trema (Gk) a hole).

(v) The *modiolus* is pierced by small canals for passage of the cochlear nerves and one larger one, the longitudinal canal of the modiolus from the base to the last half turn of the cochlea.

(vi) The *spiral canal of the modiolus* is a small canal at the base of the lamina spiralis winding around the axis and containing the spiral ganglion of the cochlear nerve.

(vii) *Scala tympani* is the lower of the two scalae commencing at the cochlear (round) window.

(viii) Near the round window is the opening of the *aqueduct of* the *cochlea*, which conveys perilymph to the aperture in the glossopharyngeal notch of the petrous bone in the jugular foramen where it communicates with cerebrospinal fluid.

(ix) *Scala vestibuli* commences at the cavity of the vestibule and communicates at the apex of the modiolus with the scala tympani by way of the helicotrema.

(x) Each scala contains *perilymph*.

4.3. The *membranous labyrinth*

4.3.1. The *membranous labyrinth* is an interconnected system of sacs and membranous canals filled with endolymph and lined by a simple squamous epithelium on a very thin lamina propria.

4.3.2. The connective tissue layer of the membranous labyrinth comprises finely fibrillated intercellular substance, pigment cells and spindle- or stellate-shaped fibroblasts.

4.3.3. From the lamina propria, thin trabeculae run through the peri lymphatic spaces to the endosteum to support the membranous labyrinth within the osseous labyrinth.

4.3.4. The spaces and endosteum are lined with a layer of flattened connective tissue cells (mesothelium).

4.3.5. The membranous labyrinth is separable into two parts, a portion concerned with static and kinetic (vestibular) sense and a portion concerned with auditory sense.

4.3.6. The portions concerned with *static sense* are:

A. The *utricle* (diminutive of uterus (L) a little womb) a small sac communicating with the saccule by the utriculosaccular duct. The *endolymphatic duct* (aqueduct of the vestibule) arises from the utriculosaccular canal, passes through the temporal bone, and ends as a blind enlargement, the endolymphatic sac in contact with the dura mater on the posterior surface of the petrous temporal bone.

B. The *saccule* (sacculus (L) a little bag) is a smaller sac located in front of the utricle and below it. Ductus reuniens is the short tube connecting the saccule with the cochlear duct. In both the saccule and utricle are specialized neuroepithelial cells in sense organs known as *maculae* (macula (L) a spot).

4.3.7. The part of the labyrinth concerned with *kinetic sense* comprises:

A. Three *semicircular ducts* whose ampullae communicate with the utricle. In the ampullae of the semicircular ducts are neuroepithelial cells in sense organs known as *cristae* (crista (L) a crest).

4.3.8. The part of the labyrinth concerned with auditory sense is the *cochlear duct* (cochlea (L) a snail), which contains specialized neuroepithelial cells in a complex organ, the spiral organ (of Corti).

4.4. Development of the membranous labyrinth

4.4.1. At 22 days, the internal ear begins to develop from a thickened ectodermal plate, the *auditory* (*otic*) *placode* at a site midway along the side of the hindbrain.

4.4.2. The paired placodes form *auditory pits*.

4.4.3. By 4 mm, the pits invaginate and close into *otocysts* (*auditory vesicles*).

4.4.4. The *endolymphatic duct* arises from the cyst as a secondary outgrowth. Its blind extremity dilates into the endolymphatic sac.

4.4.5.   By 5 weeks, the *cochlear pouch* (*future cochlear duct*) is an elongated ventral part of the otocyst.

4.4.6.   The mid portion of the *otocyst* (*vestibular pouch*) indicates the future utricle and saccule while the dorsal portion (future semicircular ducts) first appear as two flattened pouches. The superior and posterior ducts arise from a single pouch.

4.4.7.   In the seventh week, further modelling of the otocyst progresses toward a definitive system of ducts and sacs. The central walls of flattened secondary pouches flatten further until their opposing walls fuse and break down, forming the semicircular ducts which remain attached at their ends.

4.4.8.   By the eighth week, the cochlear duct has begun to coil, reaching two and a half turns by 30 mm. Its constriction connecting the cochlear duct with the remainder of the labyrinth is the ductus reuniens.

4.4.9.   Sensory areas, the *cristae* and *maculae* begin to form in the seventh to eighth weeks.

4.3.10. The *spiral organ* (*of Corti*) is at first (10 weeks) a single layer of columnar epithelium which divides longitudinally into large inner and small outer ridges.

(i) The tectorial membrane is secreted by interdental cells of the spiral limbus.

(ii) Cells of the outer ridge undergo selective autolytic involution, leaving the inner spiral sulcus.

(iii) Mesenchyme surrounding the cochlear duct differentiates into cartilage which, at 10 weeks, vacuolates, forming two peri lymphatic spaces, scala vestibuli and scala tympani.

(iv) The vestibular membrane separates scala vestibuli from the cochlear duct and the basilar membrane separates scala tympani from the cochlear duct.

(v) The lateral wall of the cochlear duct remains attached to cartilage by the spiral ligament.

(vi) The medial angle of the cochlear duct remains attached by cartilage to the modiolus (axis of the cochlea).

4.5. Detailed structure of the saccule and utricle

4.5.1. *Maculae* are neuroepithelial areas 4–6 square mm in diameter comprising part of the epithelial wall of the saccule and utricle.

4.5.2. *Neuroepithelial cells* in the maculae are:

  A. *Type I Vestibular cells* (*Sensory hair cells type I*) are pear-shaped neuroepithelial cells with an apical tuft of 40–100 hairs (*stereocilia*) which progressively increase in length toward one pole of the cell and a single non-motile kinocilium adjacent to the longest hair.

    (i) Central actin containing fibrillar cores of the hairs penetrate a cuticular plate in the apical cytoplasm which also contains actin.

    (ii) Cells lie in a chalice like enlargement of an afferent nerve ending.

  B. *Type II Vestibular cells* (*Sensory hair cells type II*) are cylindrical cells which also have 40–100 hairs (*stereocilia*) progressively increasing in length toward a single *kinocilium*. Each hair contains a central filamentous core which runs into an apical cuticular plate.

    (i) Type II cells are innervated at the base by efferent as well as afferent nerve endings.

    (ii) Synaptic bars are cylindrical cytoplasmic structures surrounded by synaptic vesicles adjacent to the basal plasmalemma of sensory hair cells facing individual afferent nerve endings.

When sensory hairs are bent in the direction of the kinocilium, both type I and II cells increase their firing rate. If hairs are bent in the opposite direction, the cells decrease their firing rate.

4.5.3. *Supporting cells* are tall, irregular cells located between vestibular cells. They contain a terminal web, bundles of microtubules, lysosomes and small secretory granules.

4.5.4. The *otolithic membrane* (*statoconial membrane*) is a gelatinous substance covering the vestibular cells of the maculae. Hairs of vestibular cells penetrate the membrane but are separated from it by a narrow space filled with endolymph.

4.5.5. *Otoliths* (*statoconia or otoconia*) are small crystals of calcium carbonate and protein 3–5 μm long and 2 μm wide overlying the otolithic membrane. Since the otoliths have a higher specific gravity than endolymph, changes in head position change the relationship between maculae and the line of gravitational force. The displacement of the otolithic membrane also bends hairs of the vestibular cells, causing their depolarisation or hyperpolarization depending on the direction of displacement.

4.6. Detailed structure of the semicircular ducts

  4.6.1. A *crista* (crista (L) a crest) or crista ampullaris is a small ridge-like sensory organ projecting into the ampulla of each semicircular duct and placed perpendicular to the axis of the duct.

  It comprises:

  A. *Neuroepithelium* (*Type I and II Vestibular cells*) identical in structure to those in maculae; however, the hairs and kinocilium are much longer in Type I cells while only the kinocilium is very long (50 μm) in Type II cells.

  B. *Supporting cells* are identical in structure to those in maculae. They secrete the matrix of the cupula.

  C. The *cupula* is an acellular flap of glycoprotein, situated above each crista arranged perpendicular to the ampulla of a semicircular duct and extending to the roof of the ampulla.

  4.6.2. Hairs of vestibular cells penetrate the cupula which, being more viscid than endolymph, is displaced during rotation of the head. Hairs are bent and vestibular cells excited (endolymph remains relatively stationary because of inertia while the cupula is deflected). Excitation or inhibition occurs in vestibular cells depending on whether hairs are displaced towards (excitation) or away from (inhibition) the kinocilium.

4.7. Detailed structure of the cochlear duct

  4.7.1. The *cochlear duct* is a diverticulum of the saccule containing the organ of hearing (the *spiral organ or organ of Corti*). It spirals two and a half times around a central axis (the modiolus), ending at the helicotrema.

  4.7.2. The *vestibular membrane* (*of Reissner*) is a thin sheet extending obliquely from the internal edge of the spiral limbus to the spiral ligament, which separates the scala vestibuli from the cochlear duct. The membrane appears to play a role in water and electrolyte transport.

A. The inner (*cochlear duct*) surface is covered by flattened epithelial cells with extensive basal infolding and micropinocytotic vesicles on a basal lamina.

B. Centrally are occasional collagen microfibrils.

C. The outer (scala vestibuli) surface is covered by attenuated fibroblast-like cells.

4.7.3. The *spiral* (*basilar*) membrane forming the floor of the cochlear duct is stretched between the spiral ligament laterally and the osseous spiral lamina medially.

A. The spiral lamina supports the spiral organ and separates the cochlear duct from the scala tympani.

B. The *arcuate zone* is the inner third of the basilar membrane, comprising a layer of flattened mesothelial cells which produce amorphous substance containing parallel auditory strings.

C. The *pectinate zone* is the outer two thirds of the basilar membrane which contains auditory strings arranged in two layers.

D. *Auditory strings* are compact bundles 8–10 μm thick of collagen-like microfibrils stretched between the spiral ligament and osseous spiral lamina. They are embedded in an amorphous mass belonging to the basilar membrane. There are about 20000 auditory strings varying in length from 0.04 mm in the basal cochlea to 0.5 μm in the helicotrema.

4.7.4. Each frequency of sound transmitted to cochlear perilymph and endolymph provokes vibration of the corresponding auditory strings. Vibrations are transmitted to hair cells whose hairs are displaced relative to the tectorial membrane.

4.7.5. The *stria vascularis* is a vascularized stratified columnar epithelium covering the inner surface of the spiral ligament. It is responsible for the secretion of endolymph.

It comprises:

A. Marginal (*dark or chromophil*) cells with a well-developed basal labyrinth.

B. *Intermediate* (*light or chromophobe*) *cells*, stellate in shape without contact with the luminal surface.

C. *Basal cells*, flattened irregular cells on the basal lamina which may be progenitors of the other epithelial cell types.

4.7.6. The stria is the only vascularized epithelium of the body carrying a rich intraepithelial capillary plexus.

4.7.7. The *spiral ligament* (prominence) is a crescent-shaped thickened vascularized endosteum of the lateral wall of the cochlea. It extends from shortly above the attachment of the vestibular membrane to below the level of the basilar membrane.

4.7.8. The *spiral limbus* (limbus (L) a border of hem) of the medially placed osseous spiral lamina is the thickened endosteum of the lamina spiralis protruding into the cochlear duct. It extends from the vestibular lip to the tympanic lip with the inner spiral sulcus between.

   A. In the upper surface of the spiral limbus are interdental cells which produce the tectorial membrane.

   B. Bundles of collagen fibers in the spiral limbus are vertically oriented, forming auditory teeth between which lodge interdental cells.

   C. Some fibers radiate into the arcuate part of the basilar membrane.

   D. The vestibular membrane is fixed to the inner edge of the spiral limbus.

4.7.9. The *spiral organ* (*of Corti*) is an epithelial ridge of highly specialized cells situated on the basilar membrane of the cochlear duct. It comprises:

   A. *Supporting cells*:

      (i) *Inner pillar cells* are tall columnar cells with a broad base resting on the basilar membrane and contacting other inner and outer pillar cells. A slender middle portion and flattened head articulates with a convexity on the head of outer pillar cells forming the inner tunnel (of Corti). The cytoplasm contains bundles of vertical parallel microtubules and microfilaments which end in a terminal web in the head of the cell. With outer pillar cells, inner pillars maintain a constant height of the spiral organ.

      (ii) *Outer pillar cells* are longer cells with a broad base, slender middle and expanded head with medial convexity.

The head fits into a concavity beneath the head of inner pillar cells. The flattened process of the head of outer pillar cells reach the free surface of the spiral organ and contact the innermost row of outer hair cells. Two bundles of microtubules and microfilaments converge from the base of the cell to end in a terminal web in the head. With inner pillar cells, outer pillars maintain the height of the spiral organ and enclose the inner tunnel (of Corti).

(iii) *Inner phalangeal cells* (*of Deiter*) are thin, tall cells which surround inner hair cells. They are arranged in two longitudinal rows between inner pillar cells and border cells. The heads of cells of the internal row reach the surface of the spiral organ, terminating as a long, narrow microvilli-bearing inner phalanx. Cells are attached at the edges of the phalanx to the border cell and inner hair cell. Non-myelinated nerve fibers pass between the bases of the inner hair cell and the inner phalangeal cell to reach inner hair cells. Inner phalangeal cells rest on the basilar membrane and are supporting elements for inner hair cells.

(iv) *Outer phalangeal cells* are tall, very irregular cells with a cylindrical body resting on the basilar membrane. They surround the base of outer hair cells enclosing nerve endings as they do so and have a long thin stalk which terminates in a rhomboid flat extension (phalanx or phalangeal process). There are 4–5 rows of outer phalangeal cells. A bundle of microtubules extends vertically from the basal cytoplasm, through the stalk and into the phalanx. Junctional complexes join the phalanx to the outer hair cell and adjacent outer phalangeal cells. Viewed from above, the contours of outer phalangeal cells form a network pattern, the reticular membrane. Outer phalangeal cells support outer hair cells.

(v) *Border* (*peripheral*) *cells* are slender cells adjacent to inner phalangeal cells delimiting the inner boundary of the spiral organ. Their height gradually decreases from the spiral organ as they become squamous cells lining the inner spiral sulcus.

(vi) *External supporting (Claudius') cells* are clear cuboidal cells lining the external spiral sulcus. Outwardly, they reach the stria vascularis and inwardly, the external limiting cells. They are a supporting cell of the spiral organ.

Böttcher Cells are polyhedral external supporting cells only found in the basal coil of the cochlea. They are interposed between Claudius' cells and the basilar membrane. They are connected to one another by interdigitations and thought to have a secretory or absorptive role.

(vii) *External limiting (Hensen's) cells* are supporting cells situated beyond outer phalangeal cells overlying Bottcher cells. Initially the same height as outer phalangeal cells, they decrease in height toward Claudius' cells. They are believed to modulate the transmission of vibrations.

B. *Cochlear hair cells*.

(i) *Inner hair cells* are large, pear-shaped mechanoreceptor cells surrounded by inner phalangeal cells. There are 3500 inner hair cells arranged in a single row along the length of the cochlea. At the apical pole of the cell are 60 hairs (stereocilia) arranged in two to six rows in a U or W pattern with its convexity directed toward the inner pillar cells (away from the modiolus). The tallest hairs are always directed towards the stria vascularis. Subsequent rows of hairs decrease in height. Each hair contains a filamentous core containing actin which penetrates a cuticular plate in the apical hair cell cytoplasm. The tallest hairs contact the tectorial membrane and their displacement relative to the membrane provokes depolarization of the cell. The basal cytoplasm contains synaptic bars facing afferent nerve endings. Efferent nerve endings from neurones in the contralateral superior olivary nucleus in the brainstem also form synapses with the basal cytoplasm. Inner hair cells form desmosomes with border cells medially and inner pillar cells laterally.

(ii) *Outer hair cells* are tall columnar mechanoreceptor cells each lying in a cup-like depression of an outer phalangeal cell. There are about 20000 outer hair cells arranged in 3–5 rows along the length of the spiral organ. The apical pole is surrounded by the reticular membrane (phalanx) of outer phalangeal cells and reinforced by an apical cuticular plate.

The apical pole of the cell bears 100–200 hairs (stereocilia) of which the tallest is oriented toward the centriole (away from the modiolus) which contact the tectorial membrane. In the basal cytoplasm, synaptic bars face afferent nerve endings while post synaptic cisternae are located beneath large efferent terminals.

4.7.10. Vibrations of the basilar membrane displace the cells relative to the tectorial membrane. The resultant distortion of hairs provokes depolarization of the cell.

4.7.11. The *tectorial membrane* is a jelly-like, acellular, cuticular structure extending from the vestibular lip of the spiral limbus to slightly beyond the outermost row of outer hair cells. The membrane consists of radial microfibrils embedded in a homogeneous matrix. The *band of Hensen* is a stripe of non-striated dark material on the undersurface of the membrane making contact with hairs of the hair cells. The membrane is secreted by interdental cells which cover the cochlear duct side of the spiral limbus.

4.7.12. *Interdental cells* are bottle-shaped cells lying between auditory teeth (regularly spaced radial ridges of vertical collagen fibers at the upper surface of the vestibular lip of the spiral limbus). Their cytoplasm contains organelles consistent with a secretory function of mucopolysaccharide which transforms into the tectorial membrane.

4.8. Nerves of the Labyrinth

A. *Spiral Organ*

(i) *Afferent nerves* are dendrites of myelinated bipolar neurones of the spiral ganglion (cochlear ganglion) situated at the base of the bony spiral lamina.

(ii) Bipolar cell dendrites radiate in parallel bundles to inner hair cells and outer hair cells. The majority of fibers innervate the relatively small population of inner hair cells. Only a minority of fibers supplies the far more numerous outer hair cells by branched processes.

(iii) The axons of bipolar neurones pass centrally to cochlear nuclei in the medulla, forming the cochlear division of the vestibulo-cochlear nerve.

(iv) *Efferent nerves* from the contra lateral superior olivary nucleus form the olivocochlear bundle which inhibits hair cell activity.

(v) Sympathetic nerves from neurones in the superior cervical ganglion supply blood vessels and the stria vascularis in the cochlea.

B. *Vestibular Receptors*

(i) Afferent nerves are dendrites of myelinated bipolar neurones of the *vestibular ganglion* located in the internal acoustic meatus.

(ii) Axons of bipolar neurones form the vestibular division of the vestibulocochlear nerve.

4.9. *Blood Supply of the Labyrinth*

4.9.1. The *labyrinthine artery* is a branch of the basilar artery or the anterior inferior cerebellar artery. It divides at the base of the internal acoustic meatus into vestibular and cochlear branches.

4.9.2. The cochlear branch subdivides into 12–14 twigs which travel in canals in the modiolus and form a capillary network in the spiral lamina and basilar membrane.

4.9.3. Vestibular branches supply the utricle, saccule and semicircular ducts.

EAR – VESTIBULAR SYSTEM

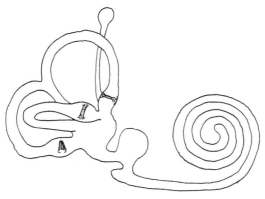

Membranous labyrinth

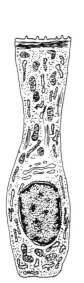

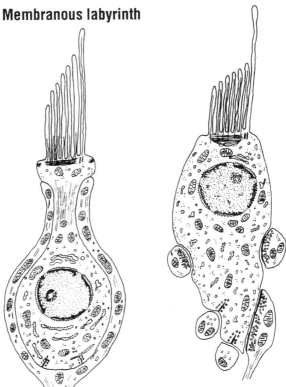

Supporting Cell

Type I Vestibular Cell
(Cell with caliciform synapse)

Type II Vestibular Cell
(Cell with disseminated synapse)

EAR – SPIRAL ORGAN

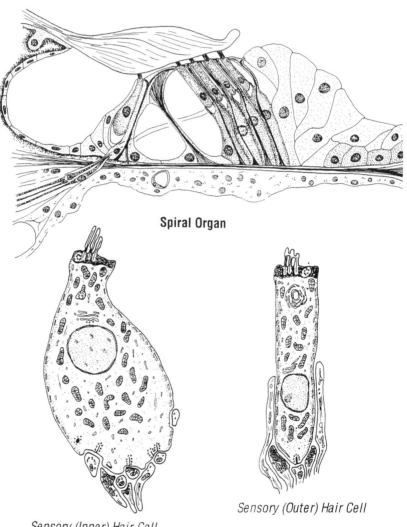

Spiral Organ

Sensory (Inner) Hair Cell

Sensory (Outer) Hair Cell

Index

vulvovaginal glands   333

white pulp   113

zona fasciculata   64
zona glomerulosa   63
zona pellucida   307
zona reticularis   64, 66